LONG-TERM CARE AND OLDER PEOPLE IN WESTERN EUROPE

Transforming Care

Series Editors: **Costanzo Ranci**, Polytechnic University of Milan, and **Tine Rostgaard**, Stockholm University and Roskilde University

---

As care and care work have been thrust into the international spotlight, the increased need for empirical, theoretical, and methodological investigation into social care and care policy and practice has been revealed. Addressing social care and care policy and practice at an international level, this series provides a crucial platform for scholars researching early childhood care, care for adults with disabilities, and long-term care for frail older people.

Also available in the series:

Care Poverty and Unmet Needs,
edited by **Teppo Kröger**, **Nicola Brimblecombe**, **Ricardo Rodrigues**, and **Kirstein Rummery**

Unpaid Work in Nursing Homes
edited by **Pat Armstrong**

Reablement in Long-Term Care for Older People
edited by **Tine Rostgaard**, **John Parsons**, and **Hanne Tuntland**

A Care Crisis in the Nordic Welfare States?
edited by **Lise Lotte Hansen**, **Hanne Marlene Dahl**, and **Laura Horn**

Find out more at:

policy.bristoluniversitypress.co.uk/transforming-care

LONG-TERM CARE AND OLDER PEOPLE IN WESTERN EUROPE

Lessons from the COVID-19 Pandemic

Edited by
Eloísa del Pino and
Francisco Javier Moreno-Fuentes

First published in Great Britain in 2025 by

Policy Press, an imprint of
Bristol University Press
University of Bristol
1–9 Old Park Hill
Bristol
BS2 8BB
UK
t: +44 (0)117 374 6645
e: bup-info@bristol.ac.uk

Details of international sales and distribution partners are available at policy.bristoluniversitypress.co.uk

British Library Cataloguing in Publication Data
A catalogue record for this book is available from the British Library

ISBN 978-1-4473-6728-4 hardcover
ISBN 978-1-4473-6730-7 ePub
ISBN 978-1-4473-6731-4 ePdf

Cover design: Robin Hawes
Front cover image: iStock/shuoshu
Bristol University Press and Policy Press use environmentally responsible print partners.
Printed and bound in Great Britain by CPI Group (UK) Ltd, Croydon, CR0 4YY

FSC
www.fsc.org
MIX
Paper | Supporting responsible forestry
FSC® C013604

Bristol University Press' authorised representative in the European Union is:
Easy Access System Europe, Mustamäe tee 50, 10621 Tallinn, Estonia,
Email: gpsr.requests@easproject.com

Contents

List of figures and tables

Figures

Tables

Notes on contributors

Marco Arlotti is a lecturer in economic sociology at the Department of Economics and Social Sciences at Marche Polytechnic University. His research interests include comparative analysis of social policies, particularly on social assistance schemes and policies for dependent older people.

Anita Böcker is an associate professor of Sociology of Law and affiliated to the Centre for Migration Law at Radboud University. Her most recent research projects dealt with retirement migration and return migration to Turkey; the emergence and significance of transnational long-term care arrangements; and the impact of the corona pandemic on labour migrants working in crucial sectors. She is currently conducting research on recruitment of skilled workers from outside the EU as a possible solution to labour shortages in the healthcare and technical sectors.

María Bruquetas-Callejo is a research fellow at the Centre for Migration Law, at the Radboud University, Nijmegen, the Netherlands. She holds a PhD in Sociology from the University of Amsterdam. She has worked as researcher and lecturer at the University of Amsterdam, Radboud University and Amsterdam University College. Since 2021 she coordinates the Spanish team at NGO FairWork, which supports victims of labour exploitation and carries out political lobby and awareness-raising on this issue.

Sara Burke is an associate professor in health policy and management at the Centre for Health Policy and Management, School of Medicine, Trinity College Dublin.

Arnaud Campéon is a professor in sociology at EHESP French School of Public Health, University of Rennes, and a researcher at the ARENES Research Centre (CNRS, UMR 6051). His work focuses on social care policies, vulnerability in old age, and professional and informal carers.

Luis Capucha has a PhD in sociology and aggregation in social work. He is the director of the Department of Political Science and Public Policies at Iscte-University Institute of Lisbon, Portugal and a researcher at the Centre for Research and Studies in Sociology (Cies-ISCTE). He has authored books, chapters, articles, and conference presentations about social policies, poverty, aging, the Welfare State, education, and popular cultures.

Stefania Cerea has been collaborating with the Social Policy Lab of the Polytechnic University of Milan. Her research interests include the condition of the elderly population and the evolution of long-term care systems. In recent years she participated in the project: 'Inclusive Ageing in Place (IN-AGE): Contrasting isolation and abandonment of frail older people living at home in Italy'.

Gibrán Cruz-Martínez is an assistant professor at the Department of Political Science and Public Administration, Complutense University of Madrid. His research focuses on comparative social policy and determinants of welfare state development in Latin America, the Caribbean, and Spain. He is co-editor of Alternautas, a member of the International Editorial Advisory Board of Social Policy & Society and co-convener of the ECPR Standing Group on Political Economy and Welfare State Politics.

Alexandre Daniel Calado is a PhD student at the ISCTE University Institute of Lisbon and a researcher at the Centre for Research and Studies in Sociology (CIES-ISCTE), Portugal. He has authored chapters of books, articles, and conference presentations about social resilience, education, poverty, and the Welfare State.

Eloísa del Pino is Senior Researcher at the Spanish National Research Council (CSIC-IPP). PhD in Political Science from the UCM and the Ortega y Gasset Research Institute (IUIOG). Degree in Political Science (UCM) and in Law (UNED). Master in Organization (ESIC). She directed the Observatorio de Calidad de los Servicios en la Agencia de Evaluación de Políticas y Calidad de los Servicios (AEVAL, Ministry of Territorial Policy) between 2009 and 2011. She was Head of Cabinet of the Minister of Health, Consumer Affairs and Social Welfare between 2018 and 2020. She has been a researcher at the Latin American Centre of the University of Oxford, the Institut d'Etudes Politiques de Bordeaux, the Pontificia Universidad Católica del Ecuador, the University of Kent, and the University of Ottawa. Her research turns around the political determinants of the reform of social policies and the Welfare State, citizen attitudes towards the State and public policies, and public administration.

Phillip Florian Schmidt studied Health Communication (BSc) and Public Health (MSc) at Bielefeld University. He is a research associate with the working group: Health Policy, Health Systems, and Sociology of Health in the Faculty of Health Sciences at Bielefeld University. His work and research cover the fields of health policy and healthcare systems.

Cristina Font Haro is a PhD candidate in social sciences at the Carlos III University of Madrid-Juan March Institute.

Thomas Gerlinger is a professor and director of the working group: Health Policy, Health Systems, and Sociology of Health in the Faculty of Health Sciences at Bielefeld University. His research interests include health policy and healthcare system development in Germany and Europe.

Caroline Glendinning is Emeritus Professor of Social Policy at the University of York, and an Academician of the Academy of Learned Societies in the Social Sciences. BA from the University of Sussex, and MPhil from the University of York, she is Member of the European Network of Independent Experts on Social Inclusion.

Michael Goudoumas is an ecological education PhD candidate. He is a certified trainer of social workers in child protection issues. He has been the Executive Assistant to the CEO of Aktios LTC Units and the Scientific Associate of Dr Prouskas. He has worked as a social worker as a coordinating team leader, project manager, and funding proposal writer in institutions and organisations in the private and the third sector. He also has qualifications in social work, BSW (Technological University of Patras, GR), consulting psychologist (ICPS), and health administration and economics MBA (NKUoA, Greece).

Jorge Hernández-Moreno works at the Spanish National Research Council (CSIC-IPP). Previously, he was a fellow at the Centro de Investigaciones Sociológicas (CIS), an FPU Fellow also at the CSIC-IPP, and a visiting researcher at the Department of Social and Political Sciences of the Universitá degli Studi di Milano. His research focuses on the territorial governance of welfare states, health and long-term care policies, comparative federalism, intergovernmental relations, and reforming the Spanish 'autonomic' State. He is Editorial Assistant and Book Review Editor of the *Journal Gestión y Análisis de Políticas Públicas* (GAPP).

Eimir Hurley is Research Fellow at the Department of Pharmacy of the University of Oslo. BA in Pharmacy from Trinity College Dublin, Master of Biostatistics from the University of Sydney, and PhD in Health Policy from Trinity College Dublin. She is the project lead of the INSPIRE-BIO project of the Norwegian Precision Cancer Medicine Implementation Consortium CONNECT.

Francisco Javier Moreno-Fuentes is Senior Researcher at the Spanish National Research Council (CSIC-IPP). He has a BA in sociology from the Universidad Complutense, MA in social sciences from the Juan March Institute, MSc in social policy from LSE, and PhD in political science from the Universidad Autónoma of Madrid.

Lennarth Johansson is a psychologist and associate professor of gerontology at the School of Health and Welfare at the Jönköping University. Currently, he is a senior advisor at the Stockholm Gerontology Research Center. He has more than 40 years of experience studying the health and social care system, informal caregiving, and social policy of care for older people.

Laura Kalliomaa-Puha is a professor of social welfare law at Tampere University. PhD in Law from the University of Helsinki, Member of the European Social Policy Network (ESPN), she is an expert in healthcare and long-term care.

Eduard Klukas initially trained as a nurse, and studied nursing and health care management (BA) and public health (MSc) at Münster University of Applied Sciences and Bielefeld University. Since 2022, he has worked as a research associate with the working group: Health Policy, Health Systems, and Sociology of Health in the Faculty of Health Sciences at Bielefeld University. His research focuses on health policy and health services.

Blanche Le Bihan is a professor in political science at EHESP, French School of Public Health, University of Rennes, and a researcher at the ARENES Research Centre (CNRS, UMR 6051). She works on social care policies focusing on long-term care policies in France and Europe, professional and informal carers.

Caspar Lückenbach studied health communication (BSc) and public health (MSc) at Bielefeld University. Since 2014, he has been a research associate with the working group: Health Policy, Health Systems, and Sociology of Health in the Faculty of Health Sciences at Bielefeld University. His work and research cover the fields of participation, health policy, and comparative health systems research.

Claude Martin is an emeritus research professor at CNRS, ARENES Research Centre (CNRS, University of Rennes, UMR 6051), is currently the director of a priority research program on autonomy, and was previously the holder of two chairs at EHESP School of Public health: on childhood, well-being, and parenting (2016–20) and on social care (2011–15). His main research fields are childcare, family, parenting, and long-term care policies. He has published extensively on these issues.

Luis Moreno (RIP) was Senior Researcher at the Spanish National Research Council (CSIC-IPP). Ph.D. in Social Sciences at the University of Edinburgh. He has been visiting scholar at the universities of Colorado (CU-Boulder), Denver (DU), Edinburgh and Rome (La Sapienza) and the

Institute for Research on Population and Social Policies (Italian National Research Council, CNR). He was Jean Monnet Senior Research Fellow at the European University Institute in Florence. His two main areas of research were Social policy and welfare state, and Territorial politics (decentralization, federalism, nationalism and Europeanization), both in comparative perspective.

Nuno Nunes is an auxiliary professor at the ISCTE-University Institute of Lisbon, Portugal. He is a researcher at the Centre for Research and Studies in Sociology (CIES-ISCTE). Nunes has authored books, chapters of books, articles, and conference presentations about social inequality, social classes, collective action, well-being, the digital society, and the Welfare State. He holds a PhD in sociology.

Manuel Pereira-Puga works at the Institute of Public Goods and Policies (IPP), Spanish National Research Council (CSIC). His research interests cover a range of topics related to health and social policy as well as science and technology systems and policies. Manuel has participated in several competitively funded research projects and has carried out public policy evaluations and consultancy work for public administrations. He has taught Sociology and Political Science at the Autonomous University of Madrid (UAM), the Carlos III University of Madrid (UC3M) and the University of A Coruña (UDC). He holds a PhD in Sociology from UDC.

Roberta Perna is Researcher at the Instititute of Public Goods and Policies of the Spanish National Research Council (IPP-CSIC). Prior to that, she was Marie Skłodowska–Curie Fellow at the University of Liège. She holds a PhD in Political Sociology from the University of Turin. Her research focuses on the welfare-migration nexus from a multi-level and comparative perspective, with a specific attention on healthcare systems, implementation gaps, and the politics of health deservingness in contemporary Europe. She is co-convenor of the ECPR Standing Group on Migration and Ethnicity.

Costis Prouskas is a psychologist with an MSc in psychological assessment in organisations (Goldsmiths, London) and a PhD in gerontology at King's College London. He has been the CEO of AKTIOS SA (Aktios Long Term Care) since 2007 and the CCO of Blocks Group since 2021. He is a founding member of the 50plus Hellas NGO and the Athens Association of Alzheimer's Disease and Related Disorders. He is also Special Secretary of the Hellenic Association of Geriatrics & Gerontology.

Costanzo Ranci is a professor of economic sociology at the Politecnico of Milano, where he chairs the Social Policy Lab. He has published many books and scientific articles on welfare, long-term care policy, and social vulnerability. He has been a visiting scholar at the University of California Berkeley, the University of Barcelona, the University of Lausanne, and Harvard University. His current research focuses on long-term care policy, the economic insecurity of the middle class, and social investment.

Monika Riedel has been a senior researcher in the Health Economics and Health Policy group at the Institute for Advanced Studies (IHS) in Vienna since 1999. She holds a doctoral degree in economics from the University of Vienna. Her research focuses on human resources in the health and care sector, international comparisons of health and care systems, and aging and care systems. She is a founding Austrian Health Economics Association (ATHEA) member. She has repeatedly served as a thematic/country expert in peer reviews for the DG Employment, Social Affairs & Inclusion of the European Commission.

Pär Schön is a senior lecturer and associate professor of social work at the Department of Social Work, Stockholm University. His research covers the health and social care system for older people, social policy implications of the aging population, and how this will affect future needs and demands for long-term care services.

Katharine Schulmann is a PhD candidate at the School of Social Work and Social Policy at Trinity College Dublin.

Christoph Stegner is a staff scientist at the Institute for Advanced Studies in Vienna. He holds an MSc in Economics from the University of Vienna. He graduated during the pandemic, and his research interests focus on the various impacts of COVID-19 on health systems, with particular attention towards improving health system resilience.

Virpi Timonen is a social and health services research and leadership professor at the University of Helsinki. PhD from the University of Oxford, she is an expert on social policies, welfare states, intergenerational relations, ageing, care, technology and research methods.

Robert Urbé is an independent social policy researcher. He a member of the European Social Policy Network (ESPN), and the former President of the Direction Committee of Caritas Luxembourg.

Satu Ylinen PhD, Social Work, she is a lecturer at the Faculty of Social Sciences of Tampere University. She works on the ethical questions of gerontological social work.

Tyyne Ylinen has an MSc in Social Work from Tampere University where she is a researcher working at the Faculty of Social Sciences on perceptions of social and health care professionals during COVID-19.

Vera Ylinen MSc in Sociology, is a Doctoral Researcher at the Faculty of Social Sciences of Tampere University. She works on the experiences of social and health professionals working with the elderly during the COVID-19 pandemic.

1

The challenge of policy integration and the complexity of care home responses to the COVID-19 pandemic in Europe

Eloísa del Pino and Francisco Javier Moreno-Fuentes

Managing nursing homes in a pandemic context: a three-ringed circus

During the first weeks of the COVID-19 pandemic, a regional health minister of a European country, responsible for purchasing masks, gloves, and other personal protection equipment (PPE) for his region, asked his fellow regional health ministers on a phone chatting app how they were calculating their purchase needs. All but one replied with formulas that only took into consideration the expected needs for the personnel of hospitals and healthcare centres. The odd one, who was in charge of both healthcare and social services in his region, asked the other regional ministers whether they considered that non-health facilities such as prisons, garrisons, or nursing homes could also need PPE. Surprised by this concern, which had not crossed his mind up to that moment, the regional minister who asked the initial question replied: 'Please, elaborate on this idea'. This telling anecdote shows how the care homes sector was completely out of the mental framework of the authorities having to deal with the initial stages of the pandemic. This lack of focus on this sector had very significant consequences for the way in which the disease expanded among the residents of this type of institution, and on the measures adopted to respond to this public health emergency in the early stages of expansion of the pandemic (del Pino et al, 2020).

On 30 January 2020, the World Health Organization (WHO) declared the outbreak of the novel coronavirus as a Public Health Emergency of International Concern (PHEIC), the highest level of alert under the International Health Regulations. During the first weeks of February, cases began appearing in many European countries, and the situation in Italy, the first European country where the pandemic was identified, was particularly aggravated. Between the end of February and the beginning of March, the number of positive cases increased, with cases that had been admitted to hospitals in previous weeks retrospectively identified as COVID related. Meanwhile, those responsible for social services received information from elderly care homes suggesting that some type of virus was affecting their residents. On 28 February, the WHO recommended drastic containment measures (such as holding all professional sports competitions behind closed doors, asking health professionals not to attend scientific conferences, and so on), but the suggested measures were not generally adopted. On 11 March, the WHO officially declared the existence of a pandemic, recognising the emergence of the largest global public health emergency in recent decades.

Governments had to confront a series of complex cross-sectoral and intergovernmental problems during the early stages of the pandemic (Paquet & Schertzer, 2020). One of the key factors in tackling such problems was to get the actors involved to work in an integrated way to improve the coherence of policy-making through negotiation, deliberation and agreement on the actions to be implemented (Tosun & Lang, 2017; Howlett & Saguin, 2018: p 6). This objective was not easy to achieve if, prior to the pandemic, there were no institutional capacities and coordination mechanisms already in place (standards, frameworks, policy tools, procedures, and other mechanisms) to find solutions to the challenges of long-term care amidst a shattering crisis such as that produced by the COVID-19 pandemic (González, 2022; Hernández-Moreno, 2022).

All problems that involve relationships among different actors are, quite logically, exacerbated during an emergency. The urgency of solving problems of a great magnitude, such as those generated by a pandemic, may have opened a window of opportunity for public policy integration, which involved understanding and addressing multiple dimensions (social, sanitary, security, or economic, among others), and the complexity of the governance structures (with different levels of government administrations, for example, central, regional or local), as well as the plurality of actors involved in this domain within the different public administrations (such as the different agencies and areas of policy responsibility from the different institutional levels, from the European, to the local, passing by the national and the regional). In that context, public and private actors are able to learn from their common experiences by finding solutions to the complex policy problems created by the emergency, in the case studied in this volume, to ensure adequate care for people living in nursing homes in the context of a pandemic. Once tested during an emergency, those formulas may endure thereafter in ways that would have been difficult to anticipate in times of normalcy.

At the outbreak of COVID-19, central governments of many European countries considered that, in the face of an emergency such as a pandemic, which seriously threatened people's health and life, urgent and forceful measures had to be adopted. However, they soon realised that many of the competencies and the management expertise needed to respond to this emergency had been in the hands of regional and/or local government for decades, that they knew much less than they thought they did about the day-to-day operations of those administrations in those policy domains, and that their ability to control them was doubtful at best.

This situation was particularly true in the case of care homes for the elderly and dependent people. Residents in care homes live collectively, something that greatly contributes to the potential spread of infections and diseases. Furthermore, their age, the frequent occurrence of concomitant chronic conditions, and the widespread lack of personal autonomy (implying the need for daily interaction with caregivers), makes this population especially vulnerable to pandemics. Anticipating this scenario would have permitted them to include these groups in national security strategies and emergency plans. Nursing homes accounted for a very significant proportion of all COVID-19-related deaths in developed countries during the first wave of the pandemic (WHO, 2020). The challenge of nursing homes for governments was colossal, at some point risking collapsing the critical care capacities of the healthcare and social systems (Armstrong & Braedley, 2023). This was due to, at least, three reasons.

First, despite the fact that there has been a generalised trend to deinstitutionalise elderly people, and to facilitate their living in the community since the 1980s, the number of long-term care beds in nursing and residential care facilities increased in years prior to the pandemic in most EU Member States (from around 2.4 million in 2010, to nearly 3 million in 2020, according to OECD data [OECD, 2023]), also in relation to population size. As it is generally well known, older adults in care homes were among the most vulnerable groups during the pandemic.

Secondly, the vast majority of European care homes and LTC systems entered the COVID-19 crisis in a weak structural situation, characterised by scarce resources and a large increase in demand in the years prior to the outbreak of the pandemic, an unclear model for their future evolution, a highly fragmented institutional system involving several levels of government, numerous public, private, and non-profit actors, all poorly coordinated with the healthcare system despite coordination being a major requirement for efficiency, and limited capacity on the part of the authorities to ensure compliance with nursing home regulations.

The COVID-19 pandemic, and its management by nursing homes, constituted a clear example of how real-world problems many times constitute thorny or wicked problems which rarely respect the boundaries of institutionally defined public policy sectors, departmental boundaries, or the jurisdiction of a single level of government (Peters & Tarpey, 2019; Capano et al, 2020). In this manner, the pandemic soon ceased to be a strict health crisis, and quickly became a serious challenge for managers responsible across a wide range of public policy sectors, including social services at all levels of public administration (central government responsibility in basic regulation with a significant role played by regional or local governments), including notably the nursing homes sector (Greer et al, 2020; Boin et al, 2021).

The key analytical dimension used in this book to study the complexity of the problem of managing the pandemic in the nursing homes of European societies is the different institutional capacity to provide an integrated public policy response, involving multiple actors, to efficiently and effectively respond to an emergency that made the structural problems of nursing homes, and the peculiarities of the populations served by those centres, more salient. The circumstances generated by the pandemic forced European public administrations to adopt innovative and unprecedented policy measures to deal with the crisis as quickly as possible. Although reaching this point in the different countries was not easy, the pressing need to solve the complex problems that arose during this emergency situation represented an opportunity to experiment with institutional and management formulas that hardly would have gathered sufficient consensus to be implemented in times of normality (Elgström & Jönsson, 2000; Maggetti & Trein, 2022), or even in subsequent waves of the same crisis.

Evolution of the crisis and complexity of its analysis

It is difficult to estimate what the weight of the management of the pandemic was in the impact of the COVID-19 pandemic in the care home sector in the early stages of the expansion of the disease. We know that other factors, such as the moment when the virus arrived in the country or region, the relative incidence in the territory around the care centre, the type of healthcare system of the country, the demographic profile of the population, the density of its main cities and/or other determinants of health, contribute to explain the impact of the pandemic in this particular sector.

The scientific literature on crisis management, after analysing the governmental response to dozens of events of different nature (terrorism, accidents and public health, natural, war, or economic catastrophes), has detected a series of phenomena that hinder decision-making and the implementation of emergency responses in situations of high pressure. Some of these problems are, for example: the underestimation of risks due to multiple factors such as disbelief, overconfidence in the system itself, and the remoteness of its origin; the transience of the initial phase in which the intervention is more certain; the possible indecision about who should be the 'owner' of the crisis and the reasons why this occurs. Among the latter can be pointed out the lack of legal provisions or the weight of electoral motives in the decisions to be taken; the so-called 'scale dilemma', referring to which level of government should be mainly responsible;

lack of capacity (resources, expertise, personnel); the lack of empathy and simplification on the dynamics of operation of other public policy sectors and actors; the unwillingness of some organisations to cooperate with others; excessive rigidity in complying with protocols, sometimes outdated, and little flexibility to adapt to the situation; the deficient dissemination of existing plans and protocols; poor communication; unnecessary overlap and conflicts between agencies and actors involved in crisis operations (the so-called 'battle of the Samaritans'); the inability to make sense of the crisis and gain credibility for the measures to be accepted; the problem of mass convergence consisting of the fact that many people and organisations want to use certain scarce resources (spaces, material); the collapse of systems and the inability to continue providing certain services because they are immersed in an emergency, for example health, education, transport, care; resistance to evaluation for fear of political consequences and poor learning, understood as an 'intentional effort to (re)examine, (re)evaluate, and (re)calibrate existing and proposed beliefs, policies, and institutional arrangements)' (Boin, 2007: p 143; Ansell et al, 2010).

Several issues appear recurrently in the analysis of the management of the COVID-19 crisis. The level of prior preparation of the centres to deal with situations of this type affected the speed with which the first reaction measures were adopted (very relevant in epidemics), as well as the availability of protection resources. The forecasts on vertical and horizontal coordination with the administrations determined the scope of the measures, the rigidity or flexibility with which they acted, or even the aid that the centres could receive (Ministerio de Derechos Sociales y Agenda 2030, 2020). The level of professionalisation of the personnel influenced the ability to protect, recruit, or train staff in the preparation and implementation of contingency plans, or the speed with which nursing homes organised health care for their residents, an element that seems crucial in the management of a public health crisis.

Intersectoral coordination between health and social services, both among administrations and between nursing homes and healthcare centres, appears central in the understanding of the effects of the epidemic in the care home sector. The consequences of the lack of coordination between the two sectors appears to have played a very significant role in the impact of the pandemic. After the 2009 H1N1 swine flu pandemic, for example, some countries reconsidered who should be responsible for handling a pandemic crisis due to the overload of demands on the health authorities. While some opted for someone with a more transversal vision and/or with greater political leadership in charge of coordinating several Ministries, others opted for the establishment of liaison mechanisms. Unfortunately, the COVID-19 pandemic placed the systems, once again, under serious problems of capacity, ability to secure resources, technology, and professionals to achieve its objectives, and not many lessons extracted from previous emergency situations were adopted.

The lack of capacity (data collection, material, testing, and analysis) conditioned public healthcare responses to the pandemic. This was particularly true for the residential care sector, where mechanisms to share information between levels of government and policy sectors were largely absent. The underdevelopment of contingency plans and the lack of training for staff proved very damaging as well. The rare existing health protocols to be applied in nursing homes had not been designed with the participation of those in charge of implementing them, so the actions that had to be adopted by nursing homes were very difficult to apply due to their architectural configuration, the organisation of the way of working, and/or the specificities of the residents, so they could not be carried out without a severe impairment of the care functions that give meaning to these centres, or even worse, contributed to more infections among the residents.

In a pandemic crisis, hospital overflow can be considered a given, so the way in which residents in care centres are treated within the triage systems to handle the limited supply of healthcare may have very significant implications for the impact of the disease in these facilities. Similarly, the availability of care professionals in nursing homes during an outbreak may be a crucial factor in the capacity of those centres to respond to the emergency. The contagion, fear, and protocols affecting workers in those centres may have played a very significant role as well in the evolution of the disease among residents.

The number of deaths from COVID-19 in nursing homes correlates positively with the initial incidence of the pandemic, as well as with the size of the care homes, their infrastructural layout, and their degree of occupancy. The literature also points out that the relative availability of health and care professionals, and the availability of ICU beds, correlates as well with mortality (Jiménez & Viola, 2020: p 39). In addition, the number of residents and staff ratios, the anticipation of the adoption of measures, and the existence of diagnostic capacity have been measures that explain the incidence of the pandemic. Other factors that appear in the debate, such as the ownership of the residence, do not seem to significantly influence the scope of the pandemic. Other studies suggest that the high mortality in care homes for the elderly could be related to the separation between the health sector and that of nursing homes, the high relative weight of the market in the sector, the complexity of policies and the system of provision of care, the inadequate regulation in the matter, and the limited economic resources available to finance this sector (Daly, 2020).

More analyses are needed that include variables such as the structure and sectorisation of the facilities, how long it took for the protective equipment to be provided, the number of tests that were carried out (and when), the time at which health personnel systematically intervened in the residences, or the prior preparation measures in the AC. These variables frequently appear in interviews as decisive factors in starting to control the epidemic in these centres.

Although much more evidence is required, these analyses do denote the complexity that, given the great heterogeneity and diversity of the residential sector in Europe, it is intrinsic to strategic decision-making and the implementation of effective public policies in an area that has become a priority due to its epidemiological importance, the social alarm generated in the citizens, and the legal consequences that the management of this crisis may imply.

'Policy integration' to face a complex policy problem

Real-world problems rarely respect the boundaries of institutionally defined public policy sectors in ministries, or in the jurisdiction of a single level of government. The COVID-19 pandemic is a clear example of this. It soon ceased to be a strictly health crisis, and became a serious challenge for the managers responsible for the rest of the public policy sectors at all levels of government (Boin et al, 2021). In many countries, the rapid spread of the virus and the severity of its consequences for people's lives led to the rapid collapse of their health systems and forced governments to adopt measures to try to contain its incidence (Greer et al, 2020).

What cross-sectoral and intergovernmental challenges occur during crisis management? What do they consist of? What consequences can they have? Can they be solved? What does an integrated policy approach consist of? Which type of institutional capacities are required for supporting policy integration in this domain? What integration problems occur during a situation of crisis management? What do they consist of, and what are their causes? What consequences can they have? To what extent have the levels of government and policy sectors developed initiatives and mechanisms for the integration of the policy responses to the situation of health emergency linked to this pandemic in Europe? To answer these questions, and thus to contribute to the literature and policy analysis on crisis management, this volume analyses the case of nursing home management during the COVID-19 pandemic in a large group of European countries.

When we analyse the first measures adopted in the early stages of the pandemic we observe how they were designed from a purely health logic, and undoubtedly had benefits for the handling of the emergency, but they also soon revealed themselves to be problematic. From a sectoral perspective, three problems emerged. Some of the initiatives presented significant difficulties to be implemented, for example, how to confine the homeless or people with precarious housing. Despite their forcefulness, they were insufficient to attend to certain groups that were suffering especially from the impact of the crisis, for example, the elderly in nursing homes. Finally, the confinement and other measures had a strong social impact and on employment and the economy in general, generating new problems that could not be solved by the agencies in charge of ensuring the health of the population.

From an intergovernmental point of view, in addition to demonstrating that crisis management has an important political dimension, the measures taken revealed administrative shortcomings related to the lack of foresight as to which level of administration should have, and had, sufficient capacity to carry out certain tasks. The worsening of the crisis, but also all the problems mentioned and the awareness that COVID-19 was not going to be a fast-burning crisis like others that had occurred previously, meant that the measures initially designed had to be reviewed. Exceptions and nuances were introduced, and new initiatives were launched with an intersectoral and intergovernmental perspective.

A situation of crisis in the form of an emergency, a disaster, or a catastrophe, poses 'a serious threat to the basic structures or fundamental values and norms of a social system, which under the pressure of time, and in uncertain circumstances, requires critical decision-making' (Rosenthal et al, 1989: p 10). The analysis of hundreds of crisis management experiences helps to identify how some of the relationships between the plurality of actors involved in different, but somehow linked, policy sectors are intensified in the event of a crises (Boin, 2007; Ansell et al, 2010; McConnell, 2020):

- Indecision about who (which level of government or ministry or department) should be the 'owner' of the crisis due to the lack of legal provisions, management difficulties, or certain political interests that make governments want to step aside or, on the contrary, take ownership of the crisis management.
- The so-called 'dilemma of scale', which refers to which level of government or ministry should be primarily responsible for certain tasks.
- The 'battle of the Samaritans', or the unnecessary overlap and conflicts between agencies and actors involved in crisis operations.
- The problem of massive convergence, whereby many people and organisations want to use certain scarce resources (space, material, and so on).
- Lack of capacity of the different levels of public administration, or different ministries, to undertake certain tasks that may range from information analysis to policy design, the management of resources (procurement, logistics, and so on), or the implementation of those measures.
- Absence of spaces for, and practice of, collaboration between governmental bodies.
- Lack of empathy and lack of simplification of the operating dynamics of other public policy sectors and actors.

- Energy, time, and resources invested in collaboration may outweigh the benefits obtained from joint efforts.
- Lack of will of some organisations to cooperate with others.
- Struggle for political gain hindering crisis management.
- Observation from the point of view of a single specific public policy sector may cause underestimation of the salience of other dimensions involved in the potential management and resolution of the crisis.

Problems related to the intergovernmental and intersectoral dimension of governance are a daily occurrence. They do not occur only in crisis contexts, but they develop in an acute manner in emergency situations. However, some authors have suggested that leaders, urged by the need to solve problems (Elgström & Jönsson, 2000), are capable of implementing institutional formulas and intersectoral (and intergovernmental) management that would be difficult to promote in normal times but that, once tested during crises, can last later (Maggetti & Trein, 2022).

If joint work is infrequent, it is very difficult for successful collaboration to take place under conditions of maximum pressure between managers who are not used to collaborating and who have different backgrounds, or when there are no institutional mechanisms and spaces to facilitate this relationship, or when these exist, but are not used. However, the pressing need to solve problems (problem solving approach) during a crisis can represent an opportunity to bet on institutional and management formulas that would be difficult to meet consensus in normal times (Elgström & Jönsson, 2000; Maggetti & Trein, 2022). From this perspective, policy integration (Tosun & Lang, 2017) involves improving the coherence of policy-making by deliberately adopting inclusive strategies that 'bring together multiple actors to negotiate, deliberate, and agree on actions to be taken' (Howlett & Saguin, 2018: p 6). The proposal of these authors is useful to analyse the case of the management of the COVID-19 crisis and to see to what extent the first government responses to the pandemic were in line with a policy integration scheme, were prepared to face intersectoral and intergovernmental management problems or, on the contrary, presented problems in this regard (ECDC, 2015; Lückenbach et al, 2021). It is also useful to see the extent to which, over time, learning and the need to respond to the crisis favoured the adoption of these policy integration mechanisms. First, at a systemic level, formal and/or informal norms are needed, as well as general provisions for intersectoral and intergovernmental action that ensure the functioning of integrated patterns of policy-making regardless of the characteristics and preferences of the individual actors operating within the system (Domorenok et al, 2021a, 2021b).

Since the 1990s, the public management literature has used different concepts to refer to formulas designed to deal with 'Complex intersectoral-intergovernmental problems' (CIIPs), and to achieve the design of what have been called 'integrated policies' (Paquet & Schertzer, 2020). The reference to CIIPs describes the challenges of managing difficult issues such as climate change, population aging, or mass immigration, problems that require the involvement of various intra- and/or supra-state levels of government to be addressed, and that defy traditional forms of collaboration among them.

On the other hand, 'wicked problems' are conceptualised in the policy literature as those in which it is difficult to isolate a single cause and therefore clearly identify solutions (Rittel & Webber, 1973; Termeer et al, 2019). These types of problems are difficult to solve, not only because of their complex nature, but also because they require the concurrence of several public policies to be adequately addressed. They imply the need to coordinate financial and human resources, knowledge, experience, interests, procedures, and processes that usually operate in largely compartmentalised silos (Peters & Tarpey, 2019; Capano et al, 2020).

Building on the concepts of 'wicked problems' and the CIIPs previously defined, a third category of problems quite common in contemporary societies, and showing specific features in times of crisis, can be pointed out. Domorenok et al (2021a, 2021b) identify and systematise the various institutional capacity components that are relevant for integrated policy designs and, based on Wu et al (2015), propose combining three levels (systemic, organisational, and individual) to achieve integrated policies that may circumvent intersectoral and intergovernmental management problems (Table 1.1):

a) The systemic level: formal and/or informal rules, as well as general provisions, for inter-sectoral and intergovernmental action are needed to ensure the functioning of integrated patterns of policymaking, regardless of the characteristics and preferences of individual actors operating within the system (Domorenok et al, 2021a, 2021b). During a crisis, difficulties increase, particularly in circumstances where the pressure to make decisions is extreme (for example, situations that may claim many victims), and where there is a clear awareness of the short time windows to adopt sound measures.

   Crisis management experts are accustomed to dealing with complex environments, and, just like in the healthcare field, to establishing protocols with the aim of reducing uncertainty in both the decision-making process, and in the subsequent actions that follow. The existence of a prior systemic framework (for example, preparedness and response plans) to guide public decision-makers is essential during the early stages of a crisis to understand what is happening (causes of the crisis, the immediate threat and the time limit for mitigating it, as well as the probable course of events, the consequences of the possible decisions, and so on), to make

Table 1.1: Institutional capacity and policy integration framework for analysing the management of nursing homes in the context of the COVID-19 pandemic

Levels	Definitions	Indicators in the pandemic
Systems and instruments	Comprehensive long-term policy framework, establishing coherent policy goals and consistent policy instruments	• Laws, strategies, and plans for preparedness and response to epidemics that would allow coordinated interventions between the health system and the social services system and among levels of government • Socio-health coordination plans and exercises prior to the pandemic and during the pandemic, which consider all levels of government • Clear rules on an integrated sectoral and territorial leadership in the pandemic crisis. Rules about how to manage territorial or sectoral differences • Interoperable information systems to monitor health in nursing homes
Organisation structures	Vertical and horizontal coordination mechanisms to ensure synergies and complementarity within and between the administrations involved	• At the political-administrative level of the organisation, sectoral or territorial coordination structures ensuring information exchange and support for action • Ad hoc expert committees • At an operational level, administrative procedures and tools introduce and systematise to manage the pandemic
Individual	Qualified staff capable to design and manage cross-sectoral and intergovernmental integrated strategies	• Empathy and perception of shared objectives between policy sectors and policy levels • Professional background, specific training, on cross-sectoral skills • Collaborative initiatives encouraging change in mind-sets and administrative practices

Source: Own elaboration based on Wu et al (2015), Tosun and Lang (2017), El-Taliawi and Van Der Wal (2019), and Domorenok et al (2021a, 2021b).

decisions, and to implement them in an integrated manner: determine which collective efforts should be made in response to the crisis, and to ensure that they are consistently applied (Weick, 1995).

b) The organisational level: one of the challenges of policy integration is to combine the different logics of the different organisations that have been working individually until then. In organisational practice, this affects the institutional arrangements, the procedures for decision-making and implementation, the mechanisms for coordination between sectors and levels of government that enhance interaction, as well as the coordination and synergies between individuals and units involved in each integrated design. Again, the possibility of discussing procedures or institutional arrangements during a crisis is considerably more complex, as it requires meeting space between the different actors at a time when the organisations themselves are under severe stress.

c) The individual level: includes the personal characteristics of the leadership and other actors involved with different expertise, skills, experiences, and motivation for integration. This follows those studies that emphasise the role of certain individual characteristics, such as managerial, technical, or political skills, to condition the degree of policy integration (Wu et al, 2015). Domorenok et al (2021b) also propose empirical indicators that help to identify the presence of different levels. Under conditions of deep uncertainty and urgency, bureaucratic organisations may not be the most adequate environments for the development of these tasks, but they have certain advantages that can be exploited to try to be more effective and efficient.

The conceptualisation proposed by these authors is useful to analyse the management of the COVID-19 crisis in Europe, and to understand the extent to which the first governmental responses to the pandemic were in line with a policy integration scheme. It is also useful to check whether emergency policy responses were adapted to face cross-sectoral and intergovernmental management problems or, on the contrary, presented problems in this regard. Finally, it is useful to analyse to what extent early learning about the nature of the crisis, and the need to respond to its effects, favoured the adoption of policy integration mechanisms as the pandemic crisis unfolded.

These conceptual tools should help us analyse in a comparative fashion the way in which initial policy responses were developed to face the emergency caused by the COVID-19 pandemic in care homes for the elderly. Also, they shall be helpful to understand the challenges faced by healthcare and social policy authorities in those situations of maximum tension and stress.

Design and methodology of the research

The information presented in this volume is drawn from the collective work developed by a group of research teams across Europe framed within the project 'Mechanisms for the coordination of the policy response to the Coronavirus crisis in the care home sector in Europe', funded by the Spanish National Research Council (CSIC).

This research was designed in the context of the emergency created by the COVID-19 pandemic outbreak, and more precisely by the realisation that the care home sector had been very particularly exposed to the consequences of this pandemic in the first stages of the spreading of the disease, and that there probably were structural and institutional aspects that seriously limited the capacity of those centres to provide an efficient response to the emergency situation.

The research focused on the European context as a way to proceed to a fruitful comparison between social protections systems that fit within the better-known typologies of welfare regimes, and that share a basic level of development of their LTC sectors, thus allowing for a more consistent focus on the policy integration dynamics that account for the diverse response of the care home sectors of these countries in front of a relatively similar pandemic shock.

The focus of this comparative analysis is specifically placed on the 'first wave' of the pandemic, which could be established to have hit Europe between March, and early July 2020. By looking at this precise time frame we aim at apprehending the circumstances that reflect the initial response of the care home sector to this emergency situation, showing not only the level of preparedness to a pandemic, or the institutional capacity of this part of the LTC sector to respond to an unexpected shock, but most importantly, revealing the degree of policy integration that framed the range of the possible responses to the challenge posed by the pandemic to this policy domain. This temporary focus obviously limits the scope of our analysis, since many other dimensions of an emergency management could be studied by looking at the response provided to the pandemic in the whole cycle of the evolution of the disease. For practical reasons, linked to the generation of the empirical evidence on which this volume is based, gathered during the first months following the outbreak of the disease, this is not possible in this book. Nevertheless, we believe the analysis of the different case studies compiled in this volume provide a rich insight into the handling of a pandemic in the early stages of the crisis in a very sensible area such as the care homes for the elderly, where a particularly frail population finds itself collectively facing the risk of contagion, and where the response provided by public administrations and the managers of the centres from minute one of the outbreak may constitute a critical factor to guarantee the wellbeing of the residents.

The first steps given by the managers of care homes revealed the governance structure of this policy domain, but also the interconnections between the healthcare and the social care sectors, the interactions between the different ministerial areas (at all levels of government), as well as the multilevel governance structures that framed the interactions between different levels of public administrations.

The research group which initiated this project established the network of research teams from the different countries included in the comparative study by relaying on well-known and reputed experts on LTC that could become responsible for the drafting of the case study of their respective country. In order to homogenise the focus of the different national case studies, a common template was established, including the different dimensions that had to be looked up in all of the countries, as well as the key analytical concepts that guided the research in order to define the basic parameters of the generation of empirical evidence, as well as to frame the analysis

Figure 1.1: Evolution of mortality in Europe due to the COVID-19 pandemic

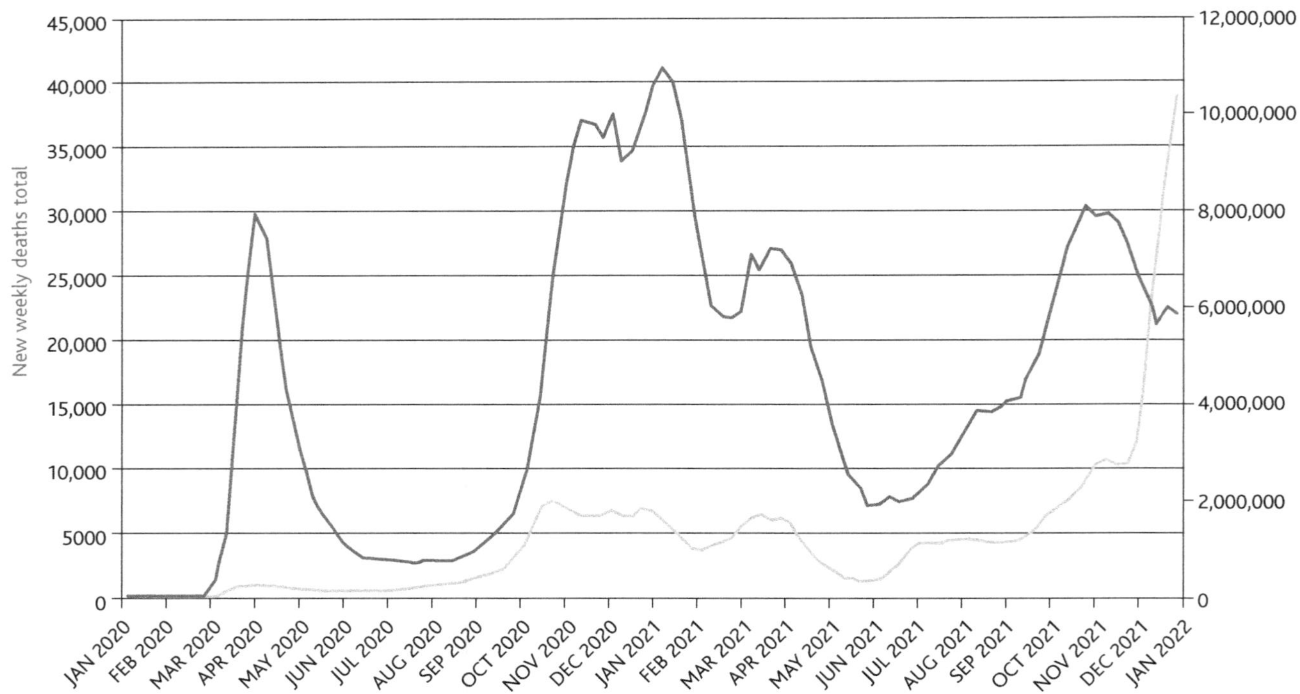

Source: WHO website (https://www.who.int/teams/integrated-health-services/monitoring-health-services/global-pulse-survey-on-continuity-of-essential-health-services-during-the-covid-19-pandemic/dashboard)

of the national case studies that form this research, and that allow for the comparative analysis which constitutes the core of this volume.

In addition to the analysis of documents issued by governmental and independent sources, together with the follow up of surveys and statistical data from their respective country, each team was responsible for generating qualitative empirical evidence by conducting in-depth semi-structured open-ended interviews with key informants including managers of care homes (directors, administrators, and/or medical supervisors), high-ranking officials responsible for social services and/or the healthcare sector (at the central and/or regional levels), as well as representatives of trade unions and/or employers' associations of the nursing homes. Key informants were identified using contacts and networks already known to the researchers, as well as internet research and analysis of previous work and documents from various official sources. Given the COVID-19 context and the mobility restrictions at the time of data collection, interviews were conducted mostly by videoconference between October and December 2020. Those interviews lasted generally between one hour and one and a half. Interview scripts were prepared according to the profile of the interviewees. In the case of experts and policymakers, the interview guide included open-ended questions related to the basic characteristics of LTC system governance (regulatory framework and main problems of the sector) and issues related to the impact of the pandemic on care home formal caregivers. Representatives of trade unions and employers' organisations in the sector were asked similar questions, as well as others related to their perception of institutional management of formal caregivers in their care homes during the COVID-19 crisis. Once all interviews were recorded and transcribed, data analysis involved a systematic review of all texts to identify patterns of ideas and concepts (Crabtree & Miller, 1999).

The final purpose of those interviews was to obtain first-hand information that would allow us to better understand the way in which care homes for the elderly handled the pandemic, and the critical consequences the decisions they adopted had over their residents. This pool of interviews, even if limited, allowed for a mix of unique points of view by each interviewee on the phenomenon under investigation, enriching the case studies written by each national team that constitute the chapters of this volume.

The empirical evidence in this volume introduces some limitations to the projection of the analysis to the evolution of the whole period of the pandemic. Nevertheless, this volume contributes to identifying the specificities of each country in the handling of the pandemic in the long-term care (LTC) sector in Europe in the early stages of a crisis of this nature. It provides a better understanding of the problems and innovative solutions that emerged in the management of COVID-19 crises in nursing homes in this region, their causes and the lessons learned from this experience.

The book also analyses in detail the institutional conditions necessary for the design of integrated policies capable of providing effective responses to the management of old people's homes in times of crisis but also in times of normality.

Structure of the volume

This book addresses the way in which different governments in Europe dealt with the coronavirus crisis in their nursing homes sector. More specifically, the research focuses on the integration mechanisms between the healthcare and social services systems for the care of the institutionalised old-age population.

Following this introduction, Chapter 2, by Roberta Perna and Luis Moreno reviews how the transformations in the demand and supply of caring, together with the need to contain healthcare costs, fostered institutional changes in the regulation, financing, and provision of old-age care in Europe in the years previous to the pandemic. Their work put forward how differences in 'national' and 'regime' visions of social risks, as a domain of state-member responsibility, shaped the context in which LTC policies evolved in different European countries over that period. This review sets the stage for the analysis of the different case studies included in the volume, as well as for the comparative analysis presented in the last chapter of the book.

Chapter 3, by Monika Riedel and Christoph Stegner, analyses the situation generated by the COVID-19 pandemic in the Austrian care home sector, which did not have an emergency plan, a specific government department, or a robust public health system, but went through the first wave of the pandemic with a relatively low infection and casualties score. According to the authors, the long tradition of consensus-finding between the social partners prevented the existing shortcomings from leading to even more significant effects across all sectors affected by the pandemic, including LTC. In that case it was soon recognised that persons in need of LTC in general, particularly residents in care homes, faced the highest risk because of the pandemic, but this understanding did not translate into a very significant change in the way in which care was provided, with the shortage of care-providing staff emerging as the clearest limitation to any significant transformation of the Austrian LTC system.

In Chapter 4, Caroline Glendinning analyses the case of England, where the pandemic made vividly explicit the multiple structural weaknesses of adult residential care, particularly compared with health services. These weaknesses notably refer to the chronic underfunding of care services, the clear prioritisation of health in national policies, the fragmented relationships between national and local government institutions and actors, the weak relationships between acute health and LTC, and the chronic shortages of paid care workers. Those fault lines had been exacerbated by a decade of financial austerity policies that had left both the residential care and the healthcare system considerably weakened, so the prospects for a coordinated response to the pandemic were not promising. The impact of COVID-19 on English residential care was devastating, and the already weakened residential home quasi-market was hit financially by a triple burden of reduced occupancy rates, extra staffing costs, and inflated PPE prices.

Chapter 5, by Tyyne Ylinen, Vera Ylinen, Laura Kalliomaa-Puha, and Satu Ylinen, reviews the evolution of the pandemic in Finland, emphasising how this country managed the pandemic period moderately well, but elderly people living in care homes were in a particularly vulnerable position throughout the pandemic, showing death rates consistently higher than the rest of the population. The country has a national emergency preparedness plan, local preparedness plans, and a special national preparedness plan for pandemics. There is also a clear governance in situations of emergency, including pandemics, and all these preventive mechanisms were put to a reality test for the first time by the COVID-19 pandemic, scoring relatively well. Nevertheless, the restrictions imposed on the living conditions of elderly people living in care homes to protect them from contagion were considered to have violated their fundamental rights, showing the complex trade-offs that have to be carefully handled in emergency situations like this one.

The case of France is analysed by Arnaud Campéon, Blanche Le Bihan, and Claude Martin in Chapter 6, showing how a strong mobilisation by public authorities tackled the direct consequences of the epidemic in care homes from the early stages of the pandemic. Considerable additional finances were allocated, and national recommendations were established to deal with this unprecedented health situation. The emergency brought to the forefront structural weaknesses in the care home sector that had been identified well before the pandemic, but had not been subject to adequate reforms. Implementing the recommendations and protocols produced by the supervisory authorities also raised numerous questions and dilemmas for the professionals responsible for applying them, since they complicated the daily work and practices of professionals working at residential care homes. Although the high death rate due to the epidemic in residential care homes can partly be attributed to the complexity of comorbidities affecting many older people, another contributory factor was the more structural difficulties endured by the sector, including the shortages in staff in residential care homes.

In Chapter 7, Caspar Lückenbach, Eduard Klukas, Phillip Florian Schmidt, and Thomas Gerlinger present the evolution of COVID-19 in the LTC sector in Germany, where the measures taken during the first months of the pandemic can be considered relatively successful as the numbers of infections and COVID-19-related deaths were kept reasonably low compared to other developed countries. Nevertheless, the public health service showed considerable technical and staffing shortcomings, and the federal structure and the decentralised responsibilities led to problems in coordinating and enforcing measures to combat the pandemic, reflected in a temporary overburdening of municipal administrative structures, numerous negotiations between the federal and Länder governments, and sometimes considerable differences in the handling of the pandemic between regions. Staff shortages in the care home sector posed a significant challenge in this country as well.

Costis Prouskas and Michael Goudoumas analyse the case of Greece in Chapter 8, where they elaborate on how the care home sector of this country scored very well in its response to the threat of the COVID-19 pandemic during the first wave of the disease. The outstanding outcome is attributed to the timely reaction of Greek authorities, the initiatives and early measures they introduced to keep low rates of infections in the community, as well as the governance structures set in place to coordinate care home managers, regional authorities and central government. The decision to isolate the residential units, regularly check employees and residents, increase protection measures, and closely observe employees' and residents' temperature and possible symptoms from the early stages of the pandemic, even before the national bodies adopted them, is also considered key to explain this positive evolution.

The case of Ireland is reviewed by Sara Burke, Katharine Schulmann, Virpi Timonen, and Eimir Hurley in Chapter 9, where they highlight how the fragmented nature of the relationship between authorities and the residential care sector led to delays in response to the crisis in nursing homes. The pandemic highlighted key weaknesses in the care home sector, especially in terms of deficits in clinical governance, the lack of skilled staff, minimum staffing requirements, and inadequate premises, especially in terms of ability to isolate suspected cases. The management of the pandemic in care homes became distinctly paternalistic and medicalised in character, to the point where all other needs of older persons were negated.

Chapter 10, by Costanzo Ranci, Marco Arlotti, and Stefania Cerea, presents the analysis of the situation in Italy, the first country where the disease was diagnosed in Europe, and in which the impact among the elderly population, notably those residing in care homes, was more acute. The authors emphasise how care homes were unable not only to prevent or limit the entry of the virus into their structures, but also to provide PPE for their workers and adequate medical care to their residents, and very often unable to send them to hospitals, so care home residents were on lockdown in institutions that could not take care of them (Hernández-Moreno & Pereira-Puga, 2021; Hernández-Moreno et al, 2023). This critical situation was not only due to the priority given to hospitals in the anti-pandemic policy, but further reinforced by the structural weaknesses affecting care homes before the pandemic. The inaction of public administrations contributed to determining those conditions of low quality in the management of services that favoured the dramatic impact of the pandemic in Italian residential institutions.

Robert Urbé and Cristina Font Haro present the case of Luxembourg in Chapter 11. This small country experienced very similar situations to the rest of the continent, since no legal framework or protocols could protect its citizens, or indicate what measures to take in front of a pandemic like COVID-19. Moreover, materially, Luxembourg was only prepared to provide medical and social care to a small fraction of the population of sick and older people, experiencing significant shortages of personnel in addition to the material constraints to respond to the exponential increase in demand for medical and social care.

The evolution of the situation in the Netherlands is analysed by María Bruquetas and Anita Böcker in Chapter 12 of the volume. The authors point out how excess mortality was exceptionally high among people receiving LTC in care and nursing homes during the first wave of the pandemic. The focus of the crisis on the hospital and ICU occupancy contributed to this situation in care homes, a situation that remained underexposed during the first months of the pandemic due to the lack of representation of this sector in the Outbreak Management Team (OMT) which advised the government on how to deal with the pandemic. The dilemma between quality of life and safety of the residents, including infection prevention, became a central concern as the handling of the pandemic was analysed at the political and institutional level.

The case of Portugal is reviewed by Luis Capucha, Alexandre Daniel Calado, and Nuno Nunes in Chapter 13 of the volume. The authors emphasise the lack of existence of links between health and social security authorities in Portugal, as well as the non-existence of emergency plans against a pandemic as some of the factors that made the handling of the pandemic in the care home sector more complex. Other dimensions specific to the situation of the care home sector, such as the insufficient levels of healthcare, the lack of rigor in the handling of residents' documentation, the absence of systems for regular assessment of the degree of dependence of users, the lack of definition of the medication circuit, and the shortage of nursing staff, were also pointed out as structural weaknesses that put the elderly population at risk.

Chapter 14 analyses the situation in Spain based on the research conducted by Jorge Hernández-Moreno, Roberta Perna, Manuel Pereira-Puga, and Gibrán Cruz-Martínez. The study conducted by this team shows how a series of structural problems of the LTC system such as the vertical and horizontal fragmentation across actors in the health and social service domains, the weak coordination, the precarious employment conditions, and the shortages of professional caregivers made the outbreak of the COVID-19 pandemic particularly problematic for the care home sector in this country. The complex governance of the sector, and the lack of coordination between the health and social care sectors, aggravated the situation in a context where protocols to address this type of situation did not exist, and where the infrastructural characteristics of care homes sometimes made it very difficult to insulate residents without seriously limiting their basic freedoms.

In Chapter 15, Lennarth Johansson and Pär Schön analyse the evolution of the situation in Sweden, a case characterised by the lack of general lockdown or harsh restrictions adopted by the authorities. Instead, the Swedish strategy was based on voluntary measures, emphasising individual responsibility to follow government recommendations. As a result, the official efforts to stop or slow the spread of infection were few, weak, and late. The healthcare system was ill-prepared for a pandemic, and took considerable time to be reorganised and adapted to the situation, or to develop routines and effective treatments for COVID-19. There was a severe shortage of PPE, hospital beds, and care personnel, as well as insufficient knowledge of basic hygiene routines among care personnel. The impact on residents of care homes was very high.

Finally, Chapter 16 provides a comparative analysis of the different case studies presented in this volume and presents some concluding remarks. The coronavirus crisis in nursing homes was a very complex policy problem, not only because of the characteristics of the affected population, the previous situation of the homes, and the nature of the crisis, but also because of the structural complexity of the relationship between the diverse actors involved in this sector which was made significantly more strained by the stressful context of the first phase of the pandemic. Nonetheless, this situation opened up a window of opportunity to successfully implement measures that mitigated the severe incidence of the pandemic among nursing home residents. Although it is not possible to establish the relative weight that the management of the care homes sector during the pandemic may have had in the death-toll vis-à-vis other factors, everything seems to indicate that had there been preventive measures and emergency plans in place to prevent the entry of the virus and its transmission within nursing homes (or at least to reduce its intensity), the number of deaths may have been sensibly smaller. To better understand what happened in these centres, and to facilitate policy learning, this study identifies the difficulties faced by institutional actors and nursing home managers between January and August 2020.

References

Amela Heras, C., Cortés García, M., and Sierra Moros, M. J. (2010) Bases epidemiológicas para la toma de decisiones sobre medidas de salud pública (no farmacológicas) durante la respuesta a la pandemia de gripe (H1N1) 2009. *Revista Española de Salud Pública*, 84(5), 497–506.

Ansell, C., Boin, A., and Keller, A. (2010) Managing transboundary crises: identifying the building blocks of an effective response system. *Journal of Contingencies and Crisis Management*, 18(4), 195–207.

Armstrong, P. and Braedley, S. (2023) *Care Homes in a Turbulent Era: Do They Have A Future?*, Cheltenham: Edward Elgar Publishing.
Béland, D. and Marier, P. (2020) COVID-19 and long-term care policy for older people in Canada. *Journal of Aging & Social Policy*, 32(4–5), 358–64.
Boin, A. (2007) *La Política de la Gestión de Crisis: El Liderazgo Público Bajo Presión*, Madrid, España: INAP.
Boin, A., McConnell, A., and t Hart, P. (2021) *Governing the Pandemic: The Politics of Navigating a Mega-Crisis*, London: Springer Nature.
Bowblis, J. and Applebaum, R. (2021) Prevalence of COVID-19 in Ohio nursing homes: what's quality got to do with it? *Journal of Aging & Social Policy*, 33(4–5), 414–30.
Capano, C., Howlett, M., Jarvis, D., Ramesh, M., and Goyal, M. (2020) Mobilizing policy (in)capacity to fight COVID-19: understanding variations in state responses, *Policy and Society*, 39(3), 285–308.
Carter Anand, J., Donnelly, S., Milne, A., Nelson-Becker, H., Vingare, E., Deusdad, B., Cellini, G., Kinni, R., and Pregno, C. (2022) The COVID-19 pandemic and care homes for older people in Europe – deaths, damage and violations of human rights, *European Journal of Social Work*, 25(5), 804–15.
Cox, R. H., Dickson, D., and Marier, P. (2021) Resistance, innovation, and improvisation: comparing the responses of nursing home workers to the COVID-19 pandemic in Canada and the United States, *Journal of Comparative Policy Analysis: Research and Practice*, 23(1), 1–10.
Crabtree, B. F., and Miller, W. L. (1999) Doing qualitative research. In B. F. Crabtree & W. L. Miller (eds) *Researching practice settings: A case study approach*, Thousand Oaks, CA: Sage Publications, pp 293–312.
Daly, M. (2020) COVID-19 and care homes in England: What happened and why? *Social Policy & Administration*, 1–14.
del Pino, E., Moreno, F. J., Cruz, G., Hernández, J., Moreno, L., Pereira, M., and Perna, R. (2020) Informe gestión institucional y organizativa de las residencias de personas mayores y COVID-19: dificultades y aprendizajes, Instituto de Políticas y Bienes Públicos (IPP-CSIC) [online], Available from: https://digital.csic.es/handle/10261/220460
Domorenok, E., Graziano, P., and Polverari, L. (2021a) Introduction. Policy integration and institutional capacity: theoretical, conceptual and empirical challenges, *Policy and Society*, 40(1), 1–18.
Domorenok, E., Graziano, P., and Polverari, L. (2021b) Policy integration, policy design and administrative capacities: evidence from EU cohesion policy, *Policy and Society*, 40(1), 58–78.
ECDC (2015) Preparedness planning for respiratory viruses in EU Member States – three case studies on MERS preparedness in the EU, Estocolmo, Suecia: ECDC [online], Available from: https://www.ecdc.europa.eu/en/publications-data/preparedness-planning-respiratory-viruses-eu-member-states

Elgström, O. and Jönsson, C. (2000) Negotiation in the European Union: bargaining or problem-solving? *Journal of European Public Policy*, 7(5), 684–704.

El-Taliawi., O- G. and Van Der Wal, Z. (2019) Developing administrative capacity: an agenda for research and practice, *Policy Design and Practice*, 2(3), 243–57.

González, A. (2022) La coordinación del Sistema Nacional de Salud en España: regulación y resultados en tiempos de pandemia, in C. Colino (ed) *Retos de la Gobernanza Multinivel y la Coordinación en el Estado Autonómico: de la Pandemia al Futuro*, Madrid: INAP, pp 73–92.

Greer, S. L., King, E. J., da Fonseca, E. M., and Peralta-Santos, A. (2020) The comparative politics of COVID-19: The need to understand government responses, *Global Public Health*, 15(9), 1413–16.

Hernández-Moreno, J. (2022) La gestión institucional de la crisis de COVID-19: coordinación intergubernamental e intersectorial en las políticas de Sanidad y Servicios Sociales, in C. Colino (ed) *Retos de la Gobernanza Multinivel y la Coordinación en el Estado Autonómico: de la Pandemia al Futuro*, Madrid: INAP, pp 93–127.

Hernández-Moreno, J. and Pereira-Puga, M. (2021) *On the Corona Frontline: The Experieces of Care Workers in Spain*, Stockholm: FES Nordic Countries.

Hernández-Moreno, J., Pereira-Puga, M., and Cruz-Martínez, G. (2023) COVID-19 and nursing homes in decentralized Spain: how governance and public policies influence working conditions and organizational responses to the crisis, *Administration & Society*, 55(9), 1651–79.

Howlett, M. and Saguin, K. (2018) Policy capacity for policy integration: Implications for the sustainable development goals, Lee Kuan Yew School of Public Policy Working Paper Series, Singapore: National University of Singapore.

Jiménez, S., and Viola, A. (2020) La asistencia residencial en España y COVID-19, *Studies on the Spanish Economy*, eee2020-20, FEDEA.

Lückenbach, C., Klukas, E., Schmidt, P. H., and Gerlinger, T. (2021) Governmental response to the COVID-19 pandemic in long-term care residences for older people: preparedness, responses and challenges for the future: Germany, MC COVID-19 working paper 06/2021 [online], Available from: https://pub.uni-bielefeld.de/record/2951007

Maggetti, M. and Trein, P. (2022) Policy integration, problem-solving, and the coronavirus disease crisis: lessons for policy design, *Policy and Society*, 41(1), 53–67.

McConnell, A. (2020) Evaluating success and failure in crisis management, *Oxford Research Encyclopedia of Politics* [online], Available from: https://oxfordre.com/politics/view/10.1093/acrefore/9780190228637.001.0001/acrefore-9780190228637-e-1633

Ministerio de Derechos Sociales y Agenda 2030 (2020) Información sobre los mecanismos de coordinación adoptados en cada territorio entre los servicios sociales y el sistema sanitario para asegurar la atención médica en los centros sociales residenciales en casos de covid-19, 7 de septiembre [online], Available from: https://www.mscbs.gob.es/ssi/imserso/docs/Coordinacion_sociosanitaria_CCAA.pdf

OECD (2023) *OECD Health Statistics 2023: Beds in residential long-term care facilities* [online], Available from: https://stats.oecd.org/wbos/fileview2.aspx?IDFile=4439d7fd-6fd3-4baa-ad56-35245def07f0

Paquet, M. and Schertzer, R. (2020) COVID-19 as a complex intergovernmental problem. *Canadian Journal of Political Science/Revue canadienne de science politique*, 53(2), 343–7.

Peters, B. G. and Tarpey, M. (2019) Are wicked problems really so wicked? Perceptions of policy problems, *Policy & Society*, 38(2), 2018–36.

Rittel, H. W. and Webber, M. M. (1973) Dilemmas in a general theory of planning, *Policy Sciences*, 4(2), 155–69.

Rosenthal, U., Charles, M. T., and 't Hart, P. (eds) (1989) *Coping with crises: The management of disasters, riots and terrorism*. Springfield, IL: Charles C Thomas.

Termeer, C. J., Dewulf, A., and Biesbroek, R. (2019) A critical assessment of the wicked problem concept: relevance and usefulness for policy science and practice. *Policy and Society*, 38(2), 167–79.

Tosun, J. and Lang, A. (2017) Policy integration: mapping the different concepts, *Policy Studies*, 38(6), 553–70.

Weick, K. (1995) *Sensemaking in organizations*. Thousand Oaks, CA: Sage.

WHO (2020) *Preventing and Managing COVID-19 across Long Care Services: Policy Brief*, Ginebra, Suiza: World Health Organization [online], Available from: https://www.who.int/publications/i/item/WHO-2019-nCoV-Policy_Brief-Long-term_Care-2020.1

Wu, X., Ramesh, M., and Howlett, M. (2015) Policy capacity: A conceptual framework for understanding policy competences and capabilities, *Policy and Society*, 34(3–4), 165–71.

2

Welfare regimes and long-term care in the 'Old Continent'

Roberta Perna and Luis Moreno

Introduction

Throughout the 20th century, dependency and the need for care traditionally constituted a neglected social risk by most European welfare states. In the Fordist society, the social division of care conceived the family as the leading actor in charge of caring for dependent family members. At the same time, state intervention was relegated to assistance measures for specific, limited circumstances, such as lack of family ties, poverty, or a very high degree of disability (Ranci & Pavolini, 2013). Entitlement to receive care 'was framed implicitly as an entitlement to be cared for by a female family member. It certainly did not result in a social right' (Saraceno, 2008: p 2).

During the last three decades, however, demographic and social transformations and economic considerations created a 'problem pressure' (Ferrera, 2005) no longer negligible for European welfare states. On the one hand, the share of older people steadily increased over the last decades (Eurostat, 2022). In 2021, people aged 65+ represented more than one-fifth (20.8 per cent) of the population in the EU, against 17.6 per cent in 2011. The old-age dependency ratio, which measures the relation between the population aged 65+ and the working-age population (15–64 years), was 33.5 per cent in January 2021, compared to 26.4 per cent in 2011. According to the latest population projections, those aged 65+ will account for 31.3 per cent of the EU's population by 2100, and the old-age dependency ratio is projected to almost double, reaching 57.1 per cent in 2100. On the other hand, the increasing participation of women in the labour market, and the redefinition of family care obligations, reduced the caregiving capacity of traditional family-based systems (Jensen & Møberg, 2011), particularly in the case of highly dependent people (Costa & Ranci, 2010).

Hence, the transformations in the demand and supply sides of caring – together with the need to contain and rationalise increasing healthcare costs associated with ageing in times of permanent fiscal austerity (Bonoli, 2006) – fostered institutional changes in the regulation, financing, and provision of old-age care in Europe (Ranci & Pavolini, 2013).

This chapter provides an overview of existing arrangements of long-term care (LTC) for older people in Europe, focusing on their differences and expected trends and challenges. As this overview will suggest, these arrangements essentially replicate and reinforce pre-existing varieties of 'welfare regimes' in Europe. Despite this heterogeneity, however, old-age care systems have faced common challenges in the last decades.

Welfare regimes and old-age care: an overview of LTC types in Europe

The 'welfare regime' approach, proposed by Gøsta Esping-Andersen (1990), has been the most influential in the conceptual and methodological debate on social policy development in the last decades. According to this approach, welfare states are characterised by a constellation of economic, political, and social institutional arrangements. Thus, to speak of a 'welfare regime' denotes that a complex of legal and organisational features are systematically interwoven in the relation between the state and the market. Based on the study of three main dimensions (state–market relations, stratification, and de-commodification) Esping-Andersen's analysis leads to the identification of three ideal-type welfare regimes: the Social-Democratic, the Liberal, and the Conservative. Various contributions have confirmed this typology since its inception, while others have challenged and expanded it from substantive and methodological perspectives (Leibfried, 1992; Sarasa & Moreno, 1996; Ferrera, 1996; Castles & Obinger, 2008; for a review of the debate on welfare regimes, see Arts & Gelissen, 2010; Ferragina & Seeleib-Kaiser, 2011). Still others have argued that Esping-Andersen's typology is quite limited to the work–welfare nexus, while it is of relatively little use for domains such as the care–welfare nexus (Lewis, 1992; Knijn & Ungerson, 1997), or for the analysis of healthcare systems (Bambra, 2005; Wendt, 2009).

Although at various paces, since the end of the century all countries in the 'Old Continent' have been confronted with increasing demands for old-age care. National responses have varied across Europe (Anttonen & Sipilä, 1996; Costa-Font, 2010), often along the paths traced by existing welfare regimes (González de Durana & Moreno Fuentes, 2009; Rodríguez Cabrero & Marbán Gallego, 2013).

The Nordic model pioneered the development of a public system for dependency and old-age care at the beginning of the 1970s, which gradually replaced women's role as caregivers in the family as they entered the labour market. As it is well known, Nordic countries represent the quintessential Esping-Andersen (1990) Social-Democratic type. In this model, social protection is sanctioned as an individual's right, leading to a generous system of universal and highly redistributive benefits for all citizens. Following this legacy, dependency and old-age care arrangements in Northern Europe have been progressively included in the municipal social services system as an additional universalistic right (Nielsen et al, 1997), primarily based on the public provision of residential care. Nevertheless, since the turn of the millennium, Scandinavian countries have gone through a progressive shift towards arrangements that combine cost-containment in public social expenditure with the externalisation of service provision to market players with less generous coverage of home and residential care (Trydegård & Thorslund, 2010). Likewise, these countries emphasised beneficiaries' freedom of choice and the provision of cash benefits to promote home care (Kröger, 2011), getting closer to countries of the so-called 'Liberal' welfare regime.

Esping-Andersen's (1990) 'Liberal' ideal type, whose features can be more clearly perceived in Anglo-Saxon countries, embodies the market's primacy in the welfare domain. This market predominance is encouraged by the state, either actively – by subsidising private welfare schemes – or passively – by keeping social benefits to a modest level and with little income redistribution across classes. Inheriting this logic, LTC in Anglo-Saxon countries has been largely conceived regarding social assistance as entirely separated from (universalistic) healthcare and care services provided mainly by private actors. In this model, LTC is structured around two basic pillars: means-tested cash benefits financed by social securitym, or transfers for family caregivers (for those who do not comply with means-tested requirements, private insurance is the only available option) for people in need; or through municipal social services whose conditions for access are – again – dependent on the situation of need (free-of-charge for those in need, subject to co-payments otherwise). Prioritising the market and fostering externalisation in service provision, the Liberal LTC model promotes beneficiaries' freedom of choice across types of care and care providers via the so-called 'Personal budget'.

Moving to continental Europe, the Conservative type is characterised by the principle of subsidiarity and the predominance of social insurance schemes. This welfare model offers a moderate level of de-commodification (social benefits mainly depend on former contributions and occupational status). At the same time, the sphere of solidarity remains corporatist, with little room for social stratification to change. When it comes to LTC, almost all countries sharing the features of this ideal type underwent significant reforms during the 1990s, shifting from pure social assistance to means-tested LTC provisions (in cash or in-kind) financed through general taxation and social security contributions, together with co-payments. Managed in coordination between the central administration, meso-governments, and municipalities, LTC in these countries is grounded on a mixed model of service provision, with a significant presence of private non-profit and for-profit actors. As is the case in Nordic countries, however, since the mid-2000s pressures towards cost-containment have triggered the externalisation of service provision, prioritising (cheaper) cash benefits instead of the provision of in-kind services, as well as the promotion of private insurance as a complement to public programmes for dependency and old-age care (Rothgang, 2010).

Extending Esping-Andersen's typology to address the distinctive features of Southern European welfare systems (for example, intra-familial pooling of resources, household solidarity, pre-eminence of values of family inclusion and life-cycle redistribution [Ferrera, 1996; Sarasa & Moreno, 1996]), implied the conceptualisation of a Mediterranean welfare regime ideal-type. While some welfare schemes are relatively generous (particularly in old-age pensions), others have been almost non-existent until recently, such as minimum income schemes, or parental leaves. Regarding LTC, the family – and women in particular – still hold a primary role, with the state assuming a subsidiary – although increasing – responsibility (Da Roit et al, 2013). During the last decades, the rapid ageing of the population, together with the acceleration in the participation of women in the labour market and the progressive changes in the traditional division of caring roles within the family, has resulted in increasing demands for the formalisation of more comprehensive dependency and old-age care provisions (González de Durana & Moreno Fuentes, 2009; Marbán Gallego, 2020).

Concerning Central-Eastern European countries, the existence of a common welfare type is still under discussion (Arts & Gelissen, 2010). Since the collapse of the Soviet Union, those countries underwent enormous social, political, and economic transformations, often under international and EU influence (Ferge & Juhász, 2004). It has resulted in a 'layering' of inherited communist elements, a revival of pre-communist, Bismarckian elements, and the entering of strongly market-oriented elements, with considerable pressure towards liberalisation and privatisation of social protection. Consequently, some scholars define these countries' welfare systems as a 'continental–liberal hybrid'. In contrast, others point out their diversification along the corresponding lines of the Liberal and the Continental types (Potůček, 2008). This heterogeneity also applies to the LTC domain, although it is challenging to identify standard features in this domain. In general, as for Southern European countries, growing care needs have increasingly pressured governments to develop new welfare arrangements for old-age care (Österle, 2011), often characterised by social assistance provision financed by a mix of (decreasing) public resources, and (increasing) private insurance.

Different arrangements, common challenges

Although embedded in different national welfare traditions, research has pointed out the existence of common trends and challenges in the regulation, financing, and provision of old-age care across Europe (Rostgaard, 2002; Pavolini & Ranci, 2008; Pfau-Effinger & Rostgaard, 2011; Spasova et al, 2018; Marbán Gallego, 2020). Three trends appear particularly significant for their policy coordination and efficiency challenges and the accessibility, availability, and quality of old-age care.

Horizontal and vertical fragmentation: policy coordination, accessibility, and equity challenges

In most countries, LTC for older people is not a policy field on its own, but competency and responsibilities for regulation, financing, and service provision which are generally scattered between healthcare and social services (Spasova et al, 2018). This horizontal fragmentation frequently hampers coordination, or even the provision of care, with detrimental effects for dependent people (extended waiting periods, complex administrative procedures, fragmentation of services).

This horizontal fragmentation is frequently accompanied by a vertical distribution of competency and responsibilities between national, regional, and municipal actors in which different levels are responsible for regulating, financing, and providing health and social services associated with LTC (del Pino et al, 2021). For instance, health-related LTC services are regulated and financed at the national level (for example in Belgium, France, Greece, Ireland, the Netherlands, and the UK), or, less frequently, at the regional level (Denmark, Italy), while social care for the elderly can be regulated and funded by the national level (Greece, Ireland, Italy, Luxembourg), the regional or local level (Denmark, Finland, the UK), or by a combination of those equilibriums (for example in Austria, Belgium, Spain, France, and the Netherlands). Likewise, the provision of social LTC services is frequently the responsibility of regions (Austria, Belgium, Spain, France, Italy, and the Netherlands) and/or municipalities (Denmark, Greece, Italy, Finland, the Netherlands, and the UK), while home care is usually a responsibility of the latter.

This puzzling distribution of competences and responsibilities may lead to weak coordination between levels and areas of intervention, which in turn may cause incoherent policy planning and inefficient allocation of resources for old-age care. Moreover, in federal countries or countries, with significant devolution of powers to subnational authorities, the decentralisation of responsibilities in LTC across regions and municipalities often results in important intra-national differences concerning care provision, eligibility criteria, and out-of-pocket payments (for example in Belgium, Spain, Finland, Italy, the Netherlands, and Sweden), which may reflect in territorial inequalities.

De-institutionalisation and commodification of care: challenges to accessibility and availability

Across Europe, home care – that is, care provided in the beneficiary's home – is usually favoured over residential care – where the dependent person lives in a residential facility (Spasova et al, 2018). However, the possibility for older people to enjoy home care highly depends on availability. While home and community-based care are most developed in Nordic and Western European countries, home care remains underdeveloped in Southern and Central-Eastern European countries and in the UK, where it is often restricted to dependent people with special needs.

However, where de-institutionalisation policies have been promoted (to a large extent in Nordic countries with a long tradition of residential care), prioritisation of home care has frequently resulted in reduced investment in – and thus shortages in the availability of – residential facilities (Kröger, 2011). On the contrary, in countries where residential care has been structurally underdeveloped (Southern and some Eastern European countries), efforts have been made to increase residential facilities. However, their availability is still limited compared to existing demand (Rodríguez Cabrero & Marbán Gallego, 2013).

Shortages in the supply of public home and residential care, together with deliberate policies to increase competition in LTC in some countries (such as Sweden and the UK), have triggered a process of commodification of care, with the emergence of a solid private for-profit care market. The establishment of 'Personal budgets' and the prioritisation towards cash-for-care schemes – allowances provided to elderly dependent people and their families which they can either pass on to informal caregivers, or use to employ a paid caregiver – represent a common trend in European countries (Da Roit & Le Bihan, 2011). However, as demand for old-age care keeps increasing de-institutionalisation may lead to shortages in the supply if it is not balanced by increased home and community care investment. Likewise, the externalisation of providing old-age care to private for-profit actors may limit care affordability, opening the door to informal care provision.

Precariousness of employment and informal care provision: quality challenges

Despite LTC being progressively formalised as an area of intervention of national welfare states across Europe, with the emergence of significant changes in the gendered distribution of care the provision of old-age care continues to rely mainly on informal or unqualified carers – female family members of the dependent person and migrant women to be employed, more or less regularly, as domestic workers – (Bettio & Plantenga, 2004; Pfau-Effinger & Rostgaard, 2011; Da Roit et al, 2013). In addition, poor working conditions and employment precariousness in LTC (low pay, limited training, high workload) are frequently identified as causes and consequences of the low attractiveness of the LTC occupational sector across countries (Spasova et al, 2018), leading to shortages of qualified professional carers.

The precariousness of employment in formal care provision and the incidence of informal care affect the quality of care provided to older people (Murphy & Turner, 2017), particularly for those in high dependence or with specific care needs.

Concluding remarks

During the last decades, the transformations in the demand and supply of care –together with the need to contain and rationalise increasing healthcare costs associated with ageing in times of permanent fiscal austerity – have fostered institutional changes in the regulation, financing, and provision of old-age care in Europe. Although LTC for older people has been increasingly regulated and recognised as a social right in Europe, the COVID-19 pandemic abruptly raised collective awareness among citizens all around Europe about this 'new social risk' (Taylor-Gooby, 2004), with older people being among the most fragile targets of the virus. Beyond age-related factors, the living conditions of older people in residential facilities (collective spaces, need for daily interactions with caregivers) made this population especially vulnerable to COVID-19.

Against these double sources of vulnerability, however, the referred-to challenges have been of dramatic importance for managing the COVID-19 pandemic, as the country case studies included in this volume point out. The outbreak of the virus exacerbated institutional problems related to coordination dynamics between levels of government and between healthcare and social services. Shortcomings in managing inter-sectoral coordination between healthcare and social services, as well as poor vertical coordination across national, regional, and local actors are systematically mentioned in the case studies included in this volume. Likewise, structural problems associated with precarious employment in the LTC sector, and shortages of professional caregivers, are often identified as aggravating elements in the difficulties related to managing the pandemic.

The common challenges brought about by the COVID-19 pandemic in all EU countries have probably added another piece of 'Europeanisation' to LTC. The EU does not have competences in these matters. However, the early 2000s dependency and old-age care have been included in a broader European social policy strategy focusing on sustainable pension systems, quality healthcare, LTC services, and social inclusion (Council of the European Union & EU Commission, 2003; European Union, 2019). Through the Open Method of Coordination (OMC) and, more recently, through the adoption of the European Pillar of Social Rights, this strategy attempts to offer perspectives for reconciling the dichotomies between economic and social issues, stimulating a common framework for development and mutual learning in social protection and inclusion.

Accordingly, there are three main dimensions involved in advancing Europeanisation within the OMC: i) the diffusion of concepts around which the proposals of EU's institutions are aimed; ii) techniques of policy implementation, which have inspired the procedures adopted by European governments in order to achieve the referred-to aims; and iii) the establishment of indicators with which governmental intervention is assessed and justified (Moreno & Serrano, 2009).

Differences in perspectives put forward by 'national' and 'regime' visions of social risks as a domain of state-member responsibility have been tempered, as evidenced by the common trends in LTC mentioned in this chapter, or the massive vaccination in all EU. The passing of time will confirm whether the COVID-19 pandemic has to be regarded as a turning point in furthering Europeanisation through sharing good practices and benchmarking objectives in the vital LTC sector of welfare development.

References

Anttonen, A., and Sipilä, J. (1996) European social care services: is it possible to identify models? *Journal of European Social Policy*, 6(2), 87–100.

Arts, W. A. and Gelissen, J. (2010) Models of the welfare state, in F. G. Castles, S. Leibfried, J. Lewis, H. Obinger and C. Pierson (eds) *The Oxford Handbook of the Welfare State*, Oxford: Oxford University Press.

Bambra, C. (2005) Cash versus services: 'worlds of welfare' and the decommodification of cash benefits and health care services, *Journal of Social Policy*, 34(2), 195–213.

Bettio, F. and Plantenga, J. (2004) Comparing care regimes in Europe, *Feminist Economics*, 10(1), 85–113.

Bonoli, G. (2006) New social risks and the politics of post-industrial social policies, in K. Armingeon and G. Bonoli (eds) *The Politics of Post-Industrial Welfare States: Adapting Post-War Social Policies to New Social Risks*, London: Routledge, pp 3–26.

Castles, F. G. and Obinger, H. (2008) Worlds, families, regimes: country clusters in European and OECD Area Public Policy, *West European Politics*, 31(1), 321–44.

Costa, G. and Ranci, C. (2010) Disability and caregiving: a step toward social vulnerability, in C. Ranci (ed) *Social Vulnerability in Europe: The New Configuration of Social Risks*, London: Macmillan, pp 159–85.

Costa-Font, J. (2010) Editorial introduction: long-term care in Europe, *Social Policy & Administration*, 44(4), 357–8.

Council of the European Union and EU Commission (2003) Joint report by the Commission and the Council on supporting national strategies for the future of health care and care for the elderly: 7155/03, Brussels, 10 March [online], Available from: https://ec.europa.eu/employment_social/soc-prot/healthcare/elderly_en.pdf

Da Roit, B. and Le Bihan, B. (2011) Cash-for-care schemes and the changing role of elderly people's informal caregivers in France and Italy, in B. Pfau-Effinger and T. Rostgaard (eds) *Care Between Work and Welfare in European Societies. Work and Welfare in Europe*, London: Palgrave Macmillan.

Da Roit, B., González Ferrer, A., and Moreno Fuentes F. J. (2013) The Southern European migrant-based care model, *European Societies*, 15(4), 577–96.

del Pino, E., Moreno, L., and Hernández-Moreno, J. (2021) Territorial welfare governance changes: concepts and explanatory factors, in Y. Kazepov, E. Barberis, R. Cucca, and E. Mocca (eds) *Handbook of Urban Social Policy: International Perspectives on Multilevel Governance and Local Welfare*, Cheltenham: Edward Elgar.

Esping-Andersen, G. (1990) *The Three Worlds of Welfare Capitalism*, Cambridge: Polity Press.

European Union (2019) *Joint Report on Health Care and Long-Term Care Systems & Fiscal Sustainability. Country Documents 2019 Update*, Institutional paper 105. Brussels: European Commission, Directorate-General for Economic and Financial Affairs [online], Available from: https://ec.europa.eu/info/sites/default/files/economy-finance/ip105_en.pdf

Eurostat (2022) Population structure and ageing, *Eurostat Statistics Explained* [online], Available from: https://ec.europa.eu/eurostat/statistics-explained/index.php?title=Population_structure_and_ageing#:~:text=The%20old%2Dage%20dependency%20ratio,person%20aged%2065%20or%20over

Ferge, Z. and Juhász, G. (2004) Accession and social policy: the case of Hungary, *Journal of European Social Policy*, 14(3), 233–51.

Ferragina, E. and Seeleib-Kaiser, M. (2011) Thematic review. Welfare regime debate: past, present, futures? *Policy & Politics*, 39(4), 583–611.

Ferrera, M. (1996) The 'southern model' of welfare in social Europe. *Journal of European Social Policy*, 6(1), 17–37.

Ferrera, M. (2005) *The Boundaries of Welfare: European Integration and the New Spatial Politics of Social Protection*, Oxford: Oxford University Press.

González de Durana, A. and Moreno Fuentes, F. J. (eds) (2009) *El Tratamiento de la Dependencia en los Regímenes de Bienestar Europeos Contemporáneos*, IMSERSO, Colección Estudios, Serie Dependencia No. 12007, Instituto de Mayores y Servicios Sociales.

Jensen, P. H. and Møberg, R. J. (2011) Tensions related to the transition of elderly care from an unpaid to a paid activity, in B. Pfau-Effinger and T. Rostgaard (eds) *Care Between Work and Welfare in European Societies: Work and Welfare in Europe*, London: Palgrave Macmillan.

Knijn, T. and Ungerson, C. (1997) Introduction: care work and gender in welfare regimes, *Social Politics*, 4(3), 323–7.

Kröger, T. (2011) Under tension: formal care work with older people, in B. Pfau-Effinger and T. Rostgaard (eds) *Care Between Work and Welfare in European Societies: Work and Welfare in Europe*, London: Palgrave Macmillan.

Leibfried, S. (1992) Towards a European welfare state?, in F. Zsuza and J. E. Kolberg (eds) *Social Policy in Changing Europe*, Frankfurt: Campus, pp 245–79.

Lewis, J. (1992) Gender and the development of welfare regimes, *Journal of European Social Policy*, 2(3), 159–73.

Marbán Gallego, V. (2020) Los (des) cuidados de larga duración en España: ¿Reforma o perfeccionamiento del SAAD?, in F. J. Moreno Fuentes and E. del Pino (eds) *Las Transformaciones Territoriales y Sociales del Estado en la Edad Digital*, Madrid: Centro de Estudios Políticos y Constitucionales, pp 331–54.

Moreno, L. and Serrano, A. (2009) The European Social Model and social policies: a formative institutional evaluation, *Gestión y Análisis de Políticas Públicas*, 2, 11–32.

Murphy, C., and Turner, T. (2017) Formal and informal long term care work: policy conflict in a liberal welfare state, *International Journal of Sociology and Social Policy*, 37(3/4), 134–47.

Nielsen, H. W., Sipilä, J., Anderson, M., Hammerqvist, S-E., Norlander, L., Rauhala, P-L., and Thomsen, K. (1997) A multitude of universal public services: how and why did four Scandinavian countries get their social care service model?, in J. Sipilä (ed) *Social Care Services: The Key to the Scandinavian Welfare Model*, London: Routledge, pp 27–50.

Österle, A. (2011) Long-term care in central and south-eastern Europe: challenges and perspectives in addressing a 'new' social risk, *Social Policy & Administration*, 44(4), 461–80.

Pavolini, E. and Ranci, C. (2008) Restructuring the welfare state: reforms in long-term care in western European countries, *Journal of European Social Policy*, 18(3), 246–59.

Pfau-Effinger, B. and Rostgaard, T. (2011) *Care Between Work and Welfare in European Societies*, London: Palgrave Macmillan.

Potůček, M. (2008) Metamorphoses of welfare states in central and eastern Europe, in M. Seeleib-Kaiser (ed), *Welfare State Transformations: Comparative Perspectives*, London: Palgrave Macmillan, pp 79–95.

Ranci, C. and Pavolini E. (eds) (2013) *Reforms in Long-Term Care Policies in Europe: Investigating Institutional Change and Social Impacts*, Cham: Springer.

Rodríguez Cabrero, G., and Marbán Gallego, V. (2013) La atención a dependencia en una perspectiva europea: de la asistencialización a la cuasi-universalización, in E. del Pino and M. J. Rubio Lara (eds) *Los Estados de Bienestar en la Encrucijada: Políticas Sociales en Perspectiva Comparada*, Nottingham: Tecnos, pp 237–61.

Rostgaard, T. (2002) Caring for children and older people in Europe: a comparison of European Policies and practice, *Policy Studies*, 23(1), 51–68.

Rothgang, H. (2010) Social insurance for long-term care: an evaluation of the German model, *Social Policy & Administration*, 44(4), 436–60.

Saraceno, C. (2008) *Gender and Care: Old Solutions, New Developments?* RSCAS Distinguished Lectures 2008/2, Florence: Robert Shuman Centre for Advanced Studies, European University Institute [online], Available from: https://cadmus.eui.eu/bitstream/handle/1814/9307/RSCAS_DL_2008_02.pdf?sequence=2&isAllowed=y

Sarasa, S. and Moreno, L. (eds) (1996) *El Estado del Bienestar en la Europa del Sur*, Madrid: Consejo Superior de Investigaciones Científicas [online], Available from: http://digital.csic.es/handle/10261/179555

Spasova, S., Baeten, R., Coster, S., Ghailani, D., Peña-Casas, R., and Vanhercke, B. (2018) *Challenges in Long-Term Care in Europe: A Study of National Policies*, Brussels: European Commission [online], Available from: https://ec.europa.eu/social/main.jsp?catId=738&langId=en&pubId=8128&furtherPubs=yes

Taylor-Gooby, P. (ed) (2004) *New Risks, New Welfare: The Transformation of the European Welfare State*, Oxford: Oxford University Press.

Trydegård, G.-B. and Thorslund, M. (2010) One uniform welfare state or a multitude of welfare municipalities? The evolution of local variation in Swedish elder care, *Social Policy & Administration*, 44(4), 495–511.

Wendt, C. (2009) Mapping European healthcare systems, *Journal of European Social Policy*, 19(5), 432–45.

3

Muddling through after a strong start: tackling the COVID-19 pandemic in Austrian nursing homes

Monika Riedel and Christoph Stegner

Introduction

In Austria, the devastating impact of the pandemic in neighbouring Italy, including an overcrowded health system and a high death toll, was covered broadly in the media and resulted in significant respect – if not fear – of the potential consequences of this novel disease already in February 2020. The Austrian government reacted quickly and imposed rather strict measures (Hale et al, 2021) to contain infections and to avoid catastrophic situations in hospitals, as observed in reports from the neighbouring country. With effect from week 12/2020, schools had to jump into 'remote teaching'. Due to the complete lack of experience and preparation for this teaching mode, most pupils had several weeks' worth of lost education. Apart from those dealing with essential goods like grocery shops and pharmacies, all shops went into lockdown. Employees were urged to work from home wherever possible. A strict curfew was imposed with a limited list of exceptions: necessary shopping, employment, help for persons in need of support, and outdoor activities like walking, running, and biking for the sake of health and sanity, given a safe distance to other people was kept (*COVID-19-Maßnahmengesetz* and related ordinances).[1] Some measures were criticised as exceeding reasonable limits, like the closure of parks and children's playgrounds, because these measures might lead to a concentration of people in accessible areas. Some regulations were later declared as not justified by the Constitutional Court. A generous public support program for short-time work was introduced to facilitate compliance with the imposed measures and to stabilise the economy (§13 (1) *Arbeitsmarktpolitik-Finanzierungsgesetz*).[2] Under this programme, working hours for employees could be reduced to between 10 per cent and 90 per cent of the agreed standard working hours. As a result, employees received total compensation of between 80 per cent and 90 per cent depending on their previous net wage, and employers only had to pay for the number of hours worked.

Figure 3.1: COVID-19 deaths among care home residents in the first wave (up to 26 June 2020), as a percentage of all COVID-19 deaths

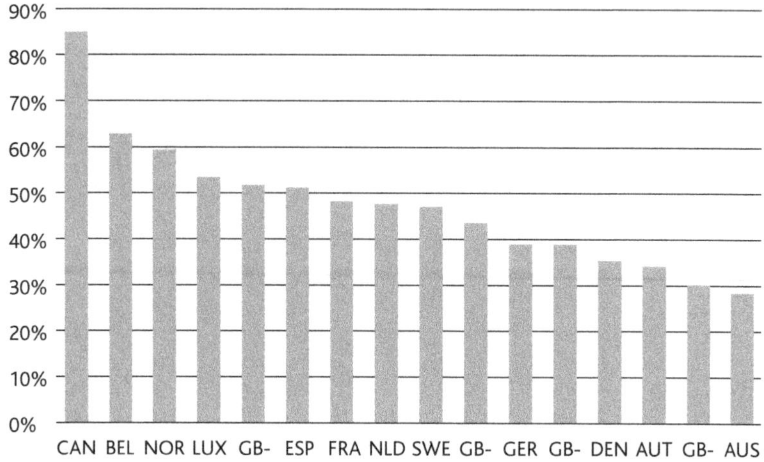

Source: Comas-Herrera et al (2022)

In light of this swift and decisive reaction, it can be seen as straightforward that the number of cases and the number and share of deaths were lower in Austria than in other countries during the first wave. About 34 per cent of all deaths due to COVID-19 occurred in care homes in Austria. Only two of the 16 countries (Australia and Wales) in an international sample achieved a lower share (see Figure 3.1; Comas-Herrera et al, 2022). It must be noted, though, that the infected population in Austria was, on average, younger than that in Italy, which may have contributed to this relatively favourable outcome.

It became apparent early in the pandemic that the infection rate in care homes correlates to infection rates in the surrounding area (Abrams et al, 2020; Shi et al, 2020). The Austrian experience corresponds with this general observation during the first wave (BMSGPK, 2020; Comas-Herrera et al, 2022). During the pandemic, Austria lost its favourable position regarding overall infection rates and regarding the overall death toll. Thus, infection rates and fatalities due to COVID-19 increased in care homes.

Two issues may have contributed to this 'lost headstart': First, the government switched from an overly strict pandemic regime to a somewhat optimistic scenario as early as the Summer of 2020, more or less ignoring warning voices from national and international scientists (Hale et al, 2021). One may assume that this contributed to the observed slack in preventive behaviour among the general population. Secondly, there was a lack of common ground among political parties concerning pandemic management, with fierce opposition against isolation measures and, later on, vaccination campaigns, predominantly from the right-wing *Freiheitliche Partei Österreichs* (FPÖ). Experts, however, criticised the preparations for a second wave in the autumn of 2020 as rather half-hearted, resulting in a steep incline in infection rates, as discussed later. Governmental optimism rather than opposition from the far right likely contributed more to the change in pandemic strategy as the next elections were scheduled to occur more than 4 years later. Moreover, at that time, polling numbers of the FPÖ were lower than they had been in years.

During the relatively favourable situation in the first wave, the COVID-19 pandemic had already highlighted several weaknesses of the Austrian long-term care (LTC) system, most prominently a lack of support for unpaid care and live-in personal carers as well as shortages of formal care staff (Brugger et al, 2021; Leiblfinger et al, 2021; Leichsenring et al, 2021). Besides, on an organisational level, the highly decentralised responsibilities with only limited governance and steering capacity on a central level resulted in inequities in access to supply. Furthermore, the lack of national emergency preparedness, including streamlined and efficient communication, led to differing interpretations of national regulations across and within the nine states (*Bundesländer*).

This chapter is organised as follows. First, background information on the Austrian LTC system in general and the care home sector is provided. Next, the legal background for actions taken during the pandemic, the measures imposed, and some effects within the care home sector are discussed. Finally, we analyse the measures taken and widen the view to also consider the pandemic's evolution over the following months.

The role of the residential care sector for the older-age population within the broader long-term care

In Austria, there is a strict separation between health care and long-term care in service provision and financing. While sickness funds with mandatory enrolment along the lines of employment provide health care, public funding for LTC originates solely from taxes. The responsibility for LTC services rests mainly with *Bundesländer* that also provide in-kind benefits (residential care homes, care at home, and smaller quantities of semi-residential care and support services). *Bundesländer* provides these directly or by tasking – mostly not-for-profit – organisations. A seven-tiered benefit-in-cash (*Pflegegeld*) was introduced in 1993, and since 2012 its regulations have been uniform across the country. From the start, *Pflegegeld* was designed as a benefit in cash, conditional only on the level of care needs but not on income, wealth, the reason for dependency, family carers, or specific use of this money. Due to its unconditional nature and the fact that one's *Pflegegeld* assessment also serves as entitlement criterion for several LTC benefits (most notably, level four or higher is usually required when applying for a place in a residential care home, and level three or higher for several support measures for informal carers), this benefit has played a major role in the Austrian LTC system. The share of *Pflegegeld* in public expenses for LTC also underlines this vital role. In 2020, public expenses for *Pflegegeld* amounted to €2.7 billion (2.6 per cent more than in 2019), compared to public expenses[3] of €2.6 billion for LTC services in kind (6.4 per cent more than in 2019; Statistik Austria, 2021).

Furthermore, *Pflegegeld* and other minor LTC benefits in cash are regulated and administered mainly on the national level, in contrast to benefits in kind. These standard regulations, therefore, to some degree exert a unifying power in an LTC system otherwise designed mainly by the individual *Bundesländer*, which place priorities in care provision differently. In 2012, a national fund (*Pflegefonds*) was introduced to cover the increasing public expenses for LTC. The rules enabling *Bundesländer* to draw money from this fund are also designed to support harmonisation in the Austrian LTC landscape.

Generally, residential care costs are to be borne by the resident and usually far exceed income – typically old-age pension plus *Pflegegeld*. However, because many people favour living at home and with increasing care needs, many families employ live-in carers, mostly from eastern neighbouring countries, to provide so-called 24-hour care. In 2007, 24-hour care was legalised, and a special additional care allowance was introduced to support this form of care at home, provided certain conditions are fulfilled (§21b *Bundespflegegeldgesetz*). In 2020, there were 24,031 persons in need of care receiving this support, while 95,263 persons received residential care in care homes and 151,582 persons received formal personal or social care at home.

Given the high costs of both forms of care (residential care, 24-hour care), and the unconditional nature of *Pflegegeld*, most persons in need of care are being cared for by family members with or without additional visits by professional care services. It has been estimated that about 19 per cent of all people in need of care live in residential care homes, 5 per cent use 24-hour care, 2 per cent use semi-residential care, and 42 per cent of all people in need of care do not receive any professional care services but rely on informal care from relatives, neighbours, and other persons (Bachner et al, 2018: p 169). A recent study estimates that about 10 per cent of all adult persons living in Austria are involved in providing informal care. A striking result of this study is that family care is an issue related to persons in need of care living at home and those in residential care. It might relate to providing actual (physical) care to residents (like helping during meals or going for a walk around the premises), and in many cases, is experienced as a burden due to the perceived responsibility for residents (Nagl-Cupal et al, 2018). The latter result might be partly explained by the high prevalence of dementia in residential care – up to 85 per cent (Auer et al, 2018).

However, demand for places in residential care homes experienced a sharp increase in recent years. Just before the parliamentary election in the fall of 2017, all political parties agreed to abandon the *Pflegeregress.* This regulation requires spending down all assets (except a small amount to cover burial costs) before social assistance steps in to help finance costs for residential care. Consequently, the number of residents increased by 10.4 per cent (2016–2017) and 15.3 per cent (2017–2018), compared to a maximum annual increase of 2.4 per cent over the 4 preceding years (BMSGPK, 2021).

Table 3.1 provides a brief overview of the numbers of care recipients and staff in the two most common settings of care, residential care, and home (nursing) care. Unfortunately, numbers on staff by qualification or private/public provider are unavailable. *Bundesländer* organises the information in Table 3.1 to point out the regional variation in capacity. For example, each FTE provides care for, on average, 2.3 residents in residential care in Vorarlberg, but for 3.3 residents in Carinthia. In Vienna, the proportion of persons aged 80 or over in residential care is almost twice the proportion in adjacent Lower Austria. In 2020, residential care facilities across Austria employed 36,558 full-time equivalents (FTE) to provide care, which corresponds to almost three times the employment in-home care and home nursing care (12,806 FTE) (Statistik Austria, 2021). Only in recent years, registration requirements for health professions were introduced in Austria. According to the first report drawing on these registration data, 15 per cent of the registered care staff in care homes (including day care centres) were registered nurses, 30 per cent were graduates of the newly developed 2-year education in *Pflegefachassistenz*, and 55 per cent were nursing aids (*Pflegeassistentin*) (Holzweber et al, 2021).

Measures adopted to address the impact of the pandemic on the residential care sector for the older-age population

Preparedness

The Austrian law on epidemics *(Epidemie-Gesetz, 1950)*[4] was amended multiple times during the COVID-19 pandemic, for example concerning specific screening programs or contact tracing. The law obliges, among others, restaurants, hotels, and care homes to document the contact information of their customers/visitors and allows the Minister for Social Affairs (MSA) to conduct screenings for the population or specific population groups.

Apart from their obligation to contribute to contact tracing, care homes are not explicitly mentioned in the *Epidemie-Gesetz*. However, the law touches them in at least two ways: (1) Healthcare professionals such as nurses are responsible for following hygiene standards and notifying the relevant offices of new infections; (2) Care homes can be understood as included in the more general term facilities.

Table 3.1: Number of care recipients and staff in two settings of care, 2020

	Number of recipients		Care staff in FTE		Recipients of care per FTE		Recipients per 100 inhabitants 80+		Population share
Bundesland	Home (nursing) care	Residential care	Home (nursing) care	Residential care	Home (nursing) care	Residential care	Home (nursing) care	Residential care	80
Austria, 2020	**151,582**	**95,263**	**12,806**	**36,558**	**11.8**	**2.6**	**30.9**	**19.4**	**5.5 %**
Austria, 2019	**153,152**	**96,458**	**12,654**	**35,971**	**12.1**	**2.7**	**33.4**	**21.0**	**5.2%**
Burgenland	6,628	2,927	344	1,050	19.3	2.8	34.0	15.0	6.6 %
Carinthia	11,670	7,996	865	2,415	13.5	3.3	31.8	21.8	6.5 %
Lower Austria	31,294	13,394	3,028	5,241	10.3	2.6	30.8	13.2	6.0 %
Upper Austria	20,799	15,216	1,253	5,854	16.6	2.6	25.2	18.4	5.5 %
Salzburg	8,151	5,789	765	2,324	10.7	2.5	27.6	19.6	5.3 %
Styria	24,764	17,886	1,434	6,511	17.3	2.7	32.0	23.1	6.2 %
Tyrol	11,821	7,894	983	3,065	12.0	2.6	29.7	19.8	5.2 %
Vorarlberg	8,505	2,921	605	1,288	14.1	2.3	42.1	14.5	5.1 %
Vienna	27,950	21,240	3,530	8,811	7.9	2.4	33.3	25.3	4.4 %

Source: Statistik Austria (2021), Pflegedienstleistungsstatistik. Note: care recipients per 100 inhabitants are calculated by simple division of all recipients by number of inhabitants in the respective age group, regardless of the recipients' actual age.

While the *Epidemie-Gesetz* does define responsibilities and capacities, it does not propose a plan of action in case of new health threats. The latter is incorporated in the Austrian *Pandemieplan* (pandemic plan), which dates back to 2006 and is only equipped to deal with influenza viruses. In January 2020, the media criticised these shortcomings. In response, the MSA stated that the *Pandemieplan* was currently being updated in cooperation with the nine *Bundesländer* and other stakeholders involved in managing a pandemic.[5]

Fundamentally, the definition and publication of pandemic plans is the responsibility of the *Bundesländer*. For instance, the plan for Vienna was adapted during the SARS crisis in 2012. Although the plan was said to be adjusted in February 2020, according to media coverage, the online version of the plan[6] still dated back to 2006 in 2021, and is now no longer accessible. It is used to assign responsibilities for managing a pandemic to different stakeholders. The relevant stakeholder for long-term care is *Fonds Soziales Wien* (FSW, an agency organising social services at the behest of the City of Vienna).

As *Bundesländer* have regulatory power for the care home sector, it was up to them to issue regulations to protect residents from infection. By mid-March 2020, all *Bundesländer* had implemented bans or limitations for visitors in care homes (BMSGPK, 2020). However, a general code of action on how to deal with COVID-19 infections among residents in care homes was not introduced until May 2021, almost 15 months after the first lockdown. In the meantime, care homes were left on their own. Several care home carriers, for example, installed their pandemic boards to deal with such situations adequately.[7]

There was no pandemic-specific training for care home staff in place before the emergence of COVID-19. During the pandemic, however, it was recommended to focus on telemedicine training, not only regarding the pandemic, but also to facilitate digitalisation in the health system (Wiener Heimkommission, 2020).

In Austria, several crisis boards provide expertise and coordination of authorities and stakeholders. The first board is the SKKM (*Staatliches Krisen- und Katastrophenschutzmanagement*, governmental management in case of crises and catastrophes). It was established in 1986, works for the Ministry of the Interior, and, in the COVID-19 crisis coordinated the activities of the relevant government ministries, the nine *Bundesländer* governments, red light organisations, and the national broadcast organisation. In addition, the 'Taskforce Corona' was established in February 2020, consisting of medical experts, and issued recommendations regarding protective measures. Finally, GECKO (*gesamtstaatliche COVID-Krisenkoordination*, general governmental COVID-crisis coordination), established in December 2021, is the latest addition to relevant Austrian crisis boards. It consists of experts from different fields and advises the government. It is part of the

Bundeskanzleramt (federal chancellery), and its reports are available online.[8] Representatives of care homes are not part of any of the national crisis boards; two representatives, however, participate in regional task forces (Leichsenring et al, 2021).

On the national level, several measures were established to avoid shortages of care staff. For this purpose, special COVID-19 acts were passed (see also Schmidt & Bachner, 2020):

- Compulsory registration in the mandatory health professional registry has been halted and was repeatedly extended. This measure aimed to facilitate retired or trained professionals working elsewhere to work in LTC during the pandemic. This regulation also helped to employ persons with foreign education.
- Individual roles and responsibilities of care staff were adapted, allowing non-trained caregivers to conduct supporting activities usually restricted to trained persons.
- Also, during school lockdowns, schools and kindergartens remained open for children with parents working in critical professions, such as the health and care sector.
- Persons in civilian service[9] during the first wave had their service period extended by 3 months to support care and emergency services. Persons who had already ended their civilian service were requested to return – with higher remuneration than their colleagues who had their average service period extended.

It is noteworthy that residential care facilities increased their staff by 1.6 per cent in 2020 compared to the previous year, and home (nursing) care by 1.2 per cent. However, we need to distinguish which measures contributed how much to the rising number of care staff. Even knowing that the number of persons living in residential care decreased slightly from 2019 to 2020, by 1.2 per cent (Statistik Austria, 2021), it could be observed that care staff increasingly suffered under the prolonged pandemic working situation. Including their constant use of PPE (personal protective equipment), constant change of rosters (for example, due to infected colleagues), longer working hours, and general uncertainty. In a survey, six out of ten respondents from care professions stated that they did not expect to be able to keep working until retirement, unless they reduced working hours or could work under improved working conditions.[10]

In recognition of their tremendous workload during the pandemic, care staff were awarded a one-time bonus of €500 per employee. This bonus, however, was criticised as being awarded only to a fraction of nursing home staff, being paid after a long waiting time, and being only a pittance compared to the duration of pandemic working conditions. So again, there remained a feeling of 'too little, too late' for many.

Management of capacity (organisational level)

Care home staff were put under severe strain with the onset of the crisis. Among other factors, understaffing due to staff shortages, increased communication needs of relatives, and correct donning of PPE – if available – led to an increased workload. Furthermore, while the fear of contracting COVID-19 and becoming a potential source of infection was an additional stressor for staff, new developments like the implementation of telehealth also posed challenges (Wiener Heimkommission, 2020; Brugger et al, 2021).

There needed to be more timely and coordinated governmental efforts to provide PPE and disinfectant for institutions. The resulting lack of PPE sometimes increased understaffing due to infected employees, and was further corroborated by the unavailability of tests. In care homes with a sufficient supply of PPE, this was often due to leftovers from previous cases of infectious diseases or recommendations for early procurements by Italian network partners. That is why some *Bundesländer* issued recommendations to stock up on PPE earlier to public facilities than private ones (Volksanwaltschaft, 2020). In addition, care homes divided workers into separate teams to minimise the spread of COVID-19 among employees (Schmidt & Bachner, 2020).

Plans to test all employees and residents in care homes across the country were announced in April 2020 by the MSA. The targeted testing program planned to carry out about 130,000 tests in 918 retirement and care facilities (Neubauer et al, 2020). Up to June 2020, there were 923 positive cases in 117 facilities, with about 79 per cent of these cases incurred between 16 March and 16 April. Few infections were registered in care homes in May and only very few clusters in June 2020 (BMSGPK, 2020).

In late October 2020, there were plans to test all staff working in care homes for a second time. However, an ordinance issued on 13 October 2020 (Testing Strategy – *Österreichische Teststrategie SARS-CoV-2*) stated that staff samples should be tested conditional on incidence parameters. The second lockdown, introduced in early November 2020, also obliged employees in care homes (and hospitals) to produce a negative test weekly or constantly wear a suitable face mask.

Testing numbers in care homes up to December 2021 are only available for five of nine *Bundesländer* (Burgenland, Carinthia, Styria, Tyrol, Vienna). Even for those *Bundesländer*, a disaggregation of tests by months is not available, according to a statement of the MSA to the Austrian parliament. In the five *Bundesländer*, about 1.6 and 0.9 million tests were registered for care home staff and residents, respectively (BMSGPK, 2022a). In per capita terms, this corresponds to about 16 tests per resident.

In November 2021, Austria introduced workplace entry requirements (*3G am Arbeitsplatz*). From then on, only convalescent (up to 6 months), vaccinated, or negatively tested (PCR within the last 72 hours, LFT within the last 24 hours) employees were allowed to enter their workplace, including staff in care homes. The entry requirements were rescinded for most workplaces in early March 2022 but are still in place for care homes. Additionally, in February 2022, a vaccine mandate for the general population aged 18 and above was introduced. It was, however, heavily disputed, never executed, and suspended following the commission's first report tasked with monitoring the vaccine mandate in early March (Kollaritsch et al, 2022a). A second report published in May 2022 affirmed the assessment of the first report. However, they also mentioned a possible reintroduction of the vaccine mandate in autumn should a worst-case scenario emerge. In any case, the commission encouraged the legislator to use the summer to prepare for various scenarios in autumn (Kollaritsch et al, 2022b).

Austria has the highest number of hospital beds (per capita) in general, particularly ICU beds.[11] Nonetheless, hospitals re-scheduled non-urgent procedures very early on to free up capacity and reserve ICU capacities for potential COVID-19 patients. ICUs, in particular, were overwhelmed with the surge of COVID-19 patients resulting in postponed surgeries in the first wave and in later waves of the pandemic. During the first wave, non-urgent surgeries were postponed quite comprehensively, while in later waves and with more experience, hospitals acted more selectively in this respect.[12,13] However, it has to be said that the Austrian hospital sector has yet to experience caseloads as large as in, for example, Italy.

There is no systematic evidence concerning the consequences on the care home sector, specifically in Austria. Nevertheless, international evidence suggests the presence of barriers to accessing health care services for care home residents during the pandemic (Heneghan et al, 2021). Due to high hospital capacities in Austria, these barriers may have been less severe than in other countries. It is still an open question how far the documented excess mortality for the 65-plus population in Austria during 2020 and 2021, also among non-COVID-19 patients, was partly caused by access barriers to hospital care (Islam et al, 2021; University of California and Max Planck Institute for Demographic Research, 2022).

Governance

In 2018, the government restructured the vertical cooperation between levels of government by shifting power and responsibilities from the central level to the *Bundesland* level. For example, this minor reform of the Austrian federal system eliminated the veto power of the federal government for some pieces of legislation.[14] However, during the COVID-19 crisis, this has been criticised by opposition parties as impeding cooperation across *Bundesländer* and complicating oversight during crises like pandemics, as opposed to the more centralised situation before.

Initiating and executing preventive and curative measures, collecting relevant information on diseases due for notification, and monitoring these measures, fall under the districts' responsibility. However, suppose diseases are more widespread (to the level of *Bundesland* or the whole country). In that case, the responsibility is shifted to the next highest level (*Bundesland* governor or minister of health – MoH, respectively), with the latter overruling the former in case of conflicting regulations. According to the *Epidemie-Gesetz*, the *Bundesländer* governments are responsible for notifying the MoH of noteworthy developments immediately and must cooperate (§43 *Epidemie-Gesetz*). Thus, in a pandemic, the national level (represented by the MoH) is the relevant regulator, but the district level executes the measures. Therefore, if ambiguities arise from national regulations, the same regulations can be executed differently in each district. It occurred in the current pandemic, for example, when some districts regarded a negative test result as sufficient to lift the quarantine. At the same time, other districts insisted that quarantine needs to be complied with until the necessary time has passed, irrespective of test results.

The central level, more specifically the MSA (currently the same person as the MoH), issued recommendations for care homes but refrained from implementing binding rules or ordinances as would have been preferred by care home managers, for example, for liability reasons (Volksanwaltschaft, 2020). Overall, six documents with relevant recommendations on the following topics were issued:

1. Mental health recommendations during the COVID-19 pandemic for caregivers of older adults (published on 25 March 2020).
2. Processes concerning critical health and key staff that came into unprotected contact with persons with COVID-19 infection (category I infection risk) (published on 29 March 2020, last update 8 January 2022).[15]
3. Stepwise easing of visitor limitations for care homes which had been issued due to the COVID-19 pandemic, starting on 4 May 2020 (published on 28 April 2020).
4. Protective measures for care staff in residential, semi-residential, and home care settings (published on 8 May 2020).
5. Stepwise return to everyday life in care homes and semi-residential institutions, starting on 9 June 2020 (published on 9 June 2020).
6. Protective measures for nursing and care: inpatient and semi-residential facilities and mobile services (published on 11 May 2021).

The responsibility for the provision of LTC and its regulation rests on the *Bundesländer*. By mid-March 2020, each *Bundesland* had implemented bans or limitations for visitors in care homes to protect the vulnerable elderly population (BMSGPK, 2020).

Intersectoral coordination

In Austria, as in many countries, the fragmentation between the health and the LTC sector is a matter of continued concern. It is mainly due to the organisational set-up described in the introduction of this chapter, with LTC being organised by *Bundesländer* in cooperation with municipalities and financed by tax revenues and medical care in the organisational and financial responsibility of health insurance.[16] Furthermore, the unrestricted right to choose one's GP does not end at the door of care homes. Thus, persons moving into residential care usually remain in the care of the same GP. As regular employees of a care home, on the other hand, GPs (and even more so, specialists in geriatric medicine) are extremely rare in Austria and more or less limited to facilities of one large residential care organisation in Vienna and few residential care facilities dedicated to residents with exceptionally high care needs.

Consequently, it is typical that several GPs visit the same care home, each caring for their patients according to their practice style. It may vary because Austria's adherence to evidence-based medicine guidelines is not very strict. This is sometimes perceived as adding to the staff's administrative burden because they sometimes must follow diverse treatment routines with otherwise similar residents. Communication, for example, to adjust medication with notoriously busy GPs, can be time-consuming (Riedel, 2017). Furthermore, laws define a broader set of competencies for registered nurses than social health insurance is willing to accept in their coverage decisions, for example, continued prescription of incontinence products is only covered by social health insurance if prescribed by an MD. Also, such regulations increase administrative burdens for nursing staff. Increased use of eHealth, as described further on, was perceived as increasing the efficiency of care provided by care staff (Riedel, 2021).

According to media coverage, some GPs discontinued their medical care in care homes. A series of phone interviews with nursing directors of care homes confirmed that medical care was reduced during the first wave of the pandemic because not all GPs were prepared to visit care homes. As of mid-May 2020, 79 per cent of interviewees reported that medical care was regular again (Volksanwaltschaft, 2020). Some care staff, however, felt that visits by GPs became increasingly sporadic and superficial and were often replaced by phone calls, creating the impression that some GPs did not take the health of residents seriously (Brugger et al, 2021). On the other hand, other staff experienced the collaboration with GPs via phone as a welcome enhancement of their professional role (Hoedl et al, 2022).

Before the pandemic, phone consultations with GPs could not be billed with health insurance. In order to reconcile physical distancing with the continuation of care, this regulation was eased during the pandemic and was extensively used for patients in care homes. This novelty (at least in the Austrian context) added tasks and responsibility to the usual role of nursing staff, which was appreciated as increased recognition by some staff members (Hoedl et al, 2022).

A further administrative change was the implementation of e-medication. These (long-time overdue) modernisations of administrative aspects in the care process are perceived to have helped provide general medical and nursing care, including patients in residential care (Riedel, 2021).

The increased use of ICT and eHealth improved or even enabled certain aspects of care, but it comes with its challenges. For example, the introduction of telemedicine to replace GP visits (meaning that a nurse uses a notebook or tablet to facilitate visual contact between resident and GP) in a group of residential homes elucidated some potential pitfalls: acceptance of this new work process relies heavily on education and prior experience with these tools, for both professions (nurse, GP), in addition to the doubtful usefulness for patients with cognitive limitations. Another problematic aspect might be a shift in professional roles. While both professions work alongside each other in case of in-person visits by GPs, some nurses felt they were partly reduced in their professional role as mere assistants to the GP, in contrast to national efforts to enhance the role of nurses. Furthermore, while most GPs felt that this version of telemedicine increased their efficiency, nurses felt an increase in workload, partly due to the higher complexity of arranging virtual as opposed to in-person visits (Plunger et al, 2022).

Concerning the transition between hospitals and care homes, no statistics are available. According to anecdotal evidence, during the pandemic hospitals released their patients back to care homes earlier than before. Furthermore, patients were only sometimes tested before returning. While hospitals reduced non-urgent care during the first lockdown and, far more selectively, also in later phases, there is no strong indicator that cares home residents faced entry barriers in case of urgent need or emergencies. There are, however, reports that some care home staff became more reluctant to send residents to hospitals in case of incidents when good recovery 'at home' could well be expected and the benefit of an emergency room visit was doubtful (Hoedl et al, 2022).

Assessment of these measures

Like many European countries, Austria was hit by the pandemic somewhat unprepared. A specific challenge in Austria resulted from the government constellation. The new government had been in office only for a couple of weeks and consisted of a new conservative–green coalition. Thus, it may have surprised observers that this new government had been able to pull through a relatively comprehensive set of measures rather quickly, but this presumably was the result of the long-standing tradition of consensus agreements in Austrian policy (Mätzke, 2021). The newly appointed MSA/MoH had announced pre-pandemic that the main focus during his term in office would be the long overdue reform of the LTC sector. As a member of the junior party (*Grüne*) in the coalition and largely lacking strong backing from either powerful stakeholder groups or *Bundesländer* governments, he had to fight complex political constellations in addition to the pandemic (Riedel, 2021). Six of the nine Austrian *Bundesländer* had/have a *Landeshauptmann/-frau* (*Bundesland* governor) of the *Neue Volkspartei*, the senior partner in the national government coalition, while there is no *Landeshauptmann/-frau* of *Grüne*. These preconditions slowed down political decisions, contributing to national regulations often being perceived as coming too late and not being sufficiently transparent.[17]

Communication of measures and provision of, for example, PPE, was perceived to be suboptimal. The initial phase was dominated by introducing fear of the pandemic and by political rhetoric rather than by scientific information. In the Summer of 2020, the rhetoric changed from overly dramatic to overly optimistic, resulting in slack concerning preparations for the second wave and steeply rising case numbers after the summer.

Low reliance on scientific knowledge relates to information of the public, but also, for example, official case definitions that did not reflect the state of knowledge (Zollner-Schwetz et al, 2021). Such weaknesses refer to most areas of crisis management during the pandemic, including the LTC sector. Specific regulations for the LTC sector were rare initially, which may reflect the low involvement of LTC professionals in the political decision-making processes. Executive power to carry out regulations on the district level created further delays, differences in interpretations of national regulations, and presumably inequities.

Evolution of the situation in the care home sector in the following phases of the pandemic and challenges for the future of the care home sector in Austria

Compared to other high-income countries, the care home sector in Austria tackled the first wave of the pandemic relatively well in fatalities: about one in three COVID-19 deaths occurred in care homes, which is a lower share than in most comparable countries.

After a summer of relatively relaxed attitudes towards pandemic preparedness, the pandemic's second wave produced far more significant infections than the first wave (see Figure 3.3). In the second wave, the

Figure 3.2: COVID-19 deaths among care home residents in the second wave (between 26 June 2020 and 26 January 2021), as a percentage of all COVID-19 deaths

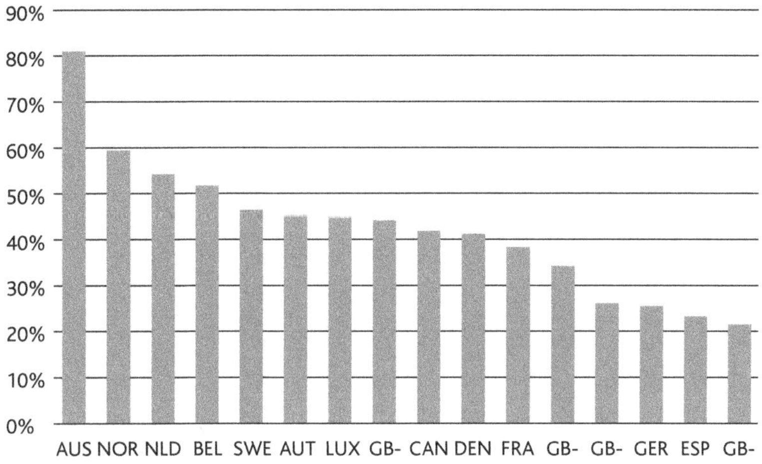

Source: Comas-Herrera et al (2022)

share of care home residents among all COVID-19 deaths increased in chronological and international comparison. Only five out of 16 countries (Australia, Norway, Netherlands, Belgium, and Sweden) reported a higher percentage than Austria (Figure 3.2). Concerning COVID-19 deaths among staff members of care homes, only two fatalities were registered in Austria up to December 2021, one each in January and February 2021 (BMSGPK, 2022b).

Across all care homes as of December 2021, 24.4 per cent of all residents had been COVID-19 positive, and 4.5 per cent of all residents died of COVID-19. Thus, the case fatality rate in care homes (18.3 per cent) is a multiple of that in the general population in Austria (1.0 per cent). Compared to residents in care homes, exactly half of that percentage had been COVID-19 positive in the population aged 85 or older (irrespective of place of residence) in the same timeframe, and 2.5 per cent of all persons in this age group died of COVID-19 (see Figures 3.3 and 3.4).

Lessons learned

After the turmoil following the spread of the virus from a Tyrolean skiing resort, Austria tackled the first months of the pandemic surprisingly well, considering that neither an up-to-date pandemic plan, a relevant government department, nor a robust public health culture was present when the first wave hit. In addition to this less-than-perfect background, the newly elected government coalition still needed time to develop a cooperation

Figure 3.3: New cases as a percentage of the respective population in care homes, the Austrian population without care home residents, and the population aged 85 and older

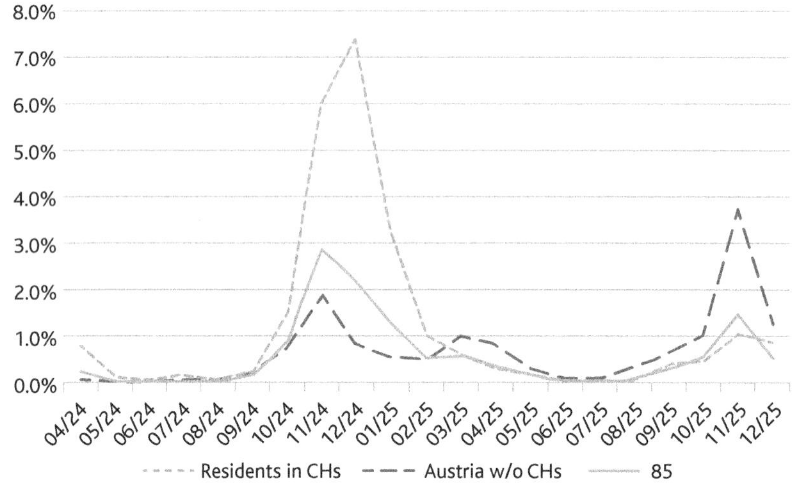

Sources: AGES (2022), BMSGPK (2022a, 2022b), Statistik Austria (2022)

Figure 3.4: New deaths as a percentage of the respective population in care homes, the Austrian population without care homes, and the population aged 85 and older

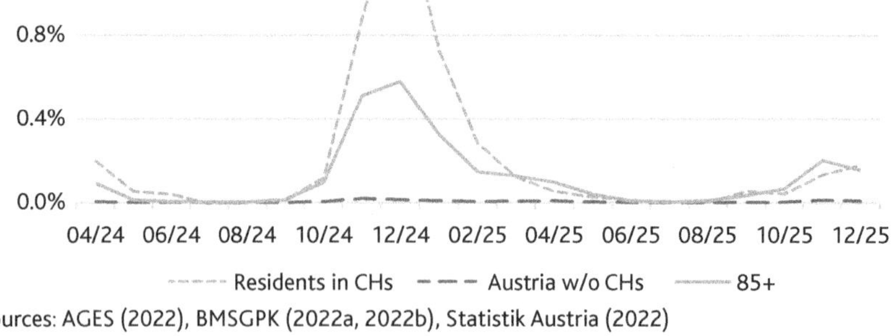

Sources: AGES (2022), BMSGPK (2022a, 2022b), Statistik Austria (2022)

routine between the two partners in the new coalition. The long tradition of consensus-finding between the so-called social partners prevented the mentioned shortcomings from leading to even more significant effects across all sectors affected by the pandemic, including LTC (Mätzke, 2021).

At least, that is the picture that emerges from the comparatively low infection and death statistics for the first wave. Behind the scenes, frontline staff, and managers of LTC provider organisations felt very much left alone (Volksanwaltschaft, 2020). Media and politicians concentrated on protecting health care providers on the one hand and the general population. On the other hand, specific groups like persons in need of LTC – but also children and students – were no particular focus of concern in the initial phase. Though it was soon recognised that persons in need of LTC in general, particularly residents in care homes, faced the highest risk, this understanding did not translate into properly representing this population group in the respective crisis boards. It may be assumed that incorporating knowledge from actual care providers would have contributed to the higher applicability of regulations. As is, regulations were often perceived as contradictory and not very usable in real life (Volksanwaltschaft, 2020).

Enacted measures underlined politicians' priority for preventing infection over safeguarding mental well-being. At the onset, the lack of a pandemic plan, lack of PPE, and in parts of the staff, lack of knowledge of the hygienic standards to apply and how to effectively prevent infections were felt as particularly burdensome (Volksanwaltschaft, 2020; Brugger et al, 2021; Hoedl et al, 2022). In these respects, much knowledge has been gained, and it may be assumed that there is increased awareness and a higher standard of knowledge, theoretical as well as in managing everyday routines. These learnings, it is hoped, will carry over to better manage other major and minor crises, like the annual flu season.

Government regulations concentrated on visitor bans or restrictions and isolation, while only very little concern was initially given to measures limiting the psychological effects of these measures. Visitor restrictions did not only apply to social visits (family, friends) but also mainly to clergy, patient rights organisations, or volunteers, such as in the palliative care context (Leichsenring et al, 2021). Surveys report that almost half of all interviewed care home residents felt lonely often (32 per cent), or occasionally (17 per cent) in 2020 (Gallistl et al, 2021). While there is evidence of residents coping well during the pandemic with steady life satisfaction (Roehner et al, 2021), there are also reports of visiting bans deteriorating the health status of residents (Hoedl et al, 2022). Efforts to counteract isolation by increasing internet use have far narrower limits in care homes than in the overall population, considering the high proportion of residents with impairments, impairments and the low pre-pandemic internet use of the current generation. Overall, Gallistl et al (2021) found that less than 10 per cent of interviewed residents used the internet to stay in contact with relatives, but almost all used the telephone for that purpose. The proportion of internet users might even be optimistic because participation in an interview already requires a minimum of cognitive abilities that residents with, for example, severe dementia, may not have anymore.

Loneliness and isolation among residents were already problematic before the pandemic. Though a digital push has been experienced throughout society, better applicability of ICT to counteract isolation and loneliness in care homes will likely need specific efforts. It refers not only to adequate infrastructure but also to the training of its users. Its uptake must be understood as a process requiring continued engagement and support rather than an individual intervention (Gallistl et al, 2021).

During the first weeks of the pandemic, two issues concerning LTC received the most media attention: infections and infection control in care homes, and the organisational problems in 24-hour care. While clients of 24-hour care make up roughly 5 per cent of all persons in need of LTC in Austria, pandemic-related problems in this sector attracted possibly the largest public attention among all settings of LTC provision. For several weeks, travel restrictions prohibited following the usual pattern of 2–4 weeks in the care recipient's place of living, alternating between two carers, most of whom come from Romania, Slovakia, or other Eastern European countries. As the replacement carer could not enter the country, or had to follow up to 2 weeks of quarantine before arriving at the client's place, most of the present carers extended their stay because the clients could not be left alone or be cared for by family. (Leiblfinger et al, 2021). Thus, the pandemic highlighted very clearly how fragile the system of 24-hour care is, and how small its resilience is towards crises. From 2019 to 2020, the number of persons receiving public support for 24-hour care decreased by 3.2 per cent. The decrease in this LTC segment is much more substantial than in-home care (1.2 per cent) and in-care homes (1.0 per cent). Furthermore, the decrease in clients of these LTC services is stronger than the overall decrease among recipients of *Pflegegeld* in the same period (0.8 per cent). This decrease stems almost entirely from the four higher levels (with more severe care needs) that comprise 32 per cent of all *Pflegegeld* recipients in 2020 (BMSGPK, 2021).

In later phases, with the increasing availability of PPE and tests and established routines that smoothed the management of the care rosters, the vulnerability of this specific mode of LTC provision has been forgotten. However, though carers need to be recruited from increasing distances because resources in nearer places have been depleted, there currently needs to be more public discussion as to how this vulnerable system might be replaced, or its resilience towards crises improved. Meanwhile, public attention returned to the more general yet most significant problem in the provision of LTC: the staff shortage.

What is next?

A participatory reform process for the LTC sector was initiated in 2020.[18] The final report on this process lists five priority areas, 17 goals, and 64 measures as the outcome, including measures to recognise the work of carers and improve their working conditions. As the most concrete outcome of this process until early 2022, the role of community nurse is being introduced to help bridge the gap between elements of health care and LTC in the highly fragmented care system.[19] However, the limited scale of this program – a total of about 150 community nurses in all pilots across Austria – leaves ample room for further endeavours. Additionally, it is planned to broaden further the entry into the nursing profession by introducing 'nursing apprenticeships', a controversial measure because many researchers and stakeholders would favour more emphasis on higher educational pathways. Another new route into the profession is pilot programs in nursing that have started in several secondary schools in *Bundesländer*.[20]

In Austria, prioritising the provision of community care over care homes is a political commitment that did not pass the pandemic stress test. The factual priority of care homes, only recently demonstrated by the abolished *Pflegeregress*, also continued during the pandemic. Many day centres were closed. Also, some providers of home-nursing care discontinued their service. Concerning the provision of PPE, some providers of home-nursing care face even more difficulties than care homes. Even the newly introduced community nurses are an uncertain gain for community care as long as it is determined where the staff for these positions will come from. If community nurses are former home-care nurses, the effect on strengthening community care will be limited.

The reform of Austria's LTC sector was announced to be the priority focus of social policy in 2020. Unfortunately, the pandemic halted this process even before it began. The re-launch by way of the so-called *Taskforce Pflege* later in 2020, set a list of priorities but did not yet specify concrete measures. In May 2022, the MoH presented an outline of 20 measures for the reform of LTC in Austria, with a budget of 1 billion euros to be spent over 4 years.[21] Some of these measures concern the education of staff, as described earlier. The most outstanding 'new' efforts are a wage increase for active nurses and financial support for students in nursing programmes. Furthermore, some measures strive to broaden the scope of professional competencies, primarily for nurses with lower qualification levels. Though touching on important issues, the reform proposal has been criticised as consisting of individual headlines instead of precisely defined measures and lacking a coherent structure.

As already mentioned, securing more staff is vital but cannot suffice alone. The fragmentation of the entire health and care system often works as an obstacle to smooth patient pathways. Bureaucratic paper flows sometimes obstruct care processes and direct carer's time and energy to unnecessary tasks like obtaining GP's prescriptions for nursing material they might as well obtain within their professional capacity (Riedel, 2021). Allowing care staff to concentrate on their core tasks instead could improve care quality and job satisfaction alike. The pandemic ironically removed some obstacles by introducing efficient digital solutions for administrative processes (e-medication, consultation via phone). Successful efforts like these should be continued and extended rather than stopped after the pandemic because they will be indispensable to supporting future care staff.

Notes

1 https://www.parlament.gv.at/gegenstand/XXVII/I/564
2 https://www.parlament.gv.at/gegenstand/XXV/I/587
3 This number refers to so-called 'net expenses', total expenses for publicly co-funded LTC services in kind minus user contributions (about 35 per cent of total expenses) and contributions from other sources (about 4 per cent of total expenses). Thus, public spending for LTC services in kind is in effect higher than the share of 'net expenses' (61 per cent) suggests, because user contributions include Pflegegeld and other sources stem partly from public funds as well, for example the hospital fund.
4 https://www.ris.bka.gv.at/GeltendeFassung.wxe?Abfrage=Bundesnormen&Gesetzesnummer=10010265
5 https://www.kleinezeitung.at/oesterreich/5761121/Coronavirus_Oesterreichischer-Pandemieplan-wird-derzeit-ueberarbeitet
6 https://www.wien.gv.at/gesundheit/sandirektion/influenza/influenza.html
7 https://www.wienerzeitung.at/%20nachrichten/politik/oesterreich/2068607-In-die-Pflegeheime-kehrt-der-Alltag-zurueck.html
8 https://www.bundeskanzleramt.gv.at/themen/gecko.html
9 In Austria, 18-year-old males either have to join the military for 6 months or, alternatively, become a civilian servant for 9 months and perform duties in health and social care.
10 https://ooe.arbeiterkammer.at/service/presse/Arbeitsklima_Index-_Pflege_am_Limit-.html
11 https://www.oecd.org/coronavirus/en/data-insights/intensive-care-beds-capacity
12 https://kurier.at/chronik/oesterreich/corona-spitaeler-fahren-operationen-zurueck/401092026
13 https://www.derstandard.at/story/2000129536711/wien-verschiebt-wegen-corona-erste-planbare-operationen
14 https://www.wienerzeitung.at/nachrichten/politik/oesterreich/977353-Von-Bundes-und-Landessachen.html
15 https://www.sozialministerium.at/Informationen-zum-Coronavirus/Coronavirus---Fachinformationen.html
16 A noticeable exception of this straightforward fragmentation is that the hospital sector is organised and financed by specially set-up organisations, Landesgesundheitsfonds, in each of the nine Bundesländer, see Bachner et al (2018).
17 https://www.derstandard.at/story/2000134583214/zu-langsam-gebremst-zu-frueh-geoeffnet-wie-ex-minister-anschober
18 https://goeg.at/taskforce_pflege
19 https://orf.at/stories/3246670/
20 https://www.land-oberoesterreich.gv.at/248006.htm
21 https://www.sozialministerium.at/Themen/Pflege/Pflegereform.html

References

Abrams, H. R., Loomer, L., Gandhi, A., and Grabowski, D. C. (2020) Characteristics of U.S. nursing homes with COVID-19 cases. *Journal of the American Geriatrics Society*, 68(8), 1653–6.

AGES (2022) AGES-Dashboard COVID-19, Agentur für Gesundheit und Ernährungssicherheit [online], Available from: https://COVID19-dashboard.ages.at/data/data.zip

Auer, S. R., Höfler, M., Linsmayer, E., Beránková, A., Prieschl, D., Ratajczak, P., Šteffl, M., and Hol-merová, I. (2018) Cross-sectional study of prevalence of dementia, behavioural symptoms, mobility, pain and other health parameters in nursing homes in Austria and the Czech Republic: results from the DEMDATA project. *BMC Geriatrics*, 18(1), 178.

Bachner, F., Bobek, J., Habimana, K., Ladurner, J., Lepuschütz, L., Ostermann, H., Rainer, L., Schmidt, A. E., Zuba, M., Quentin, W., and Winkelmann, J. (2018) Austria: health system review, *Health Systems in Transition*, 20(3), 1–256.

BMSGPK – Bundesministerium für Soziales, Gesundheit, Pflege und Konsumentenschutz (BMSGPK) (ed) (2020) *COVID-19 in Alten- und Pflegeheimen*, Endbericht Stand: Juli 2020, Available from: https://www.sozialministerium.at/dam/jcr:0889c607-9583-4d65-b965-5a1a53b678db/COVID19_APH_final_Stand%204.8.2020.pdf

BMSGPK (2021) Österreichischer Pflegevorsorgebericht 2020. Wien: Bundesministerium für Arbeit, Soziales, Gesundheit und Konsumentenschutz, Available from: https://www.sozialministerium.at/dam/jcr:788ac2e7-9238-47a6-9125-d6f49d6a896a/BMSGPK_Pflegevorsorgebericht_2022.pdf

BMSGPK (2022a) Anfragenbeantwortung 8648/AB vom 31.01.2022 zu 8833/J (XXVII. GP)

BMSGPK (2022b) COVID19-Fälle je Altergruppe [online], Available from: https://www.data.gv.at/katalog/dataset/3765ed62-0f9d-49ad-83b0-1405ed833108

Brugger, M., Hengalova, R., and Stefan, J. (2021) *COVID-19 and the Perceived Stressors of Austrian Long-tem Care Workers*, Vienna University of Economics and Business [online], Available from: https://www.gpa.at/content/dam/gpa/downloads/kollektivvertrag/gesundheit,-soziales,-kirchen/sw%C3%B6/2021/COVID-19%20and%20the%20perceived%20Stressors%20of%20Austrian%20Long-Term%20Care%20Workers.pdf

Comas-Herrera, A., Marczak, J., Byrd, W., Lorenz-Dant, K., Patel, D., Pharoah, D. (eds), and LTCCOVID contributors (2022) *LTCCOVID International Living Report on COVID-19 and Long-Term Care*, LTCCOVID, Care Policy & Evaluation Centre, London School of Economics and Political Science, DOI: 10.21953/lse.mlre15e0u6s6

Gallistl, V., Seifert, A., and Kolland, F. (2021) COVID-19 as a 'digital push?' Research experiences from long-term care and recommendations for the post-pandemic era, *Frontiers in Public Health*, 9, 660064, DOI: 10.3389/fpubh.2021.660064

Hale, T., Angrist, N., Goldszmidt, R., Kira, B., Petherick, A., Phillips, T., Webster, S., Cameron-Blake, E., Hallas, L., Majumdar, S., and Tatlow, H. (2021) A global panel database of pandemic policies (Oxford COVID-19 Government Response Tracker), *Nature Human Behaviour*, 5(4), 529–38.

Heneghan, C., Dietrich, M., Brassey, J., and Jefferson, T. (2021) CG Report 6: effects of COVID-19 in care homes – a mixed methods review, Collateral Global [online], Available from: https://collateralglobal.org/wp-content/uploads/2022/03/CG_Report_6_Effects_of_COVID_19_in_Care_Homes.pdf

Hoedl, M., Thonhofer, N., and Schoberer, D. (2022) COVID-19 pandemic: burdens on and consequences for nursing home staff, *Journal of Advanced Nursing*, 78(8), 2495–506.

Holzweber, L., Zach, M., Gruböck, A., Juraszovich, B., Mathis-Edenhofer, S., Rappold, E., and Wallner, A. (2021) *Jahresbericht Gesundheitsberuferegister 2020* [online], Available from: https://jasmin.goeg.at/1823/1/GBR_Bericht_2020_fin_bf.pdf

Islam, N., Shkolnikov, V. M., Acosta, R. J., Klimkin, I., Kawachi, I., Irizarry, R. A., Alicandro, G., Khunti, K., Yates, T., Jdanov, D. A., White, M., Lewington, S., and Lacey, B. (2021) Excess deaths associated with COVID-19 pandemic in 2020: age and sex disaggregated time series analysis in 29 high income countries, BMJ, 373(1137) [online], Available from: https://www.bmj.com/content/373/bmj.n1137

Kollaritsch, H., Schernhammer, E., Stöger, K., and Wendehorst, C. (2022a) *Erster Bericht zum begleitenden Monitoring der Impfpflicht gegen COVID-19*, 8 March [online], Available from: https://www.ris.bka.gv.at/Dokumente/Mrp/MRP_20220309_9/006_001.pdf

Kollaritsch, H., Schernhammer, E., Stöger, K., and Wendehorst, C. (2022b) *Zweiter Bericht zum begleitenden Monitoring der Impfpflicht gegen COVID-19*, 23 May [online], Available from: https://www.parlament.gv.at/dokument/XXVII/SONS/24/imfname_1447681.pdf

Leiblfinger, M., Prieler, V., Rogoz, M., and Sekulová, M. (2021) Confronted with COVID-19: migrant live-in care during the pandemic, *Global Social Policy*, 21(3), 490–507.

Leichsenring, K, Schmidt, A. E., and Staflinger, H. (2021) Fractures in the Austrian model of long-term care: what are the lessons from the first wave of the COVID-19 pandemic? *Journal of Long-Term Care*, 33–42, DOI: https://doi.org/10.31389/jltc.54

Mätzke, M. (2021) Political resonance in Austria's coronavirus crisis management, in S. L. Greer, E. J. King, E. M. da Fonseca, and A. Peralta-Santos (eds) *Coronavirus Politics: The Comparative Politics and Policy of COVID-19*, Ann Arbor: University of Michigan Press, 280–94.

Nagl-Cupal, M., Kolland, F., Zartler, U., Mayer, H., Bittner, M., Koller, M., Parisot, V., and Stöhr, D. (2018): Angehörigenpflege in Österreich. Einsicht in die Situation pflegender Angehöriger und in die Entwicklung informeller Pflegenetzwerke. Universität Wien.

Neubauer, S., Habimana, K., and Schmidt, A. (2020) COVID-19 Health System Response Monitor. Austria, European Observatory on Health Systems and Policies, Available from: https://eurohealthobservatory.who.int/monitors/hsrm/hsrm-countries/hsrm/austria/preventing-transmission/physical-distancing

Plunger, P., Eitenberger, M., Kletecka-Pulker, M., Wochele-Thoma, T., Klager, E., Ruf, A. K., and Eibensteiner, F. (2022) Using telemedicine in nursing homes during the COVID-19 pandemic: a multi-perspective view on the implementation process, *Nursing Open*, 9, 1155–63.

Riedel, M. (2017) Medizinische versorgung in pflegeheimen, *Health System Watch*, 3, 1–16.

Riedel, M. (2021) *MC COVID-19. Governmental Response to the COVID-19 Pandemic in Long-Term Care Residences for Older People: Preparedness, Responses and Challenges for the Future*, MC COVID-19 working paper 1/2021 [online], Available from: https://digital.csic.es/bitstream/10261/227263/3/210216_CSIC_COVID_AUSTRIA.pdf

Rohner, R., Hartman, V., Heidinger, T., and Gallistl, V. (2021) COVID-19 Care. Auswirkungen der Corona-Pandemie in der Langzeitpflege. Projektbericht, Available from: https://link.springer.com/article/10.1007/s00391-022-02116-5

Schmidt, A. and Bachner, F. (2020) Ensuring sufficient infrastructure and workforce capacity, *COVID-19 Health System Response Monitor – Austria*, https://eurohealthobservatory.who.int/monitors/hsrm/hsrm-countries/hsrm/austria/ensuring-sufficient-physical-infrastructure-and-workforce-capacity/physical-infrastructure

Shi, S. M., Bakaev, I., Chen, H., Travison, T. G., and Berry, S. D. (2020) Risk factors, presentation, and course of Coronavirus disease 2019 in a large, academic long-term care facility, *Journal of the American Medical Directors Association*, 21(10), 1378–83.

Statistik Austria (2021) Pflegedienstleistungsstatistik 2020, Vienna [online], Available from: https://irihs.ihs.ac.at/id/eprint/4414/1/hsw-health-system-watch-III-2017-medizinische-versorgung-in-pflegeheimen.pdf

Statistik Austria (2022) Bevölkerung zu Jahresbeginn 1982–2022 nach Bundesländern und Staatsangehörigkeit [online], Available from: https://www.statistik.at/web_de/statistiken/menschen_und_gesellschaft/bevoelkerung/bevoelkerungsstand_und_veraenderung/bevoelkerung_zu_jahres-_quartalsanfang/108123.html

University of California and Max Planck Institute for Demographic Research (2022) *Human Mortality Database* [online], Available from: www.mortality.org

Volksanwaltschaft (2020) Pflegeeinrichtungen in zeiten der Corona-pandemie, *Pressekonferenz*, 1 July 2020.

Wiener Heimkommission (2020). Bericht der bei der Wiener Pflege-, Patientinnen-und Patientenanwaltschaft eingerichteten Wiener Heimkommission 2020 [online], Available from: https://www.digital.wienbibliothek.at/wbrup/download/pdf/3302317?originalFilename=true

Zollner-Schwetz, I., König, E., Krause, R., Pux, C., Laubreiter, L., and Schippinger, W. (2021) Analysis of COVID-19 outbreaks in 3 long-term care facilities in Graz, Austria, *American Journal of Infection Control*, 49(11), 1350–3.

4

Lessons not learned: the impact of the COVID-19 pandemic on the residential care sector in England

Caroline Glendinning

Introduction

The COVID-19 pandemic threw into stark profile the multiple structural weaknesses in English adult residential care, particularly compared with health services. These weaknesses include: the chronic underfunding of care services; the prioritisation of health in national policy priorities, governance, and leadership; fragmented relationships between national and local government institutions and actors; fragmented relationships between acute health and long-term care sectors, nationally and locally; the complex relationships between local government and local private residential care home quasi-markets; and chronic shortages of paid care workers. All these weaknesses are well known, so the publicity they received during the pandemic was little surprise. However, since the initial crisis of early 2020, few steps have been taken to address them. From April 2022, an increase in payroll taxes will generate more funding that is, in due course, intended to be ring-fenced for adult care services; and there are plans to improve local joint strategic planning and service commissioning between National Health Service (NHS) and local authorities. Most other institutional and governance weaknesses laid bare by the pandemic remain unaddressed.

This chapter focuses on England (containing 84 per cent of the United Kingdom population). Within the UK, responsibilities for health and care services are devolved to the English, Scottish, Welsh, and Northern Ireland governments. There is increasing divergence between countries in the structures, funding, and governance of their services; differences were also apparent in how the four countries responded to COVID-19.

It is important to remember that residential care constitutes only a very small fraction of the total care provided to older people. Across the UK, approximately 418,000 older people live in residential care – only 2.5 per cent of the total population aged 65-plus and 15 per cent of those aged 85-plus (MHA, no date). Some people only spend a short period in residential care, typically for extended convalescence after hospital discharge. Many more older people receive domiciliary services at home. Exact numbers are difficult to estimate because there are extensive private markets in both residential and domiciliary care services. Around half of English residential placements are now fully funded by older people themselves; more than 50 per cent (£7.7 billion/€9.22 billion) of total annual income across the sector (£15.2 billion/€18.19 billion) comes from private purchasers and their families. Additionally, between 6 and 25 per cent of those receiving personal care at home (estimated to be between 145,000 and 249,000 people) purchase this privately and a further 200,000 pay privately for non-personal help with domestic tasks (Henwood et al, 2019). Both residential and domiciliary care sectors are vastly outnumbered by informal care-giving; over one third (38 per cent) of older people receive all their care from family and friends (Age UK, 2019). Across the UK, 8.8 million unpaid family care-givers contribute the equivalent of 4 million full-time paid care workers to the social care system (Kings Fund, 2022). Even more striking, a third of older people in England experiencing difficulties with personal care receive no help; 1.4 million older people do not have access to the care and support they need (Age UK, 2019). These contextual factors are important when considering the impact of the pandemic on English residential care. While residential care received considerable public and media attention as the most visible aspect of social care provision, it constitutes only the 'tip of the iceberg' of the vast amount of largely invisible, privately purchased and/or privately provided care. Indeed, the predominant focus during the pandemic on residential care may actually have eclipsed policy attention to, and public awareness of, the severe challenges also faced by organisations and care workers providing support for older people in their own homes, as well as the millions of relatives and friends who took on increased unpaid care responsibilities, often with reduced support.

Two main themes characterise the early response to the pandemic by the English government. First, the focus in the early months was almost exclusively on the NHS. The stated priority was to avoid hospitals becoming overwhelmed by very seriously sick patients. Consequently, elderly patients were discharged rapidly to residential care without being tested for COVID-19; most routine health treatments and elective (non-urgent) surgery were cancelled; and Personal Protective Equipment (PPE) supply chains and COVID-19 testing prioritised NHS staff and patients. There was little awareness or understanding on the part of government – or, indeed, of NHS leaders – of the fragmented and substantially privatised residential care market, or of local authorities' statutory responsibilities and the funding challenges they had long experienced.

A second theme was delay. Despite early evidence of the likely disproportionate impact of COVID-19 on older people, the risks of transmission in residential care premises were repeatedly discounted. Guidance for residential home managers on allowing visitors access to PPE and regular testing for staff and residents were all slow to emerge. When guidance did eventually appear, guidance came from multiple sources and was often contradictory. A full national lockdown was announced in March 2020 (when around 400 hospital deaths had already occurred), but it was another 3 weeks before any plan for residential care was published. Similarly, residential care providers began issuing urgent calls for regular testing for staff and residents in March 2020, but this was not put in place until July 2020.

This chapter will first describe the residential care sector and relationships with health services in England. It will then describe the early months of the pandemic, covering, in turn, preparedness; initial policy responses; and the impacts on care home residents and staff. The chapter will argue that, although the pandemic starkly revealed major funding and structural weaknesses in the English residential care sector, subsequent policy actions have failed to address these. In particular, residential care remains at the uneasy intersection of the private market and local authorities' statutory responsibilities. At the same time, the NHS, which has no legal or funding responsibilities for the sector, remains dependent on residential care capacity to discharge medically fit but frail older people.

Residential and health care in England – the wider context

There are structural divisions between the NHS and adult social care services, of which residential care forms part. At a national level, NHS policy is the responsibility of the Department of Health and Social care (DHSC); funding comes from national taxation, with national strategic management and accountability structures. Locally, NHS services are highly fragmented, reflecting numerous reforms and extensive marketisation. NHS England (NHSE) is responsible for national coordination, policy direction and performance management and has strategic oversight of the local Clinical Commissioning Groups (CCGs) of managers, clinicians, and lay representatives that plan and commission local hospital and community health services. Hospital and community nursing services are provided by a patchwork of semi-independent local NHS Trusts.[1] General Practitioners (GPs) and pharmacists are independent NHS contractors, although salaried posts are increasing.

Significantly, NHS services are largely free at the point of need. All older people are entitled to free prescriptions, treatment by GPs, nurses, therapists, and clinical specialists in hospitals and the community. Low-income older people can also receive help towards the costs of dental and optical treatment.

Although closely linked to healthcare planning and service delivery, responsibility for public health currently lies with local authorities. Each local authority has a director of public health (DPH), responsible for environmental health, health protection and reducing health inequalities. Local DPHs are supported by Public Health England (now the Health Security Agency, HSA), an autonomous, national agency accountable to DHSC. HSA is responsible, among other things, for responding to public health emergencies.

Local authorities are legally responsible for assessing and meeting individual and aggregate needs for social care, including residential care. Local authority governance is divided between DHSC, responsible for health and care policy, and the Ministry of Housing, Communities and Local Government (MHCLG)[2] which oversees local authority financial and accountability arrangements. The quality-of-care services is regulated by the semi-independent Care Quality Commission (CQC). CQC conducts regular inspections of all NHS and care services, whether operated by commercial, non-profit or public authorities. In the early days of the pandemic there was considerable confusion over the respective roles and responsibilities of the two government Ministries, CQC, and PHE in supporting residential care.

Over time, the NHS has withdrawn from providing long-term care for older people. Major reforms in 1994 aimed to: reform funding arrangements that had incentivised institutional over community and domiciliary care; and create quasi-markets in care services (Means et al, 2002). Local authorities have since developed extensive domiciliary and community-based services to reduce or delay needs for expensive residential care; and introduced stringent assessments restricting publicly-funded residential care only to older people with the highest levels of need. Local authorities also largely ceased providing their own services; by 2019, 84 per cent of residential care beds were owned by private (for profit) providers, 13 per cent by charitable/non-profit providers and just 3 per cent by the public sector (IPPR, 2019). Many providers are small businesses, but over 30 per cent of residential beds are owned by large international companies (CHPI, 2019).

Local authorities are legally responsible for ensuring adequate supplies of local care services (market oversight and commissioning); assessing the care and support needs of individual older people (and, separately, of family care-givers); and arranging and funding appropriate care for those meeting current eligibility criteria. Local authority funding for care comes from central government grants, most of which are not ear-marked or ring-fenced for care; local taxation (again, most is not ring-fenced for care); and user charges. A small proportion of local authority care funding is transferred from NHS budgets; this is generally ringfenced for specific initiatives such as speeding up hospital discharge.

Each local authority decides what it spends on care – there is no national budget allocation related to levels of local need. Public funding for care has been severely restricted since 2010, as local authorities have borne the brunt of 'austerity' policies which cut public spending. Government funding for English local authorities fell by 49.1 per cent in real terms in 2010–11 and 2017–18: a 28.6 per cent real-terms cut in spending power (NAO, 2018). Although local authorities tried to protect care services from cuts, their ability to do so has been increasingly limited; the percentage of local authority budgets spent on adult care actually fell during 2019–20 and the number of older people receiving local authority-funded care dropped by 5.7 per cent, despite demographic pressures actually increasing demand (Amin Smith and Phillips, 2019). Local authorities nevertheless remain the largest funders of care services on behalf of their eligible local populations and thus have major impacts on the size, shape and financial sustainability of the sector. A series of short-term policy responses to the growing care funding crisis has increased the proportion of revenue from local taxation and decreased that coming from national, redistributive grant allocations. Local tax-raising capacity is inversely related to local levels of need, thus potentially increasing geographical inequity in public funding for care services (Amin Smith et al, 2018).

Overall, most older people receive care outside the publicly funded system. Over a third (37.5 per cent) receive most of their help from family and friends and a further 12.5 per cent pay for help privately. Just 21 per cent of older people are estimated to receive most of the help they need from (or funded by) their local authority.

The range of publicly-funded services varies locally, depending on authority budgets, commissioning policies and practices, and local care provider markets. Around 70 per cent of homes provide personal care and supervision, including for people with dementia. They employ care staff with basic training; all health care (such as injections, changing dressings) apart from oral medication is provided by visiting NHS community health services. Thirty per cent of homes provide basic nursing as well as personal care and employ one or more qualified nurses. The NHS pays a standard amount to nursing homes towards the cost of this basic nursing care. Specialist nursing (such as enteral feeding, intravenous injections) is provided by NHS community services. In both care and nursing homes, all medical care is provided free by the NHS – GPs in the community and specialist clinicians in hospitals. In some areas, short-term, intensive, outcome-focused rehabilitation services are provided in care homes; in other localities there is specialist housing for older people, with care and support staff available round the clock.

Following a decade of austerity policies, local authorities fund residential care only for those who meet stringent care, income, and wealth criteria. There are broad national eligibility criteria: care needs must arise from, or be related to, a physical or mental impairment or illness; have a significant impact on wellbeing; and be reflected in an inability to carry out two or more personal care activities, maintain a habitable home, remain safe at home, maintain family or other personal relationships, and/or use local services and facilities. Anyone with assets over £23,250 (€26,415) (including the value of a house) is not eligible for any publicly-funded care, regardless of level of need. Below this asset threshold, an additional income test determines levels of co-payment charges. Around half of English residential placements are fully funded by older people themselves because their incomes and/or assets are above eligibility thresholds. There is no private insurance. Over 50 per cent (£7.7 billion/€9.22 billion) of total annual residential home income (£15.2 billion/€18.19 billion) comes from private individuals; this varies regionally, reflecting growing regional socio-economic inequalities. There are significant and growing gaps between the fees paid by local authorities – up to 10 per cent below the actual cost of residential care – and the fees paid by 'self-funding' private payers, on average 40 per cent higher for identical facilities in the same home.

Before the pandemic the residential care market was already fragile. Although local authorities pay below the actual cost of care, they remain the largest purchasers of residential care. Residential care providers' financial sustainability increasingly depends on their client mix; in a quarter of homes over 75 per cent of residents are local authority-funded and these are at high risk of financial failure or market exit (CMA, 2017). Over the past decade, providers have had to absorb significant new payroll costs arising from increases in the statutory minimum wage. Workforce shortages, particularly of registered managers and nursing staff, were already major challenges for providers and have worsened significantly since. Staff themselves have long complained of low pay; high pressure and stress; casualisation, zero-hours contracts and lack of sick pay; and the generally low social esteem of care work.

'Care deserts' are emerging in parts of England where adequate social care services are no longer reliably available, even where older people fund this themselves (Age UK, 2019).

In summary, residential care is located in a 'no-mans-land' between the public and private sectors, and between state and market modes of governance. Local authorities have overall statutory responsibility for ensuring local supply and funding care for the poorest older people; the NHS contributes nursing and clinical care. However, the allocation of public funding is not related to local need; supply is almost entirely located in the private sector; and older people themselves (and their families) fund over half of all beds.

Preparedness for the pandemic

In October 2016, the UK government conducted a simulation exercise, Operation Cygnus (PHE, 2017) on readiness for a pandemic. It involved Local Resilience Forums (multi-agency groups convened to deal with local emergencies), NHSE and PHE at local, regional, and national levels, DHSC and other government departments. Operation Cygnus concluded that both preparedness and responses were inadequate. It recommended more detailed national guidance to assist local responses; identifying and 'scaling up' effective local responses to national level; and more regional-level planning, to bridge the gap between local and national actions and promote multi-agency working.

Specific concerns were raised about residential care. It was assumed that hospitals would need to discharge patients to increase bed capacity, but Operation Cygnus found it was not possible to identify spare capacity in residential care or where this was located. There was also confusion over whether responsibility lay with DHSC (responsibility for NHS and care policy) or MHCLG (responsible for local authority finance and governance). Recommendations for residential care included requisitioning hotels and negotiating contingency contracts with larger residential provider companies. Ring-fenced funding was recommended so the NHS could purchase additional beds in residential care, staffed by returning recently retired nurses and care workers. Significantly, residential care was considered only in respect of its role in relieving pressure on hospitals; little attention was given to the potential pressures and challenges within the sector that could arise as a result of resident infections, illness, and mortality.

Local authority Directors of Adult Social Care responded with proposals to improve pandemic planning. These included improving the purchase and supply of personal protective equipment (PPE); better infection control; and recruiting volunteers from families, charities, and local communities to work in residential homes. A spokesperson for the Directors commented in *The Guardian* newspaper on 14 May 2020 'We are not aware of whether government departments picked up on any of the recommendations'. In summary, despite the simulation exercise, there is no evidence of any preparation to support residential homes in protecting or looking after seriously ill or dying residents, including those discharged from hospital, in the event of a pandemic.

Operation Cygnus modelled the impacts of a seasonal influenza pandemic. COVID-19 differed in several important respects including its speed of transmission; the vulnerability of normally healthy people to severe illness; and the availability (at that time) of a vaccine (CDC, 2020). These differences may not have been fully appreciated in the early stages of the pandemic.

Policy responses to the pandemic and the impacts on health and residential care

Like social care, the NHS had experienced a decade of funding restraint, so at the start of the pandemic there was little spare hospital capacity and low staffing levels per hospital bed. Early policy focused exclusively on slowing COVID-19 transmission rates to allow time for the NHS to increase critical care capacity. This was largely successful. During March 2020, hospitals rapidly reorganised to cope with the expected surge in COVID-19 patients, cancelling routine outpatient appointments, postponing planned treatments, moving outpatient appointments online and redeploying staff. New emergency critical care hospitals were created in under 3 weeks, in a London exhibition centre and six other English localities, with a total capacity of 3,000 beds.

Protecting the NHS – hospital discharges

In March 2020, and reflecting experiences of Northern Italy and Spain, there was considerable anxiety among policy-makers and politicians that the NHS would be overwhelmed. In response, 'very strict and tough guidance' was issued on 19 March 2020 to discharge as many patients as possible, predominantly to residential homes:

> acute and community hospitals must discharge all patients as soon as they are clinically safe to do so … Discharge from hospital should happen as soon after that as possible, normally within 2 hours … Implementing these Service Requirements is expected to free up to at least 15,000 beds by Friday 27 March 2020. (HM Government, 2020)

However, no complementary guidance or support was issued to residential homes looking after discharged patients. Most seriously, patients were not tested for COVID-19 before discharge. This was defended by PHE on grounds that it was 'very unlikely that people receiving care in a care home … will become infected' – a claim widely reproduced on care home websites. It was only in mid-April that DHSC recommended all patients should be tested before discharge from hospital to residential care. By then over 28,000 hospital patients had been discharged to residential homes; it was apparent that asymptomatic transmission could occur; and there had already been 5,700 resident deaths. A subsequent Inquiry by an influential committee of MPs concluded that this was an 'appalling error … Our care homes were effectively thrown to the wolves' (Public Accounts Committee, 2020). Care home managers were pressured to accept discharged patients who had not been tested or were known to be COVID-19 positive; some were offered additional funding to do so:

> astonishingly, neither the government nor the CQC have shown any interest in understanding the impact and consequences of those urgent

> discharges from hospitals to care homes … DHSC did not collect data on the extent to which homes successfully isolated residents with confirmed or suspected COVID-19 and did not require local authorities to collect data either. (Amnesty International, 2020: p 19)

Legislative and regulatory changes

In order to effect rapid hospital discharge, legislation temporarily relaxed local authorities' legal duties to conduct detailed assessments of individual care needs and financial circumstances before admission to residential care and to prepare and review individual care plans. The 2020 Care Act easements came into effect on 31 March. Local authorities remained under a duty to meet needs where failing to do so would breach human rights under the European Convention, such as rights to life, to freedom from inhumane and degrading treatment, and to private and family life (DHSC, 2020a). Nevertheless, the Act effectively suspended the rights of older people (and their families) to choose their destination on discharge from hospital, including returning home with added domiciliary support or moving to a specific preferred residential home.

A month after the onset of the pandemic, on 15 April 2020, an Action Plan for Social Care was published (DHSC, 2020b). This contained guidance on controlling infection; supporting the workforce; supporting residents, including at end of life; and supporting local authorities and care providers. The Action Plan strongly discouraged residential homes from applying blanket 'Do Not Attempt Resuscitation' policies and advocated personalised Advanced Care Plans, including end-of-life care preferences, for each resident. A policy of testing everyone discharged from hospital to a residential home was announced.

By the end of April 2020, after COVID-19 had spread to half the residential homes in the worst-affected areas, PHE recommended a radical lockdown of all homes to stem rising infection and death rates. PHE urged ministers to 'use NHS facilities and other temporary accommodation to quarantine and isolate residents', and 'consider whether staff can move into the care home for the next four weeks'. The proposal was rejected by DHSC (*The Guardian*, 2020a).

In mid-March 2020, CQC suspended routine inspections of residential homes. Within 2 months there was a 55 per cent increase in complaints to CQC from residential home staff about poor workplace practices, especially relating to infection control, social distancing or PPE (*The Guardian*, 2020). Suspending routine inspections, at exactly the same time that visits from relatives to care homes were also suspended, increased risks of resident abuse that remained unidentified, unreported and not investigated (Amnesty International, 2020).

Access to healthcare in residential homes

In April 2020, a geriatrician highlighted the lack of healthcare expertise in residential homes:

> many homes now have on site far more acutely ill residents who would normally have been conveyed to hospital, which is putting further strain on care homes – not least those that don't employ registered nurses or don't have quick access to general practice, district nursing, or geriatrician support. And, if residents are dying and need end-of-life care or are breathless and need oxygen, there can be problems sourcing medicines, skilled palliative care support, or masks and cylinders. (Oliver, 2020)

Pre-pandemic, there were already plans to improve health care support for residential homes. These were due to come into effect in October 2020, but implementation was brought forward. Guidance issued in May 2020, required weekly reviews of residents identified as clinical priority, including those with suspected or confirmed COVID-19, by multi-disciplinary medical and nursing teams. Clinicians were instructed to support the use of oxygen and other equipment in residential homes and, with home staff, create personalised treatment escalation plans, including for end-of-life care. Pharmacy teams were to ensure medication was delivered and reviewed; consistent access to out-of-hours medical services was to be established; and hospitals were required to admit care home residents 'where clinically appropriate' (NHS England, 2020). Two weeks was allowed for implementation.

However, GPs expressed concern about the additional staffing and costs involved (HSJ, 2020). Residential homes and relatives continued to report GPs refusing to visit regardless of residents' symptoms (Amnesty International, 2020) and levels of healthcare support remained variable. For example, although many residential homes could give low flow oxygen to residents with chronic obstructive pulmonary disease (COPD), this was not the case for subcutaneous fluids, and it was unclear whether staff could take on extended roles in the midst of a crisis (Gordon et al, 2020). Multiple reports persisted of residents' rights to NHS services being denied, including hospitals refusing admission. NHSE guidelines in April advised that some residents should not be routinely admitted to hospital; these were controversial and soon withdrawn, but the perception remained that hospitalisation was not an option (Amnesty International, 2020).

Emergency funding for residential care

By the end of April 2020, emergency funding of £6.6 billion (€7.9 billion) had been allocated to support health and social care services and £3.2 billion

(€3.8 billion) to local authorities. Of the £6.6 billion, £1.3 billion (€1.56 billion) was ringfenced for rapid hospital discharge (NAO, 2020). In May a further £600 million (€700 million) was allocated to care homes for PPE, decontamination, cleaning, isolation facilities, and infection control. Infection control measures included hiring additional staff; sick pay for existing staff to self-isolate when infected; and supplementing wages to deter staff from taking additional shifts in multiple homes, thereby increasing transmission risks (DHSC, 2020c). Additional PPE supply chains for care homes were to be piloted.

Local authorities were expected to deliver the funding quickly to their residential homes. They were also instructed to protect homes' cashflow by making planned payments early and increasing fee payments to cover new costs. Around half of local authorities temporarily increased their fees to residential homes, most commonly by 10 per cent; others set aside emergency funding or offered a single upfront lump sum.

Local authority finance leaders judged the emergency funding to be inadequate and responded that £4 billion (€4.79 billion) was needed to properly fund residential care (CIPFA, 2020). Representatives of residential home owners also reacted angrily to offers of a temporary 10 per cent fee increase for state-supported residents; some pointed out that this would not even cover their additional PPE costs (*The Guardian*, 2020b):

> I have been told about the money and had to complete a questionnaire but have not been told when or if I will be getting any money.
>
> They said we have to apply with justification to why we need funds and supply evidence to support additional costs incurred in a time where bureaucracy is not needed. We don't have time to analyse and report. (NCA, 2020)

Obtaining PPE

Operation Cygnus had found low stocks of PPE. Normally residential homes use only small quantities and source their own supplies; they do not have established supply chains and are weak purchasers, compared to the large, centralised NHS PPE procurement and supply systems. Yet even in the NHS, demand escalated exponentially at the start of the pandemic; an emergency telephone ordering system was overwhelmed (NHS Providers, 2020).

There was a critical shortage of PPE for residential homes (and many NHS staff as well). Workers in one home described how paper masks were saved solely for looking after symptomatic patients (Reuters, 2020), despite the fact that staff also had COVID-19 symptoms.

From April 2020, residential homes were able to use the NHS supply chain; PHE announced it would train care home staff in appropriate PPE use; and additional logistics capacity was purchased to speed up PPE distribution (DHSC, 2020b). Even so, some care homes still had difficulty obtaining adequate supplies or paid inflated prices in a market dominated by NHS purchasers:

> Gloves from national supplier gone up from £2.50 per box of 100 to £4.00, now £5.00…
>
> We have spent about 600 per cent more than we normally do due to masks and other gear.
>
> Our average monthly spend before COVID-19 £50 a month, last 3 months we have spent £4,000. (NCA, 2020)

Testing for residents and staff

Initially testing capacity was well below what was actually needed by residents and staff and there was confusion over who was responsible for testing in residential homes. Until mid-April 2020, tests were rationed to five symptomatic residents in any home (NAO, 2020). The Adult Social Care Action Plan promised that everyone moving to a residential home would be tested, regardless of symptoms, starting with those discharged from hospital and tests would be available for all residential home staff, for example if they were in a self-isolating household. At that point, just 1,000 home staff had been tested out of an estimated 0.5 million workforce.

By the end of April 2020, testing was extended to all staff and residents, regardless of symptoms. However, reports continued of difficulty obtaining sufficient tests even for symptomatic residents (Reuters, 2020). Tests for staff and residents were capped at 30,000 a day (Amnesty International, 2020); sector representatives estimated that at least 200,000 tests daily were required to track infections (*The Guardian*, 2020a).

There was confusion over whether PHE, CQC, or DHSC was responsible for overseeing testing in homes. The Action Plan for Adult Social Care assigned lead responsibility to CQC working with local authority Directors of Adult Social Care, DPHs, and LRFs. However, CQC claimed it was only responsible for contacting care homes and offering to order test kits; subsequently DHSC, PHE, and the NHS took lead responsibility. Eventually lead responsibility was transferred to local authority DPHs in tacit acknowledgement that a national testing system had failed (*The Guardian*, 2020a). Even by August 2020, regular testing for staff and residents was still not fully operational (*Sunday Times*, 2020).

The impact of the pandemic on residential care

Despite the Minister for Health and Social Care claiming to 'throw a protective ring' round residential care, the impact of the pandemic was disastrous.

The impact on residents

At the start of the pandemic, residential home deaths attributable to COVID-19 were seriously underestimated, partly because few residents had been tested (*Financial Times*, 2020). Moreover, infected residents frequently had atypical symptoms such as fever or loss of mobility, rather than the more common respiratory problems (Gordon et al, 2020), again leading to underestimates of COVID-19 deaths.

Evidence of the rapid spread of COVID-19 and its impact on frail older people was available from early February 2020. By late March 2020, there were almost 800 residential home outbreaks. One home tried to isolate symptomatic residents in separate rooms, but the virus still spread, killing 10 residents in 3 weeks (*The Guardian*, 2020c). From early April 2020, CQC started collecting data on COVID-19 deaths in residential homes; this showed 1,009 outbreaks and a sharp rise in resident deaths (*The Guardian*, 2020a). Official figures showed a doubling of COVID-19 deaths in residential homes between 19 and 24 April (Gordon et al, 2020). By mid-May, as many deaths were occurring in residential homes as hospitals. By late May 2020 over 16,000 residents had died – over 40 per cent of known COVID-19 deaths.

Deaths due to COVID-19 only partly reflected the pandemic's impact. Isolating residents to prevent infection also had psychological and physical costs. Residents were also prevented from seeing visitors; many homes introduced this restriction in advance of the national guidance. Eighty per cent of home managers surveyed in May 2020 reported the absence of visitors had led residents to feel isolated; a third reported reduced oral intake; a third reported it was not always possible to isolate residents (Rajan and McKee, 2020). The prolonged isolation of residents was described as 'devastating', causing significant deterioration in physical and mental health and wellbeing (Amnesty International, 2020). As the pandemic progressed and guidance became more advisory, home managers were left to make extremely tough choices, balancing responsibilities for protecting residents from risk against residents' rights and freedoms.

The impact on staff

Before the pandemic, social care staff vacancies were already rising; sickness absences and the extra staff needed to care for quarantined residents created additional pressures. The April 2020 Adult Social Care Action Plan announced the ambition of recruiting 20,000 care staff over the next 3 months, but by early June, DHSC was unable to estimate what progress had been made (NAO, 2020). The Action Plan also extended access to a website and telephone helpline providing emotional and psychological support for NHS staff to care workers.

Care workers are notoriously low paid; average hourly pay is under £10, only just above the statutory minimum wage. Since 2012–13, sector pay has increased more slowly than for other comparable occupations such as retail (Kings Fund, 2022). Zero-hours contracts with few employment benefits are common. Many staff cannot afford to self-isolate and lose pay if they are unwell; some work extra shifts across multiple homes to increase their income, thereby transmitting infection.

The Adult Social Care Action Plan did not mention staff moving between homes or between floors within homes, despite PHE having identified this infection risk. The risks to care staff were amplified by difficulties in obtaining adequate PPE. One home reported a PPE delivery of 300 masks but needed 400 every day; during its worst outbreak the home had no appropriate masks, gowns or visors; 48 staff contracted COVID-19. In a few homes, staff moved in to live with residents (*The Guardian*, 2020c). By mid-April, reports of residential care staff being overwhelmed were mounting (Oliver, 2020).

A survey of nurses working in residential homes found poor employment conditions; 80 per cent felt unvalued; others felt blamed for resident deaths, pressurised to admit residents with unknown COVID-19 status and lacking clear guidance. Over half reported worse physical or mental health: 'The two weeks of daily deaths during an outbreak were possibly the two worst weeks of my 35 year nursing career' (Queens Nursing Institute, 2020). Another survey of residential home managers in May 2020 found widespread concern over staff morale, mental health and wellbeing. Managers reported frustration at the lack of parity between the NHS and residential care and the struggle to maintain morale. Two-fifths of managers described staff shortages and reluctantly having to employ agency staff at inflated prices to fill gaps: '[We are] paying for agency staff; agency attempted to increase fees by 25 per cent. We could put double the number of staff on [to barrier nurse effectively] and still struggle and we don't have that amount of money to use for wages' (NCA, 2020).

Overall impact on residential care sustainability

The pandemic created multiple simultaneous cost pressures:

- Staff sickness and self-isolation required more use of expensive agency staff.
- Because staffing levels assume residents spend time in communal areas, additional staff were needed to care for sick or isolated residents.
- Agencies providing temporary staff increased their fees.
- Homes paid staff bonuses to deter them working extra shifts elsewhere.
- Additional PPE had to be purchased at inflated prices.
- Enhanced cleaning was needed for infection control.

At the same time, homes' income decreased. Occupancy rates dropped because of resident deaths, the additional space (for example, in shared rooms) needed to isolate infected residents and reduced admissions because of perceived infection risk. In May 2020 a large residential home business reported occupancy rates dropping from 90 to 70 per cent (*The Guardian*, 2020c): 'This business model relies on occupancy and when there are COVID-19 people in we are extremely reluctant to take [new] people in due to massive strain on resources and safety surrounding the effort of trying to barrier nurse anyone affected by a dementing type of illness' (NCA, 2020).

Some residential home businesses increased fees for self-funding privately paying residents by up to 15 per cent (BBC, 2020) to make up the income shortfall. Some 27,000 smaller residential homes (fewer than 20 beds) became highly vulnerable financially, with widespread closures expected over the next few years (Brindle, 2020).

Reflections and analysis: the pandemic in retrospect

Failure to prepare

Despite Operation Cygnus, no steps were taken to improve the preparedness of residential care for a pandemic. The simulation exercise revealed significant gaps in knowledge about the sector and structural weaknesses in governance. There was no central source of information on overall capacity, vacancy levels or residents' characteristics and needs and it was not even clear which Government department was responsible for collecting this. Recommendations – clarifying Government responsibilities, developing regional-level planning and coordination, improving training and awareness in infection control and improving access to PPE – were apparently ignored.

Perhaps the most egregious shortcoming was the exclusive focus on the role of residential care in facilitating hospital discharge, rather than understanding it to be the home and workplace of thousands of older people and care workers. Yet even this narrow focus made unrealistic and inappropriate assumptions about residential homes' capacity to cope with a highly infectious pandemic. Many smaller homes are located in older, converted houses and a decade of 'austerity' had restricted investment in infrastructure, staff training and pay, and facilities. Staffing levels assume at least some communal activities, not separate care for individuals isolated in their own rooms; moreover, conventional staffing levels do not cover high proportions of seriously ill and dying residents who also need additional specialist equipment and care.

Structural weaknesses – between national, local, and market governance

The pandemic revealed the multiple fault lines between central and local governments; between the centralised structures of NHS England, with its 'command and control' capabilities, and the diverse local authorities responsible for commissioning and purchasing services for (some) older people in their areas; and between local authority purchasers, growing numbers of older people funding their own care and the diverse private markets of competing providers. These fault lines were exacerbated by a decade of 'austerity' policies that had left residential care (and to a lesser extent the NHS) desperately weakened. The prospects for a coordinated response to the pandemic were not promising.

Among government and NHS leaders there was little understanding of this diversity and complexity. The historical low priority of social care within government and a resulting lack of senior social care voices embedded in decision-making processes rendered social care largely invisible in the early months of COVID-19, resulting in a slow and inadequate response. It was not even clear who or what organisation was responsible for different aspects of residential care, such as ensuring adequate PPE supply. Policy priorities were to protect the NHS; there were consequent delays in issuing guidance and emergency funding for social care, including residential care. When social care did finally feature in response plans, the restricted awareness of Government ministers and operational knowledge of civil servants meant the complexity of the sector was underestimated. Blanket guidance, often written with the NHS in mind, was inappropriate or difficult to interpret within residential care. Guidance was often released late on Friday evenings for implementation the following Monday, giving providers and commissioners little time to understand the implications or communicate sometimes significant changes.

There was a lack of clarity about the respective responsibilities of central government departments, arms-length regulatory bodies and local government; and between local government and the privately-owned providers of residential care. Again, recommendations from Operation Cygnus for greater attention to relationships between central and local governments were apparently ignored. Indeed, tensions between central government and local expertise and knowledge became increasingly apparent. For example, contracts were awarded to private commercial companies to establish national call centre-based testing and contact-tracing, marginalising local DPHs and denying them the information they needed for effective tracing, quarantine compliance, and preventive interventions.

The impact of COVID-19 on English residential care was devastating. Because testing was initially only available for hospital patients with suspected COVID-19, data on COVID-19 residential home deaths did not become available until late April 2020. In a market dominated by large NHS procurement chains, residential homes struggled to obtain PPE at reasonable cost. Death rates in residential homes were as high as those of hospital patients. After adjusting for age and sex, residential sector workers were over twice as likely to die from COVID-19 as the general population

(Health Foundation, 2020b). The already weakened residential home quasi-market was hit financially by a triple burden of reduced occupancy rates, extra staffing costs and inflated PPE prices.

A highly critical Inquiry by an influential group of Members of Parliament (Public Accounts Committee, 2020) concluded that the fragmented governance of the sector, with responsibilities divided between DHSC, local authorities, private care providers, and regulators, had led to inconsistent and incoherent guidance, poor central control, inadequate testing, and problems in PPE supply. Discharging 25,000 hospital patients into residential care between mid-March and mid-April 2020 without testing was an 'appalling error'. The Inquiry also criticised the month's delay between the publication of COVID-19 response plans for the NHS and social care. This 'stark contrast' illustrated the 'tragic impact' of delaying much-needed reform to social care and its continued treatment as the poor relation of the NHS. Amnesty International (2020) concluded that the English government, NHS, and other national and local organisations had directly violated the human rights of older care and nursing home residents, notably their rights to life, health, and non-discrimination, to private and family life, and may have violated their rights to protection from inhumane or degrading treatment.

The residential care workforce crisis

Of particular concern, the largely private residential care sector entered the pandemic with a poorly trained and poorly paid workforce and widespread difficulties recruiting and retaining staff. Low pay, chronically high vacancies creating reliance on transient agency staff, and frequent use of zero hours contracts were common, contributing to high levels of staff movement and insecurity. In some instances, wider COVID-19 policies actually adversely affected the care workforce. For example, unlike NHS staff, care staff were given the same advice as the general public and told to isolate for 14 days if symptomatic (DHSC, 2020b) – apparently unaware that staff employed on zero hours contracts had no access to sick pay. Additional funding released in May 2020 aimed to address this and appears to have had some impact, with a majority of homes now paying full wages to self-isolating, directly employed staff (Curry et al, 2023).

Even locally there was limited knowledge about the care workforce and this created delays in preventing infection outbreaks in local communities from being transmitted via care workers into residential homes. Residential care work continued to be regarded as low skilled and low status, despite the fact that some of the tasks care centre workers undertook during the pandemic – verifying deaths, dressing wounds, installing catheters, and giving insulin – would normally have been done by other professions such as GPs, nurses, and social workers.

Policy measures since the pandemic

In autumn 2021, proposals to reform adult social care funding were published – but these were mainly in response to an election promise rather than the weaknesses revealed by the pandemic. From April 2022, payroll taxes have increased by 1.25 per cent.[3] Until 2025 most of the additional revenue will be allocated to the NHS, to fund the pandemic legacy backlog in routine and elective care. Just £1 in £7 will go to social care. In England, from October 2023 new eligibility rules will raise both the lower and upper assets limits on eligibility for publicly-funded care; people with savings up to £100,000 will become eligible for some support. No one will pay over £86,000 (€102,270) for care over their lifetime; once the cap is reached, local authorities will take over all care funding. This will cost £3.6 billion (€4.3 billion); the remaining £1.7 billion (€2.02 billion) additional funding will go to implementing a '10 Year Vision' for social care, including: £300 million (€357 million) to expand housing-based care options; funding for housing repairs and adaptations to help people continue living at home; £150 million (€178 million) for new technology and digitisation; £500 million (€595 million) to improve care worker training and career progression; £25 million (€30 million) for family carer support; and £100 million (€119 million) towards better planning. Overall, the measures fall far short of the £5.9 billion (€7.02 billion) needed each year up to 2025 that local authority leaders estimate will stabilise a collapsing sector; more will be needed to address unmet needs, increase care worker pay and improve residential and domiciliary care.

Additional measures were announced in December 2021 to address the acute workforce crisis: a short-term fund to boost staff recruitment and retention over the winter through redeployment, incentive and overtime payments; a 'Made with Care' publicity campaign to boost recruitment; and the designation of care work as a 'shortage occupation', to be placed on a 'fast track' immigration visa list to facilitate inward workforce recruitment previously hit by Brexit. However, there are no proposals to improve care workers' basic pay, so care employers will continue to compete with other, less demanding, minimum wage sectors (Kings Fund, 2022).

Conclusions

Some (relatively minor) lessons do seem to have been learned about the need for better coordination between the NHS and care sectors, and about the need for greater clarity over responsibilities for residential care. The pandemic accelerated plans to collect data about residents and bed capacity, laying the foundations for a more robust standardised data set. As the pandemic developed, some progress was made to reduce staff movement between homes, and to improve access to sick pay, although underlying issues of low pay and insecure contracts remain.

The pandemic revealed the uneasy location of residential care between the governance regimes of a nationally funded and managed NHS; highly variable local government funding and responsibilities; and a failing private market. At the same time, the NHS remains highly dependent on the residential sector to achieve the prompt discharge of clinically fit patients who still need care and support. Commentators have therefore argued that the state needs to play a much bigger role in the residential sector, and for new legal powers to coordinate and protect the fragmented and highly precarious care market and protect residents, whether privately or publicly funded (Rowland, 2020). Others have promoted the potential benefits of operational parity between NHS and care services, with staff in both sectors seeing collaborative working as the 'new normal' (Gordon & Goodman, 2020).

However, these pleas appear to have gone unheeded. The planned reforms to social care funding are likely to yield only a small fraction of the additional resources needed to stabilise the residential care market including, as a priority, increasing care worker pay and esteem. An influential cross-party committee of MPs has called for increases of £7 billion per year simply to cover demographic changes, increase staff pay and protect people facing catastrophic costs – a third higher than the projected 2023–24 budget (Health and Social Care Select Committee, 2020). Increased funding is also recognised as an essential prerequisite for closer collaboration between the NHS and care sectors. The Health and Social Care Select Committee (2020) recognised their interdependence and noted that this was significantly weakened by the failure to match longer-term planning and investment in residential care with that of the NHS. Proposals published in early 2022 (DHSC, 2022) aim to increase collaboration, by ensuring joint strategic planning through new Integrated Care Systems, local delivery of shared outcomes and accountable local leadership. Achieving these goals is acknowledged to depend on better data sharing, pooling of resources and robust regulatory mechanisms. However, no timescale is given for implementation and, while the proposals aim to bring together local government and local NHS organisations, it is far from clear how they will bring in the fragmented, private residential care markets as equal partners with NHS and other service providers.

Notes

1. Legislation is currently being introduced which will replace these with Integrated Care Systems – dual structures that recognise the need for integration both between different NHS organisations and between NHS and local government partners.
2. Subsequently renamed the Department for Levelling Up, Housing and Communities.
3. The additional payroll levy has been withdrawn from April 2023, although the funding commitment remains.

References

Age UK (2019) *Later Life in the United Kingdom 2019* [online], Available from: https://www.ageuk.org.uk/globalassets/age-uk/documents/reports-and-publications/later_life_uk_factsheet.pdf

Amin Smith, N. and Phillips, D. (2019) *English Council Funding; What's Happened, What's Next*, Briefing Note, Institute for Fiscal Studies [online], Available from: https://ifs.org.uk/publications/14133

Amin Smith, N., Phillips, D., and Simpson, P. (2018) *Adult Social Care Funding: A Local or National Responsibility*? IFS Briefing note BN227, Institute for Fiscal Studies.

Amnesty International (2020) *As If Expendable. The UK Government's Failure to Protect Older People in Care Homes during the COVID-19 Pandemic* [online], Available from: www.amnesty.org

BBC (2020) Coronavirus: Care home residents face steep hike in fees, BBC News, 6 June [online], Available from: https://www.bbc.co.uk/news/uk-52944751

Brindle, D. (2020) As COVID-19 decimates our confidence in care homes, what are the alternatives? The Guardian, 26 May [online], Available from: https://www.theguardian.com/society/2020/may/26/as-covid-19-decimates-confidence-care-homes-what-alternatives-older-people

CDC (2020) *How is Pandemic Flu different from Seasonal Flu?* Centres for Disease Control [online], Available from: https://www.cdc.gov/flu/pandemic-resources/basics/about.html

CHPI (2019) *Plugging the Leaks in the UK Care Home Industry*, London: Centre for Health and the Public Interest.

CIPFA (2020) *Social Care: The Forgotten Front Line*, Chartered Institute of Public Finance and Accounting [online], Available from: https://www.cipfa.org/cipfa-thinks

CMA (2017) *Care Homes Market Study: Final Report*, Competition and Markets Authority [online], Available from: https://assets.publishing.service.gov.uk

Curry, N., Oung, C., Hemmings, N., Comas-Herrera, A., and Byrd, W. (2023) Building a resilient social care system in England: What lessons can be learnt from COVID-19? Research report, Nuffield Trust and Care Policy and Evalun Centre, Available from: https://www.nuffieldtrust.org.uk/research/building-a-resilient-social-care-system-in-england-what-lessons-can-be-learnt-from-covid-19

DHSC (2020a) *Care Act Easement: Guidance for Local Authorities*, 20 May [online], Available from: https://www.gov.uk/government/publications

DHSC (2020b) *COVID-19: Our Action Plan for Adult Social Care*, 15 April [online], Available from: https://www.gov.uk/government/publications

DHSC (2020c) *Coronavirus (COVID-19): Care Home Support Package* [online], Available from https://www.gov.uk/government/publications

DHSC (2022) *Joining up Care for People, Places and Populations: The Government's Proposals for Health and Care Integration*, CP573 [online], Available from: www.gov.uk/official-documents

Financial Times (2020) *Deaths in UK Care Homes from Coronavirus May be 6,000, Study Estimates*, 18 April [online], Available from: https://www.ft.com/content/9d6b46e2-55f4-4de1-ba21-f1ab9f14bcbf

Gordon, A. and Goodman, C. (2020) *Tackling the COVID-19 Outbreak in Care Homes: Messages from a Geriatrician and a Health Services Researcher About How the NHS Can Help* [online], Available from: https://www.kingsfund.org.uk

Gordon, A., Goodman, C., Achterberg, W., Barker, R., Burns, E., Hanratty, B., Martin, C., Meyer, J., O'Neill, D., Schols, J., and Spilsbury, K. (2020) Commentary: COVID in care homes – challenges and dilemmas in healthcare delivery, *Age and Ageing*, 49(5), 701–5.

Health and Social Care Select Committee (2020) *Social Care: Funding and Workforce*, Third Report of Session 2019–2, House of Commons HC206 [online] Available from: https://committees.parliament.uk/publications.

Health Foundation (2020b) *What Has Been the Impact of COVID-19 on Care Homes and the Social Care Workforce*? [online], Available from: https://www.health.org.uk/news-and-comment/charts-and-infographics/what-has-been-the-impact-of-COVID-19-on-care-homes-and-social-care-workforce

Henwood, M. et al (2019) *From Bystanders to Core Participants? A Literature and Data Review of Self Funders in Social Care Markets,* HSMC, University of Birmingham.

HM Government (2020) *COVID-19 Hospital Discharge Service Requirements*, 19 March [online], Available from: https://assets.publishing.service.gov.uk/government/uploads/system/uploads/attachment_data/file/880288/COVID-19_hospital_discharge_service_requirements.pdf

HSJ (2020) *Contentious NHS Scheme to Bolster Care Homes Brought Forward,* 29 April [online], Available from: www.hsj.co.uk

IPPR (2019) *Who Cares? The Financialisation of Adult Social Care*, London: Institute for Public Policy Research.

Kings Fund (2022) *Social Care 360* [online], Available from: https://www.kingsfund.org.uk/publications/social-care-360

Means, R., Morbey, H., and Smith, R. (2002) *From Community Care to Market Care*, Bristol: Policy Press.

NAO (2018) *Adult Social Care At a Glance*, London: National Audit Office.

NAO (2020) *Readying the NHS and Adult Social Care for COVID-19*, London: National Audit Office.

NCA (2020) *Care Provider Impact Study*, National Care Association [online], Available from: https://nationalcareassociation.org.uk

NHS Providers (2020) *Briefing: Confronting Coronavirus in the NHS: The Story So Far*, 15 April [online], Available from https://nhsproviders.org

Oliver, D. (2020) Let's not forget care homes when COVID-19 is over, *BMJ*, 369(m1629).

PHE (2017) *Exercise Cygnus Report Tier One Command Post Exercise Pandemic Influenza 18–20 October 2016*, Public Health England [online], Available from: https://assets.publishing.service.gov.uk/government/uploads/system/uploads/attachment_data/file/927770/exercise-cygnus-report.pdf

Public Accounts Committee (2020) *Readying NHS and Social Care for the COVID-19 Peak* [online], Available from: https://publications.parliament.uk/pa

Queens Nursing Institute (2020) *The Experience of Care Home Staff during COVID-19* [online], Available from: https://www.qni.org.uk/explore-qni/icno

Rajan, S. and McKee, M. (2020) *Learning From the Impacts of COVID-19 on Care Homes: A Pilot Survey* [online], Available from: www.ltcCOVID.org

Reuters (2020) Special Report Health: Coronovirus Britain, 10 May [online], Available from: https://www.reuters.com/investigates/special-report

Rowland, D. (2020) To protect older people from COVID-19, state coordination of the social care sector is urgently needed [online], Available from: www.blogs.lse.ac.uk

Sunday Times (2020) Care home Coronovirus testing pledge abandoned, 2 August [online], Available from: https://www.thetimes.co.uk/article/care-home-coronavirus-testing-pledge-abandoned

The Guardian (2020a) Government rejected radical lockdown of England's care homes, 28 May [online], Available from: https://www.theguardian.com/world/2020/may/28/government-rejected-radical-lockdown-england-care-homes-coronavirus

The Guardian (2020b) England care providers say 10% council fee rise is "too little too late", 10 April [online], Available from: https://www.theguardian.com/society/2020/apr/10/england-care-providers-say-10-council-fee-rise-is-too-little-too-late

The Guardian (2020c) Coronavirus fears leading families to remove relatives from UK care homes, 5 May [online], Available from: https://www.theguardian.com/society/2020/may/04/coronavirus-fears-leading-families-to-remove-relatives-from-uk-care-homes

5

Protecting older people's lives, forgetting about their other rights? Managing the COVID-19 pandemic in the care home sector in Finland

Tyyne Ylinen, Vera Ylinen, Laura Kalliomaa-Puha, and Satu Ylinen

Introduction

Throughout the COVID-19 pandemic, the general aim in Finland was to protect older people and other at-risk groups. In the first phase of the pandemic (in the spring of 2020), multiple measures were adopted to protect older people and prevent the spreading of the virus in the social welfare units. The measures were adopted rapidly. In general, Finland coped relatively well with COVID-19. Nevertheless, the disease was fatal to older people, especially in the social welfare units. Older people living in care homes suffered in different ways. They were the most likely to die of COVID-19. For that reason and beyond, their rights were restricted during the pandemic in ways violating their fundamental rights.

Finland already had relatively new legislation governing emergencies when the COVID-19 pandemic started. Even though it turned out that the laws needed some alterations during the pandemic, the legislation gave the authorities the power and tools to act from the start. There was also both national and local contingency planning – which turned out to be inadequate and not sufficient, but did provide some preparedness. Nationwide, the number of cases and the number of hospitalised COVID-19 patients were moderate throughout the first phase of the pandemic. The first COVID-19 case was confirmed in late January 2020. By mid-March, the number of cases was 150 in total. The Finnish government announced a state of emergency, introduced the Emergency Powers Act on 16 March and ordered several measures to prevent the spread of the virus. Public meetings of over ten people were banned, and people aged 70 years or older were advised to live in quarantine-like conditions. National and municipal culture and leisure services were closed. Visits to older people and other at-risk groups housing services were prohibited. Many functions of society were moved to remote connections, which led to a (risk of) digital divide among older people.

Finland is a sparsely populated country. There were remarkable regional differences in the spread of the infection. Quite rapidly, the cases concentrated in Helsinki's capital city and the relatively populous surrounding counties. However, the national guidelines for restrictions were similar throughout the country (Forma et al, 2020; Ylinen et al, 2021).

The restriction measures imposed in March curbed the spread of the pandemic, and in May 2020, the government announced a plan to move to a hybrid strategy: 'test, trace, isolate and treat'. Because of the new strategy, many services and activities were opened, but the services for older people remained closed. As a result, throughout the first phase of the pandemic, the total cumulative incidence of COVID-19 per 100,000 population in Finland was 124.4, and cumulative deaths 5.7. Most of the infected were working-aged people, but deaths among the working-aged have been exceedingly rare.

Since the restrictions remained heavier for older people and their services remained closed, the inclusion of older people was undermined, and their fundamental rights were violated (Ylinen et al, 2022). In addition, isolation from social relations and the abolition of leisure activities debilitated the well-being of older people (see Pirhonen et al, 2021). Older people themselves saw diminished social relationships as a cause of loneliness related to depression, feelings of insecurity, and experiences of worthlessness. Still, in Finland, older people, in general, reported fewer adverse changes during the first phase of the pandemic than expected. The older people who were most socially isolated, such as the oldest people and those living alone, seemed more susceptible to negative changes. They experienced more serious negative physical and mental impacts than others (see Koivunen et al, 2021; Lehtisalo et al, 2021). Especially older people living in care homes were isolated (see Forma et al, 2020).

COVID-19 was relatively fatal for older people since morbidity has been rather low, but the mortality rate was relatively high. The median age of the deceased was 84. Of all the deceased, over 90 per cent had one or more long-term illnesses. Of the deaths, 45 per cent occurred in long-term care, 34 per cent in primary health care units, 19 per cent in specialised medical care, and 2 per cent at home or elsewhere. COVID-19 was relatively fatal in care homes since, of all first-phase deaths, 45 per cent occurred in 24-hour social welfare units (AVI, 2020; THL, 2020). By the end of May 2020, less than 1 per cent of all residents in housing services had died of COVID-19 during the pandemic. (Forma et al, 2020; Ylinen et al, 2021). COVID-19 has had much impact on health care and has increased medical debt. Elective care was withdrawn and referred to future assignments. Before the pandemic, Finland's ICU bed numbers were relatively low. The number was then increased, and the adequacy of the ICU beds stayed at a reasonable level throughout the first phase of the pandemic. The vulnerability of older people concerning the virus led to a situation where they were restricted in ways that violated their fundamental rights. Despite various contingency plans made, no one was well enough prepared for this kind of situation, and older people and other fragile groups were not taken into account in the plans as well as they should have been.

In the next section of this chapter, we will briefly describe the history of elderly care in Finland. In the third section, we describe the background of Finland's preparedness for pandemics with a particular focus on the measures taken to protect the residential care sector. We then sketch out how the situation evolved in the care home sector in the following phases of the pandemic. We will also reflect on the lessons to be learned from the COVID-19 pandemic and the measures taken specially to protect older people in residential care.

Elderly care in Finland: from family care to a public responsibility and individual right

Finnish elderly care has evolved from family care to public responsibility and individual rights. During the 19th century, the focus was on subsistence: providing food and shelter. In particular, the conditions of the older people of the rural poor population were marked by misery and social decline. Protection for old age came in the form of poor relief; the elderly services aimed to help; and the form of helping was institutional care (almshouses). When moving towards the 20th century, the number of older people increased. Urbanisation changed perceptions of old age. It gave rise to the old age working class and increased the number of older people living alone. At the same time, old age became a social problem. For the first time, the need for care, not only for subsistence, was recognised. The form of helping was mainly institutional care, together with the care offered by families – younger generations still taking care of their older relatives. Moving towards the 1970s, the emphasis shifted to services provided by the welfare state under construction. Elderly services aimed to support the personal initiative. The form of helping was institutional care, but the emphasis started being on bringing home services (Ylinen, 2008).

From the 1970s to 1990, the concept of the older population started to be seen as quite heterogeneous. New concepts such as seniority, competence, and older people as a defined social group became part of the general discourse. Protection for old age was formed through the pension policy and the health and social services system. The aims of elderly services were rehabilitation and activation. The forms of helping were home care and institutional care. From 1991 to today, the older population has been seen as a heterogeneous group that plays an active part in society. Features important to the social status of the older population were, and still are, seen to be empowerment and access to the resources necessary in old age. During recent decades, the national ageing policy has aimed at ensuring older people have the living conditions that enable them to receive community care. Community care includes home care, support services, and care provided at day centres, service centres, and sheltered housing facilities with and without 24-hour assistance. Institutional care consists of long-term care (LTC) provision in older people's homes and primary health care (see Ylinen et al, 2021). Sheltered housing with 24-hour assistance is often like institutional care regarding residents' needs (see Linnosmaa & Sääksvuori, 2017).

The current welfare system in Finland is based on universalism, where all citizens in need are entitled to basic social security and services, mainly financed by taxes and administered by the local authorities. The Finnish care regime is a mixed one, combining public, private, and individual provisions. The services are provided by a network of actors, including public and private providers, and the responsibility for organising the services rests with the municipalities (STM, 2012). Municipalities can produce services via public facilities in cooperation with other municipalities or purchase the services from the state, other municipalities, or private providers. Municipalities may also grant a voucher to a service user. The voucher can be used to purchase the service from a private provider (see Linnosmaa & Sääksvuori, 2017). LTC services in Finland are part of the universal health and social care system, which provides services to all citizens in need of care. A network of actors, including public and private providers, provides the services. The state government and municipalities are the two most important funding sources for LTC care (see Ylinen et al, 2022). Although taxes mainly cover costs, some of the costs (in 2014, 18.5 per cent) are collected through client fees (see Seppälä & Pekurinen, 2014). The client's payment ability defines client fees – property is not considered. In addition, the monthly fee may not exceed 85 per cent of the client's net income. Social protection for older people consists of income security and services in kind arranged as a part of social and health care. The Social Insurance Institution of Finland (Kela) provides social security coverage for Finnish residents and many Finns living abroad. Among the social security benefits are family benefits, health insurance, rehabilitation, basic unemployment security, essential social assistance, housing benefits, financial aid for students, disability benefits, and basic pensions. Kela also pays a care allowance to persons in institutional care (Kalliomaa-Puha & Kangas, 2018; Ylinen et al, 2023).

Emphasis on the national ageing policy in Finland is on home care and family care (Pirhonen, 2017), and most Finnish older people live in home-like conditions with community care support. If home-like living is not an option, an older person can apply for a place from LTC. The service needs of the person applying are assessed by municipal health and social care professionals by reviewing the applicant's functional abilities, health state, and other factors related to the need for round-the-clock service. The assessment and decision are carried out as multidisciplinary cooperation following the IAS operational model (investigation, assessment, service guidance). After the assessment, the municipality is responsible for drawing up a service plan that defines the services required to support the aged's well-being, health, functional capacity, and independent living. The views of the individual in need of care should be recorded in the service plan. The municipality makes the final decision about the provision of services (see Linnosmaa & Sääksvuori, 2017). According to the Social Welfare Act, after learning of a person's need for services, the municipality has to provide for the services within 3 months.

On paper, the system seems reasonable. However, research shows that there are only sometimes enough services for older people, or the services differ from those they wish for (THL, 2019a). LTC can also be organised by informal care support, which is a combination of a benefit in kind and a cash benefit. Informal care support is paid to a relative who provides care at home for an older person or a person with a disability or chronic disease. Municipal informal care support requires a contract between the municipality and the caregiver. The amount of support is linked to the intensity of the care needed (see Linnosmaa & Sääksvuori, 2017). In Finland, both the eldercare professions and family care are female-dominated (Karsio et al, 2020). Family caregivers are often women who have to manage both their own careers and the care of their older parents or relatives (Begum et al, 2021).

Extensive preparedness provided tools, but more was needed for a pandemic like COVID-19

About preparedness and legislation

Finland is well prepared for crises such as pandemics from the national level to every care home – at least on paper. Finland has a national emergency preparedness plan, local preparedness plans, and industry-specific preparedness plans in place. Also, the legislation provides tools for the authorities. However, the COVID-19 pandemic put them to a real test for the first time.

Nationally, the Ministry of Social Affairs and Health (later MSAH) directs, controls, and is responsible for emergency and pandemic preparedness in social and health care. It cooperates with the Finnish Institute for Health and Welfare (THL) and regional state administrative agencies (AVI). The Communicable Diseases Act (1227/2016, Tartuntatautilaki) guides national preparedness for a pandemic. The act lays out the obligations of the authorities and the principles of cooperation between the authorities to prevent communicable diseases. There was also a special national preparedness plan for pandemics. It was last updated in 2012 when the WHO instructed its member countries to update their pandemic preparedness plans after the H1N1 pandemic. The National Preparedness Plan aims to limit the harm caused by a pandemic to human health, to ensure the continuity of society's activities as well as possible, to set up the guidelines for influenza pandemic preparedness at all administrative levels of health care, and to support preparations in other administrative branches (STM, 2012: pp 24–5). However, it soon became evident that the plan from 2012 needed revisions, and the work started in the spring of 2020. The updated plan is reported to be completed in early 2023 (STM, 2022).

The Emergency Powers Act (Valmiuslaki 1552/2011), meant to provide adequate powers for national and regional authorities during war or other exceptional situations, obliges the local authorities to anticipate exceptional circumstances through contingency plans. Each social and healthcare organisation must plan for preparedness from two perspectives. First, the organisation must ensure the continuity of its services and tasks in all situations as well as possible (continuity management). Second, the organisation must be prepared for the different threat models identified together, as well as exceptional events and disruptions, which require greater and closer cooperation and communication between authorities and other actors (such as a significant accident or a pandemic) (Kuntaliitto, 2019). To help draw up such plans, the MSAH has provided a handbook on emergency planning in social services (STM, 2008). The handbook acknowledges the residential care sector by guiding social services to pay special attention to guaranteeing the safety of older people and other relatively fragile groups in their contingency plans (STM, 2008: p 14). What comes to the National Preparedness Plan for Pandemics stresses the duties of health care but also acknowledges the importance of social services by referring to the handbook on emergency planning in social services. For example, the plan points out that if the potential epidemic reaches the housing service for the elderly, it will become more challenging to care for the residents. The plan also remarks that in case of a pandemic, sending residents to the hospital is problematic if the hospitals are full of infected patients (STM, 2012: p 35).

The National Preparedness Plan for Pandemics lays out the critical actors at the local level. In social services, the municipalities carry out the responsibility. In health care, a key responsibility lies with municipalities within a regional organisation, where the regional state administrative agency and the local government groups in medical districts collaboratively guide the planning of primary public care, social care, and private health care equipment and enforcement. The role of the regional organisation is to create an arrangement, management procedure, and plan for the region that considers regional and local specifics (STM, 2012: p 24). In addition to such emergency planning, self-monitoring plans are also obliged by legislation, for example, the Social Welfare Act (1301/2014).

Even though the residential care of older people is usually considered a part of social services, the personnel of residential care of older people come from both health professionals and social care professionals, most often trained nurses, practical nurses, bachelors of social sciences, geriatricians, or gerontological social workers. The legislation (professionals working in social services act 817/2015 and healthcare act 559/1994) guides the qualifications of those professionals. This legislation also obligates the regular maintenance of professional skills. Also, the law prescribes the number of workers. However, the nurse-client ratio in long-term care has also aroused doubts, mainly because it has been difficult to recruit personnel (Kalliomaa-Puha & Kangas, 2018).

Besides the obligation to contingency plans, the Emergency Powers Act provided the authorities means to restrict people's rights to unrestricted movement. The Government put the Act's provision into service by, for example, isolating southern Finland from other parts of the country for weeks in March 2020, closing restaurants, or prohibiting gatherings of people. Also, the Communicable Diseases Act provided the right to place individuals into quarantine, even against a person's will, providing proof or reasonable doubt that a highly contagious disease posing a public health risk, such as COVID-19, existed.

In addition to these legally grounded restrictions, the Government and local authorities also recommended proper rules of conduct. Such suggestions were directed mainly to older people, for example, urging them to stay at home and not to meet friends or relatives.

It is noteworthy that there was no legislation – and there still is none, despite ongoing plans – on restrictions in elderly care, even though restricting especially people with memory illnesses is necessary for their protection even in a normal situation. According to the tenet, restricting one's right to free movement violates human rights unless there is justification in the legislation. Such legislation exists, for example, restricting the rights of the mentally disabled, mentally ill, children in need of protection, people with substance abuse problems, or people with an infectious disease – but not in residential care of older people.

Organisational level management capacity in social and healthcare

One of the Finnish COVID-19 strategy's top priorities was to limit the healthcare system's burden. That is why one of the first concerns was the adequacy of beds in intensive care units (ICU). Before the pandemic, the number of ICU beds in Finland was approximately 300, and the number of intensive surveillance beds was about 150–200 (STM, 2022), one of the lowest levels in the EU (Eurostat, 2020). In the first phase of the pandemic, hospital districts began working to increase the number of beds. That was made by shutting down non-urgent operations and reorganising hospital facilities. Elective surgeries were postponed, and operating theatres and recovery areas were converted into intensive care units. In addition, surgical and ward staff were trained in treating COVID-19 patients and in working in ICUs (Tiirinki et al, 2020). In Finland, the worst scenarios did not come true; due to these actions, there were enough ICU beds. Also, the number of hospitalised COVID-19 patients was moderate throughout the first phase of the pandemic. On average, the intensive care period lasted 13.7 days, and 13.6 per cent of intensive care unit treatment periods ended with the patient passing away. By the end of May 2020, COVID-19 infection was confirmed for 286 intensive care periods, of which 209 were in the Helsinki University hospital district (KYS, 2020).

When hospital districts postponed non-urgent care to increase COVID-19 healthcare capacity, most elective surgeries, medical rehabilitation, therapies, and counselling services were suspended nationwide. Annual health checks were cancelled, and at the beginning of the epidemic, patients were even advised not to come to the health centres. Even though some health checks and services were done remotely, it led to constant delays in treating non-COVID-19 related diseases. The situation worsened the therapeutic equilibriums in many long-term illnesses, and non-COVID-19 related, initially non-urgent cases turned urgent. In addition, due to the abolition of elective functions, some cancers may have gone undiagnosed. It is later reflected as a growing medical debt. These delays will not be fixed rapidly and have a wide range of cumulative effects (Mankki et al, 2021). The same goes for social services, many vital to the older population. For example, closing day activities and moving them to remote services made coping especially hard for older people. It caused them loneliness, depression, and helplessness (Ylinen et al, 2022).

While health care was managed through the first phase moderately, the situation in long-term care could have been better. The virus was prevented from reaching care homes despite restriction measures. Instead, the virus passed into care homes, often through workers or new residents. Authorities recommended that when a new resident enters a social welfare unit or returns from home holiday, they should be treated for the first 2 weeks under quarantine conditions. This recommendation was not universally followed, partly because of the lack of a formal recommendation or guidance. In addition, restricting the movement of a resident with a memory illness is challenging since memory disease prevents the implementation of self-sufficient quarantine. In a situation where there is no evidence of actual exposure, limitations are difficult to justify. As described, part of the problem is the legislation – or the lack of it. Since the strict rules on restricting the rights on the grounds of infectious disease (positive test results) did not exist, the doctors did not have legal grounds to order any quarantine.

Even though some protective equipment was stored for crises by the National Emergency Supply Agency, the amount and quality were inadequate. The treatment of actual COVID-19 patients and the ICU was prioritised; therefore, there were shortages of personal protection equipment in care homes during the first phase of the pandemic. From 15 May 2020, staff needed to use face masks in LTC units. However, due to the shortage of masks in the municipalities, there were varying practices in using masks between LTC units. Municipalities were innovative and made their masks with the help of volunteer residents (see Forma et al, 2020).

There were reported personnel shortages in residential care of older people even before the pandemic. However, as COVID-19 hit Finland moderately, there were no significant problems in elderly care – the personnel did not get sick in vast amounts. As the other services of the municipalities have been closed or reduced (for example daycare centres, early childhood education, libraries), the staff have been relocated to care for older people (Ylinen et al, 2021). Also, retired care staff, who did not belong to the risk group, and students have been recruited as necessary (Eurohealth, 2020: p 80).

Overlapping and conflicting instructions for LTC units were problematic

At the end of March 2020, the authorities gave several guidelines for care homes and home care. The main goal was to prevent infections in LTC units. It was stated that staff and new residents should be tested if they have symptoms. In May, it was recommended that if a coronavirus case has been confirmed in the unit, testing of all employees and residents should be considered. However, there were reports showing shortcomings in testing among both groups (Forma et al, 2020).

The 24-hour social welfare units received guidance from different levels of authority. Instructions were given by the government, the MSAH, municipalities, private providers, hospital districts, and the Finnish Institute for Health and Welfare. New instructions were given frequently, and sometimes they were conflicting. The MSAH is the highest authority for the 24-hour social welfare units. In addition, hospital districts can give guidance on healthcare matters. The hospital district must also guide 24-hour social welfare units if instructions are obscure (AVI, 2020). New instructions came frequently, and the previous ones quickly expired (Ylinen et al, 2021).

Frequently given, overlapping instructions and their contradictions were perceived as problematic. It was laborious to follow constantly changing guidance from several different sources. Instructions have also come in various forms, with some recommendations and some commands. It was also impossible to get hold of the authorities to check the instructions or ask further questions (Ylinen et al, 2021).

Intersectoral coordination: older patients received adequate medical care whether they were transferred to the hospital or not

Residential care of older people is at the intersection of social and health care. Most of the help needed by older people could be labelled social, but many older people also need health care, sometimes predominantly. Even though the fluent cooperation of both sectors is the starting point of the legislation, the different ideals might collide in everyday life. For example, ideas of a good life, self-determination, or participation may vary (Ylinen et al, 2023). As explained previously, the personnel of care homes can come from both social and health professions, often from both. Care homes vary in how they provide doctor services as the needs of older people in each care home vary. The Act on older people (Vanhuspalvelulaki 980/2012) calls for adequate services, be they social or health services.

During the pandemic, one fundamental guideline was to avoid resident transfers between the care sites, such as between care homes and hospitals, whenever possible. Transfers were allowed only for medical reasons, and the new treatment site had to be notified of whether the person had respiratory symptoms (Forma et al, 2020). The plan was to treat COVID-19 in older people in residential care, even in palliative care cases. All 24-hour social welfare units – even those not usually providing medical services – were required to be able to give symptomatic treatment in their units with support from home nursing and emergency medical service units. The units needed to make sure that they have a 24-hour doctor service available in case of a need for medical consultation. The units had to prepare to provide palliative treatment for COVID-19 by training their staff and obtaining the medicines necessary. However, any resident needing hospital-level treatment, like intensive care, was transferred to the hospital. The ICU decision was and is always made by a physician, and there is a guideline to follow. Decisions have been made according to the same principles as before the pandemic.

Every patient's assessment was made to evaluate whether the treatment provides more benefit than harm (Kari et al, 2020). Because of the excellent adequacy of ICU beds in the first phase, all patients requiring intensive care could be treated (Ylinen et al, 2021).

Physical distances were maintained where possible by limiting mobility within the care unit (Forma et al, 2020). In some care homes, the movement of residents with dementia was restricted by locking residents in their rooms (for example, EOAK/5463/2020).

Inadequate preparedness and lack of legislation concerning older people

Even though there were national, local, and even care unit-level contingency plans and relatively new legislation to cater to crises and even pandemics, they proved to be inadequate. However, the Emergency Powers Act proved to be decisive in providing the possibility of quick manoeuvres for the government. The planning beforehand provided some help to the professionals even though none of those foresaw a situation like COVID-19.

The plans considered more common seasonal epidemics such as influenza or norovirus (Ylinen et al, 2021), as did the framework provided by the MSAH – it considered only commonplace hazards. A study from 2014 found that the planning was carried out quite adequately by the municipalities. However, it discovered statistically significant differences in the quality of the preparedness plans between small and large service areas and how they considered the elderly. Overall, older people and other fragile groups were not noted in the plans as well as they should have been (Rapeli & Ritola, 2014). There is a need for a comprehensive common preparedness plan and more local and unit-specific planning. Common rules are needed to ensure equal treatment of people, but on the other hand, local situations vary and cannot be considered nationally. As has also been shown during the pandemic, the situations have been very different in different parts of Finland. Perhaps there was too much national guidance: was it, for example, necessary to cut the treatment of all non-COVID-19 related diseases in areas where there were no COVID-19 patients?

Since no one was prepared to protect the elderly in a pandemic situation, decisions had to be made on the run at every level. That led to contradictory guidance, which led to inadequate and reactive leadership. There were situations where authorities did not respond to professionals' inquiries, and they had to make decisions about the measures on their own (Ylinen et al, 2021). For example, the MSAH ordered social and welfare units via the municipalities to ban visits to care homes. The orders were given so that they seemed obliging, although the communicable disease act did not include the right to obliging orders to ban visits. The recommendations for the general public were communicated in a way that was interpretable as an order.

Courts, the parliamentary ombudsman, and the national non-discrimination ombudsman have already evaluated many local solutions. The case law is quite unanimous, stating that individual discretion should have been used instead of general, overall restrictions. The restrictions were not proportionate, since some of them violated human dignity. As personal freedom guaranteed in the Constitution s. 7, is also understood to protect self-determination and autonomy, it can only be restricted to fulfilling the requirements. Just being old or disabled does not, as such, entitle anyone to restrict one's rights – not even for protection (Ylinen et al, 2023).

Since there were remarkable regional differences in the spread of the infection, an individual estimate of the needed measures would have revealed whether heavy restrictions were needed. However, the national guidelines were similar throughout the country (Forma et al, 2020). Individual assessments were often forgotten at the care homes. As a result, visits to care homes stopped almost entirely (Forma et al, 2020). Banning visits to LTC may also have implications for accessing rights in general. Often older residents need the help of their friends or relatives to fulfil their autonomy, for example. That goes especially for people with memory disorders. If residents cannot speak for themselves, their opinions should be clarified with the help of their intimates according to legislation (see Forma et al, 2020; Pirhonen et al, 2021; Ylinen et al, 2022). Isolation from loved ones and broader social networks decreased the well-being of older people living in care homes (see Pirhonen et al, 2021). Isolation is known to impact emotional and psychological well-being and physical health. It can also lead to an increased risk of mortality (see Holt-Lunstad et al, 2015; Taylor et al, 2018; Cox, 2020).

The parliamentary ombudsman, for example, took the standing that forbidding one to attend the funeral of one's spouse violated the right to family life protected in the Constitution s. 10 (protection of privacy) and the UN convention of human rights article 8. Some of the restrictions were also violations of domiciliary peace since the institutions are the homes of long-term clients. On the other hand, the courts and the ombudsman understood the exceptional circumstances. There was genuine anxiety about the wellbeing of older people, and the situation was new, unforeseen, and frightening. It concerns Finnish legislation's profound gap even in normal circumstances: there is no legislation on restricting persons with memory illness, for example. In addition, the personnel in older people's homes might not be accustomed to 'thinking legally' to recognise that their deeds have consequences for human rights. The health care professionals may need to recognise that it is not only providing medical care, but the well-being of older people is also dependent on other things such as social contacts. Now, all of a sudden, the personnel found themselves in a situation in which they should have been able to apply a law previously unfamiliar to them (the Communicable Diseases Act) and to recognise they were – while trying to protect their clients – restricting the human rights of their clients in an unlawful manner. The employees also mentioned the difficulty of coping with contradictory guidance (Ylinen et al, 2021). It must have been challenging to realise that there have not been legal grounds for all of the restrictions.

Shortages in preparedness plans and in protecting the human rights of older people

In the fall of 2020, care homes received guidance from the National Supervisory Authority for Welfare and Health (Valvira) that clients' meetings with their loved ones cannot be categorically prohibited. The clients cannot, without legal reason, be restrained from exiting the unit as long as they are not isolated or quarantined under the Communicable Diseases Act. In addition, it was reiterated that employees working in the care home must know the fundamental rights safeguarded by the clients' constitution and act in such a way that they are realised. When the availability of protective equipment improved by the fall of 2020, it got easier for care homes to organise safer meetings for the clients and their loved ones. Since then, in most care homes, pandemic-related quarantine and isolation practices have complied with the Communicable Diseases Act. However, at the end of 2020, there were still units restricting clients' rights without justification under the Communicable Diseases Act or a doctor's order. In addition, at the time, absolute visitation bans were still in place in a few units.

The COVID-19 vaccinations started in early 2021 in Finland. Older people living in care homes were one of the first groups vaccinated (right after social and health care personnel). In the spring of 2022, the fourth vaccine was offered to people living in care homes. No official statistics are available on the average share of deaths at long-term care facilities after the first phase. During the pandemic, a total of 3,638 COVID-19 related deaths were reported in Finland. The majority, 85 per cent, of the deceased have been over 70 years old. During the pandemic, the median age of all the deceased has been 83. It is estimated that the average share of deaths related to COVID-19 taking place at long-term care facilities at the beginning of October 2021 was 42 per cent in Finland.

As of now, the chain of command is unclear. There needed to be more clarity about which authority's instructions to follow in situations where new instructions came daily (see Ylinen et al, 2021). Communicating the recommendations and rules should be more precise in future crises. During the first phase of the pandemic, it was unclear to professionals and the general public whether they could use their discretion. Also, the national contingency plans should better consider protecting older people. However, we do not think drawing up a national contingency plan that is suitable for all areas, and every care home, is possible. As laborious as it may be, every unit should make up its risk assessments and plans. At the same time, it is simply impossible to prepare for all possible situations. Therefore, the possibility of the legislation to act and limit the rights of people if needed is essential. As explained, now the legislation needs to be more straightforward. That goes especially for elderly care. It must be clear whose responsibility it is to act and what the powers are. Such powers can also be misused; therefore, rights to appeal and assess the limitations of the rights of people must also be provided for. Although, as we see, crises such as pandemics are inevitably unpredictable, the personnel of care homes for older people should be trained to make decisions at the unit level. It calls for both legal and ethical know-how. The present COVID-19 situation showed that individual evaluation was often forgotten in many care homes. However, individual evaluation is the starting point for access to one's rights.

As each older person has the right to self-determination and participation, how should it be considered if, for instance, an older person living in a care home would like to take a conscious risk and meet her close ones despite the risk of getting contaminated? If the person would only be putting herself at risk, the situation is easy, but since she might also risk others, if they (including workers) are willing to take the risk, the solution is again accessible. It is also relatively easy when the older resident taking the risk could stay in quarantine in her room afterward. But if she cannot? Or if she is suffering from a memory illness or other illnesses affecting her cognition? In addition, regardless of the state of cognition, it is difficult for an individual to make decisions where one must choose between instantly visible and inevitable harmful consequences and uncertain but potentially much worse consequences. That is not only an individual-level question but also a sociological problem and ethical issue. What if every person taking conscious risks needs intensive care and only limited beds are available? Who should then be treated? If the doctor estimates that the treatment would not be effective, not all older people would be treated in ICU. Should they at least be able to take the risk, then? These, indeed, are challenging questions to answer. In a crisis, we can say that each person has an individual and collective responsibility to protect themselves and each other. However, where other adults could decide about the risks they took during the pandemic, older people living in care homes lacked such freedom. Unit-specific preparedness plans should consider how to protect the residents without unnecessarily violating their self-determination. It can be promoted by securing the continuation of contact to close ones, by providing, for example, digital meeting places or gadgets, or providing secure meetings inside or meeting places outside. It should be considered how to organise such conditions so the client can still choose to go outside, exercise and practice other hobbies, and otherwise participate in society, even in exceptional circumstances. These kinds of questions should be taken into account in future preparedness plans.

In Finland, the policy aim is to reduce institutional care and encourage older people to live in their own homes for as long as possible. That stresses that the needs of older people still living at home should be better considered while preparing for future crises. It also has to do with designing housing – how older people should be considered while planning houses, intermediate housing before existing care homes, and how pandemics should be considered in architecture (Verma, 2024). Older people who live on their own often count on the help of family and friends even more than those who live in care homes. Restricting people from seeing each other makes meeting care needs difficult or even impossible, as well as limiting self-determination. Finnish researchers emphasise the importance of social relationships. Keeping in touch might be even more critical during crises than at other times. Developing ways to secure the possibility of visiting older people during future crises is essential. It also means considering suitable and accessible digital means and taking care of working connections. Interpersonal relationships are strongly related to health and well-being (Aaltonen et al, 2021; Kulmala et al, 2021; Pirhonen et al, 2021).

As explained, the level of Finnish ICU beds is relatively low. Even though the hospitals did not need to prioritise patients this time, greater ICU beds would have reduced the pressure on elective health care and medical debt accumulated by it. Finland has managed the pandemic period moderately well. However, older people, especially those living in care homes, have been in a special position throughout the pandemic. The restrictions imposed on protecting them have violated their fundamental rights. At the same time, the statistics reporting COVID-19 related deaths have been over-represented. Therefore, in the future, contingency plans need to take better account of all older people, those living at home, and those living in care homes. In addition, the people taking care of older people should have a good understanding of clients' fundamental rights so that their rights will also be realised in times of crisis.

References

Aaltonen, M., Pulkki, J., Teräväinen, P., and Forma, L. (2021) Ikääntyneiden kokemukset hoivan ja avun saamisesta Koronapandemian aikana, *Gerontologia*, 35(4), 326–41.

Aluehallintovirasto (AVI) (2020) Usein kysytyt kysymykset [online], Available from: http://www.avi.fi/web/avi/usein-kysytytkysymykset;jsessionid=11CA933D769BAB5531C9784DB04C0628#Vanhus

Begum, S., Naskali, P., Zechner, M., Outila, M., Svensson, E-M., Wennberg, L., Harbison, J. R., Halla Arnórsdóttir, A., and Kvitberg, T. (2021) Exploring gender equality among caregivers: a sub-study based on the Nordic network, *Current Developments in Arctic Law*, 9, 97–133 [online], Available from: http://urn.fi/URN:NBN:fi-fe2021120759310

Cox, C. (2020) Older adults and COVID 19: social justice, disparities, and social work practice, *Journal of Gerontological Social Work*, 63(6–7), 611–24.

Eurohealth (2020) Health Systems Responses to COVID-19; 26(2), Available from: https://eurohealthobservatory.who.int/publications/i/9999-12-31-eurohealth-health-systems-responses-to-covid-19-26-2

Eurostat (2020) Health in the European Union – facts and figures [online], Available from: https://ec.europa.eu/eurostat/statistics-explained/index.php/Health_in_the_European_Union_%E2%80%93_facts_and_figures

Forma L., Altonen M., and Pulkki J. (2020) COVID-19 and clients of long-term-care in Finland: impact and measures to control the virus. LTC COVID, International Long-Term-Care Policy Network, CPEC-LESE, Available from: https://ltccovid.org/2020/06/14/new-report-covid-19-and-clients-of-long-term-care-in-finland-impact-and-measures-to-control-the-virus/

Holt-Lunstad, J., Smith, T. B., Baker, M., Harris, T. and Stephenson, D. (2015) Loneliness and social isolation as risk factors for mortality: a meta-analytic review, *Perspectives on Psychological Science*, 10(2), 227–37.

Kalliomaa-Puha, L. and Kangas, O. (2018) ESPN Thematic Report on Challenges in Long Term Care, Finland; European Union [online], Available from: https://ec.europa.eu/social/main.jsp?catId=22&langId=en

Kari, A., Reinikainen, M., and Valtonen, M. (2020) Tehohoidon uudet eettiset ohjeet, *Duodecim*, 136(3), 597–8.

Karsio, O., Näre, L., Olakivi, A., Soitu, L., and Zechner, M. M. (2020) Vanhuus, vaiva ja tasa-arvo [Old age, ailment and equality], in J. Kantola, P. K. Sandberg and H. Ylöstalo (eds) *Tasa-Arvopolitiikan Suunnanmuutoksia*, Helsinki: Gaudeamus, pp 227–42.

Koivunen, K., Portegijs, E., Sillanpää, E., Eronen, J., Kokko, K., and Rantanen, T. (2021) Maintenance of high quality of life as an indicator of resilience during COVID-19 social distancing among community-dwelling older adults in Finland, *Quality of Life Research*, 31(3), 713–22.

Kulmala, J., Tiilikainen, E., Lisko, I., Ngandu, T., Kivipelto, M., and Solomon, A. (2021) Personal social networks of community-dwelling oldest old during the COVID-19 pandemic: a qualitative study, *Frontiers of Public Health*, 9, Article 770965.

Kuntaliitto (2019) Kuntien Turvallisuus ja Varautuminen [online], Available from: https://www.kuntaliitto.fi/yhdyskunnat-ja-ymparisto/turvallisuus-ja-varautuminen

Kuopion Yliopistollinen Sairaala (KYS) (2020) *Tehohoidon Tilannekuva: COVID-19 Teho-osastoilla*, Kuopio: Viikkoraportti, 3 June.

Lehtisalo, J., Palmer, K., Mangialasche, F., Solomon, A., Kivipelto, M., and Ngandu, T. (2021) Changes in lifestyle, behaviors, and risk factors for cognitive impairment in older persons during the first wave of the Coronavirus Disease 2019 pandemic in Finland: results from the FINGER study, *Frontiers in Psychiatry*, 12, 624125.

Linnosmaa, I. and Sääksvuori, L. (2017) *Long-Term Care Policy in Finland: Policy Brief, Country Report*, CEQUA Study [online], Available from: https://www.julkari.fi/handle/10024/135807

Mankki, L., Lehto, I., Hirvonen, H., and Jokinen, E. (2021) *The Economic Impact of COVID-19 on the Finnish Regional Health Care Services*, UEF [online], Available from: http://codel.scot/wp-content/uploads/2021/06/UEF-Impacts-on-Finnish-health-care-sector-Feb21.pdf

MSAH (2013) *Health Care in Finland*, Brochures of the Ministry of Social Affairs and Health [online], Available from: https://julkaisut.valtioneuvosto.fi/handle/10024/69930

Pirhonen, J. (2017) *Good Human Life in Assisted Living for Older people: What the Residents are Able to Do and Be*, Tampere: Tampere University Press.

Pirhonen, J., Blomqvist, K., Harju, M., Laakkonen, R., and Lemivaara, M. (2021) Etäläheiset – hoivakotien koronaeristys asukkaiden läheisten kokemana, *Gerontologia*, 34(3), 178–92.

Rapeli, M. and Ritola, V. (2019) Sosiaalitoimen Varautuminen Suomessa: Kartoitus Sosiaalitoimen Valmiussuunnitelmien Tasosta 2014, Sosiaali- ja Terveysministeriön Raportteja ja Muistioita, 58/2018.

Seppälä, T. and Pekurinen, M. (eds) (2014) Sosiaali- ja terveydenhuollon keskeiset rahavirrat, *THL*, Raportti 22 [online], Available from: https://www.julkari.fi/handle/10024/116653

Sosiaali- ja terveysministeriö (STM) (2008) Sosiaalitoimen Valmiussuunnitteluopas, Publications of the Ministry of Social Affairs and Health, 2008, 12.

STM (2012) Kansallinen Varautumissuunnitelma Influenssapandemiaa Varten, Publications of the Ministry of Social Affairs and Health, 2012, 9.

STM (2019) Suositus Palliatiivisen Hoidon Palveluiden Tuottamisesta ja Laadun Parantamisesta Suomessa, Palliatiivisen Hoidon Asiantuntijaryhmän Loppuraportti, Raportteja ja Muistioita: 2019, 68.

STM (2022) Varautuminen Pandemiaan [online], Available from: https://stm.fi/valmiusasiat/pandemia

Taylor, H. O., Taylor, R. J., Nguyen, A. W., and Chatters, L. J. (2018) Social isolation, depression, and psychological distress among older adults, *Aging Health*, 30(2): 229–46.

THL (2019a) Kahdeksan Faktaa Vanhuspalveluiden Tilasta [online], Available from: https://thl.fi/fi/-/8-faktaa-vanhuspalvelujen-tilasta

Tiirinki, H., Tynkkynen, L-K., Sovala, M., Atkins, S., Koivusalo, M., Rautiainen, P., Jormanainen, V., and Keskimäki, I. (2020) COVID-19 pandemic in Finland – Preliminary analysis on health system response and economic consequences, *Health Policy and Technology*, 9(4), 649–62.

Verma, I (2024) Design for well-being in older people's residential environments, Fraunhofer IRB [online], Available from: https://www.irbnet.de/daten/iconda/CIB_DC23049.pdf

Ylinen, S. (2008) Gerontologinen sosiaalityö: Tiedonmuodostus ja asiantuntijuus, Kuopio: Kuopio University Publications E: Social Sciences, 155.

Ylinen, T., Ylinen, V., Kalliomaa-Puha, L., and Ylinen, S. (2021) Governmental response to the COVID-19 pandemic in Long-Term Care residences for older people: preparedness, responses and challenges for the future. MC COVID-19 working paper, Available from: https://digital.csic.es/handle/10261/227266

Ylinen, T., Ylinen, V., Kalliomaa-Puha, L., and Ylinen, S. (2022) Ethical challenges experienced by gerontological social workers in Finland during the COVID-19 pandemic, *Journal of Comparative Social Work*, 17(1), 94–122.

Ylinen, T., Ylinen, V., Kalliomaa-Puha, L., and Ylinen, S. (2023) in S. Raitakari, T. Harrikari, M. Hekkala, and M. Kivipelto (eds) Itsemääräämisoikeuden ja Suojelun Välinen Jännite Gerontologisessa Sosiaalityössä Koronapandemian Aikana: Sosiaalityö Poikkeuksellisissa Olosuhteissa ja Kriiseissä, SoPhi: Jyväskylä.

6

Impact of the French top-down management of the COVID-19 pandemic on residential care homes

Arnaud Campéon, Blanche Le Bihan, and Claude Martin

Introduction

In French residential care homes,[1] the epidemic evolved in the same way as it did in the general population, with a first wave from March to July 2020 and a second one starting in October/November 2020. In total, 224,500 care home residents were infected, with 29,300 deaths in 2020. The two waves in 2020 led to just under 15,000 deaths (Miron de l'Espinay & Richroch, 2021).

As for the general population, the studies available about the French case point to wide local disparities, with high impacts in some regions (the north, the Paris region, and the east) and lower impacts in others (the west). The pandemic was the cause of 2.5 per cent of deaths in residential care homes, but non-representative surveys, such as one carried out on 52 residential care homes all over the country, identified variations ranging from 2.3 per cent to almost half of the residents dying following contamination (Plateforme de Recherche sur la Fin de Vie, 2021).

On a national scale, during the second wave of the COVID-19 pandemic in the autumn of 2020, the incidence rate of the epidemic in residential care homes was about 1,600 residents per week for every 100,000 residents, compared to 500 people per 100,000 for the over-70s, and 450 for the general population (Miron de L'Espinay & Pinel, 2021). However, this gap began to shrink considerably in the spring of 2022 thanks to the vaccination campaign, which brought down the incidence rate to 200 for every 100,000 people in residential care homes, making it almost identical to the level for the over-70s, compared to 140 per 100,000 for the general population.

The research and statistics department at the French ministry of health and social affairs confirmed different contamination rates depending on the region. The percentages of residential care homes impacted by the pandemic ranged from 88 per cent in the Ile de France region (Paris area) to 64 per cent in the Grand-Est, and 35 per cent in Brittany. However, this difference was even wider when only looking at residential care homes confronted by critical episodes, in other words, care homes in which over 10 per cent of residents died due to the pandemic. These rates ranged from 45 per cent in Ile de France, to 23 per cent in the Grand-Est and 1 per cent in Brittany (DREES data quoted on Plateforme de Recherche sur la Fin de Vie, 2021).

This chapter looks back at these trends and considers the impact of the health crisis on residential care homes in France, focusing on the first wave of the pandemic in the spring of 2020. A strong mobilisation initially marked the health crisis by public authorities tackling the direct consequences of the epidemic in care homes. Considerable finances were allocated, and national recommendations were established to deal with this unprecedented health situation. On the one hand, the situation brought to the forefront structural weakness in the French care home sector that had been identified well before the pandemic but had not been subject to adequate reforms. On the other hand, implementing the recommendations and protocols produced by the supervisory authorities raised numerous questions and dilemmas for the professionals responsible for applying them. It was partly because they were disseminated progressively but mostly because they changed over time to adapt to the evolving situation. These frequent changes to guidelines on handling the pandemic often complicate the daily work and practices of professionals working at residential care homes.

After presenting the LTC policy in France and the situation of the residential care sector prior to the health crisis, this chapter sets out to identify the successive stages of managing the health crisis that began to impact residential care homes in February 2020. During the first pandemic wave, the health crisis management was highly centralised and based on producing numerous successive national recommendations for strict application by residential care homes; however, it came up against difficulties within care homes and in the relations between the different local actors involved. Considering these difficulties, crisis management gradually evolved to adapt to different situations, giving more room to local and institutional actors and healthcare professionals.

Role of residential care homes in the French LTC system

Traditionally characterised by a familial approach to elderly care, with a legal obligation for families to care for their older parents, since the 1990s, France has developed several LTC policy measures and evolved towards a mixed model, combining public measures and family care. As a result, LTC policy in France cuts across different policy sectors – health, social, and medico-social – and includes home-based care and residential care, public support through 'cash-for-care' benefits, and tax deductions for families that employ carers, not to mention the crucial contribution of informal caregivers within families. An analysis of the trajectory of LTC policy identifies an essential step in the late 1990s: introducing a cash-for-care benefit financed by taxes and allocated to people cared for in the home or institutions. The objective at that time was to externalise support for older people in need of care by allowing families to buy services (home-based or institutional care), pursuing a de-familiarisation approach. This cash-for-care benefit was reformed in 2002 – it became the Personal Autonomy Allowance (*Allocation Personnalisée d'Autonomie* – APA) – and is still one of the mainstays of French LTC policy.

LTC policy involves several territorial levels of governance. Regional administrations execute national health policies defined at the central level by the government, whereas the decentralised French local authorities – *départements* – are responsible for social policy. They have a crucial role in LTC regulation: they define local policy orientations in their territory, finance and manage the national cash for care benefit, and regulate care services. Although some territorial disparities exist, social care policy is subject to national regulations as national laws define the different schemes, and the government closely monitors local variations (Le Bihan & Sopadzhiyan, 2019). In addition, municipalities can develop specific voluntary support measures. Along with this territorial organisation, two major institutional actors are involved:

- the CNSA (national solidarity fund for autonomy – *caisse nationale de solidarité pour l'autonomie*), created in 2004, is a national institution responsible for implementing policy measures aimed at older and disabled people; and
- the ARSs (regional health agencies – *agences régionales de santé*), introduced in 2009, are the regional representatives of the central government, extending the regional agencies' traditionally health-sector-only intervention to the social care sector.

From the early 2000s, several reforms were initiated to improve support for older people in need of care and their families, with priority given to home-based care; however, they still need to be successfully implemented (Le Bihan & Martin, 2010). Following a wait of several years, in 2015, the Act on adapting society to ageing (*loi d'Adaptation de la Société au Vieillissement* – 2015 ASV Act) proposed a new comprehensive approach to the ageing issue centred on prevention. It also featured concrete measures to meet the needs of older people:

- an increase in APA benefits
- recognition of the role of informal carers
- closer coordination between the health and social care sectors

Despite these measures, the 2015 ASV Act was considered by professionals as insufficient, as the financial resources made available (around €700 million) remained insufficient to tackle the many challenges identified. Besides, this legislation mainly concerned home-based care, leaving aside the issue of residential care. In 2015, 728,000 older people lived in residential care (whatever their status[2]), an increase of 4.8 per cent compared with 2011 (Muller, 2017). The recent *Capacités, Aides et Ressources des Seniors* (CARE) survey (Brunel & Carrère, 2017) estimates the number of older people living at home as between 0.4 million (including only high-level dependency cases) and 1.5 million (also including mid-level dependency cases). Concerning the balance between formal and informal carers, the CARE survey established that almost 50 per cent of the elderly in need of care receive support from their relatives, and 20 per cent receive only professional support. A third gets formal and informal support (Brunel et al, 2019).

The major guidelines of a deep-seated reform, including home-based and residential care, were finally presented in a report dating from March 2019 – the Libault Report – which estimated that the additional budget needed due to demographic trends would reach €9.2 billion by 2030. Initially announced for 2019, the Old Age and Autonomy Plan has been delayed. However, following one of the recommendations of the Libault Report, two laws were promulgated on 7 August 2020, introducing a new social risk and a new social security branch. These laws strongly expressed political and institutional recognition of the need to support the loss of autonomy by creating a single autonomy sector, which includes disabled people and older people.

Managed by the CNSA, the action of this new social security branch has been set out in an agreement on targets and management (*Convention d'Objectifs et de Gestion*), which defines three priority areas: (1) the guarantee of a high-quality public service for the autonomy of older people, people with disabilities, and their families, thanks to a simplified administrative process; (2) adapted support to meet the needs of people and ensure freedom of choice in the organisation of their support (remain in their homes or move into an institution); and (3) the organisation of the new autonomy branch to ensure more efficient services and provide resources to beneficiaries.

These evolutions do not, however, bring to an end debates on LTC policy. First, the financing of the autonomy branch is not stable. It includes various types of funding aimed at older people and people with disabilities that already existed and were formerly managed by other branches of the social security system. Although this move makes public investment in this sector clearer and more efficient, it is judged to be insufficient (Ferras, 2020), as these resources are likely to increase constantly in the coming years. Besides, other significant challenges must be met: 'better coordination between the state and local authorities is needed to optimise and adjust supply according to the individual situation of older people and their families. The need to reorganise residential care is also a main policy priority' (Le Bihan & Sopadzhiyan, 2019).

Before the COVID-19 crisis, France featured 7,547 residential homes (EHPADs), offering 622,000 places, with 606,400 occupied (Miron de l'Espinay & Ricroch, 2021). These institutions cared for 10 per cent of older people aged 75 and over and one-third of those aged 90 and over. EHPAD accommodation costs range from €51 to €71 per day (Muller, 2017). These institutions take different forms (Le Bihan & Sopadzhiyan, 2019): private for-profit EHPADs (22 per cent of places), private not-for-profit EHPADs (28 per cent of places), and public EHPADs (50 per cent of places). The latter may or may not be hospitals. Despite an increase in staff-to-patient rates from 2011 to 2015 (from 59.7 to 62.8 full-time employment [FTE] for 100 places [Bazin et al, 2018]), the number of professionals remains insufficient to ensure quality care. At the end of 2015, the average age of residents was 85 years and 9 months, and more than half were highly dependent (Muller, 2017).

The cost of residential care homes is a major problem for families. This cost is divided into three components: health care, social care, and housing. One month's accommodation in a residential care home costs an average of €2,450 (Mutualité Française, 2018), with an average of €1,850 remaining to be paid by the user (after allowances and tax relief) (Le Bihan & Sopadzhiyan, 2019). While the French LTC system covers 100 per cent of healthcare costs and about two-thirds of 'dependency' costs, accommodation services are the responsibility of families, except very low-income households, which are eligible for social assistance for accommodation.

The institutions' lack of qualified staff and difficult working conditions at residential care homes have been identified as crucial issues since the mid-2010s. As a result, measures to renovate residential care homes and increase the supervision rate with the recruitment of 80,000 employees were announced back in 2019 (Le Bihan & Sopadzhiyan, 2019).

Top-down crisis management methods and their limits

The organisation of the alert system

A string of catastrophes, including an explosion at the AZF factory in Toulouse in 2001, the outbreak of SARS, the 2003 heat wave, and the risk of an avian influenza pandemic, led the French government to initiate a policy of drawing up emergency intervention plans (Torny, 2012). As a result, the first pandemic plan was elaborated in 2004 (and regularly updated until 2011) on the recommendations of the WHO (1999). However, activated during the 2009 H1N1 flu episode, it was associated with the failed management of this crisis and was therefore not activated during the COVID-19 pandemic. This non-activation, which was analysed as an 'organisational drift' by Bergeron et al (2020), has been the subject of intense controversy and led to the observation that the crisis management preparedness system was unsatisfactory (Deroche et al, 2020).

Nevertheless, specific measures have centred on planning and rationalising risks. As defined by Halpern et al (2019), various regulatory instruments for public action have been mobilised, such as the ORSAN plan (*Organisation de la Réponse du Système de Santé en Situations Sanitaires Exceptionnelles*), which was activated on 13 February 2020. ORSAN only operates in emergencies, intending to ensure optimal regional cooperation between the existing outpatient, hospital, and medico-social services. Managed by the Regional Health Agency (ARS), the ORSAN plan is based on an inventory of hospital resources likely to be mobilised during a health emergency. It defines the conditions of their use and establishes the terms by which personnel can be recalled. It was partially applied during the summer of 2014 to anticipate the entry of the Ebola virus in France and has since been activated three times: in 2014–15, for the seasonal influenza epidemic; in November 2015, following the Paris terrorist attacks; and in July 2016 after the terrorist attack in Nice. On 23 February 2020, Olivier Véran, minister for solidarity and health, announced the implementation of ORSAN – REB (to care for patients in a known or emerging epidemic or biological risk) to contain the progression of the SARS-CoV-2 coronavirus epidemic and facilitate patient treatment.

Since 2014, the ORSAN plan has included 'white plans'. Specific to each healthcare facility, the latter are organisational arrangements devised to manage 'exceptional' emergencies (accidents, climate events, biological incidents, epidemics). When emergencies occur, the impacted organisations are undermined and cannot operate normally.[3] White plans are activated by hospital directors or at the request of the local prefect (representing the ministry of the interior at the local level). The objective is to avoid services becoming overwhelmed by planning 'the fast, rational implementation of necessary means in the case of an influx of victims'. In concrete terms, this measure resulted in the reorganisation of the working conditions of social and health carers (extension of working hours, reassignment of staff to care homes in difficulty, call on the 'health reserve'), the deprogramming of non-urgent activities in hospitals, and the redistribution of beds between territories (*départements*) to increase the number of intensive care beds.[4]

In the medico-social domain, the decree of 7 July 2005 obliges all residential care homes for older people to draw up a crisis management plan called a 'blue plan', which must be part of the healthcare facility's general plan. The blue plan is produced under the responsibility of the care home's director, taking a cross-cutting approach (involving the coordinating physician, coordinating nurse, care staff, and non-care staff). It must enable the facility concerned to take an operational quality approach by producing an exhaustive overview of its regular operating capacities and evaluating its responsiveness to crises of all kinds (fire or floods, toxic clouds, food shortages, staff absenteeism). It is triggered by any event threatening public health, such as an unusual pathology with epidemic potential. In such a case, the prefect can activate an emergency plan. The regional health agency (ARS) must alert the healthcare facilities concerned, whose directors then activate their blue plan. In the case of an epidemic threat, it aims to anticipate the risks of propagation, improve reactivity in the case of contamination of a resident or employee, manage alerts by mobilising all of the means available, and protect vulnerable residents and staff. The blue plan is revised annually to reflect experience and feedback from residential care homes. Following the proliferation of the coronavirus, blue plans were activated in France on 6 March 2020. As a result, many residential care homes were able to react more quickly (in particular through individual and collective preventive measures, such as raising awareness of hand washing and social distancing, possible division of the care home premises, limitation/suspension of visits, interruption of collective activities, stock management, monitoring of the implementation of anticipated measures, and an increase in staffing levels). Following these initial measures, a multidisciplinary scientific council,[5] chaired by Jean-François Delfraissy, professor of clinical immunology and, in addition, president of the *Comité Consultatif National d'Éthique* (CCNE), was also set up on 10 March to explain the government's decisions and legitimise its action (Starck, 2020).

Fragile management capacity

The crisis highlighted several structural weaknesses affecting the medico-social sector. First, the crisis revealed shortages of human resources and a very uneven distribution of medical resources, as illustrated by the very heterogeneous presence of 'hygiene nurses' or 'coordinating doctors',[6] whose presence may have been decisive in limiting the spread of the virus in some institutions. The lack of protective equipment and insufficient mastery of specific hygiene issues in a crisis also had consequences for human resources: several thousand health staff were contaminated by the virus in their workplace (Olivier et al, 2020) and were placed on sick leave, while others exercised their right to withdraw from work for fear of the virus. In addition, some institutions faced unprecedented situations (absenteeism, burn-out) and major ethical dilemmas (Clause-Verdreau and Weil-Dubuc, 2022). Thus, the organisation of work teams and the sharing of responsibilities were disrupted, and professional practices were redefined in terms of the pace of work and the new procedures to be applied: sorting bedding, disinfecting premises, serving meals, establishing dressing and undressing codes for carers.

This new work organisation intensified exhaustion among the teams. In particular, it required significant human resource management to compensate for absences, raise awareness and inform carers about the new protocols, and boost the morale of professionals on the job. These delicate situations were particularly difficult to manage in isolated institutions that were not well integrated into a wider network of residential care homes.

The second significant difficulty concerned managing stocks of personal protective equipment (surgical masks, gowns, gloves, hydroalcoholic gel, tests), which harmed care homes: the disappearance of suppliers, sharp price increases, equipment requisitioned by the state, and excessively long delivery times. Although stocks were variable from one residential care home to the next, significant problems made it difficult to manage reserves and get hold of the equipment needed. During the first few weeks, professionals had to show remarkable ingenuity (including calling on local solidarity) to obtain the essential equipment necessary for their daily work. They also improvised makeshift solutions to protect themselves from the risk of the epidemic: making their own cloth masks and protecting themselves with bin bags. The delayed management of supplies or stocks also created uncertainty in the work of professionals due to changing instructions on the use of protective equipment.

Finally, professionals in residential care homes had to follow the recommendations of their supervisory institutions or federations, but without a clear regulatory framework or the means to do so. The information from the government, care home headquarters, the *département* council, and other organisations (national public health council) was abundant and sometimes contradictory. This tangled web of instructions, characteristic of crises where the emergency bypasses traditional channels, added confusion to the existing complexity and revealed an evident lack of coordination. Even when instructions were the same, this mass of information needed to be sorted, priority-ranked, and then assimilated to apply the protocols correctly. That is one of the significant difficulties of a health crisis: the evolving knowledge of COVID-19 and the epidemic situation led to the continuous updating of directives applied to residential care homes. Added to this came the impression of a constant lag between the arrival of official recommendations and the reality of situations experienced on the field.

During the first wave of the virus (February to July 2020), these shortages and gaps in the system significantly impacted the spread of the virus and the exhaustion of care teams, the unease of residents, and the distress of families. It should be noted that these initial malfunctions were significantly mitigated during subsequent waves of the virus (August 2020–April 2021) as care protocols became more operational, protective equipment more available, and testing more accessible. Vaccination uptake during this period was also rapid and significant, particularly for nursing home residents.[7]

Centralised management called into question

Implementing these numerous measures required a division of roles between the different institutional actors concerned. The French centralised administrative system meant that the organisation went from the central ministry for health to the regional level, with a central role for ARSs (in charge of implementing the national health policy) in piloting crisis management in each region (Ramel & Autès-Tréand, 2021). Thus, as established in the circular of 2 January 2012, the ministry's *health crisis centre* is run by the general directorate for health (DGS), with the general directorate for social affairs and inclusion (DGSC) responsible for overseeing the social care sector.

During the health crisis throughout France, each ARS had the mission of setting up a special unit for older people the ARS regional headquarters and at the level of the ARS departmental delegations. Numerous national recommendations were transmitted daily (in the form of a 'MINSANTE' document) to the ARSs, who were then entrusted with relaying the information efficiently and pertinently to those concerned on the field. Federations of residential care homes were mobilised from the very start of the health crisis in close association with the Ministry for Health and contributed to decisions made by the government. The federations of institutions also played an important role since they actively contributed to the reflections and decisions taken by the government and transmitted the information to residential care homes.

In addition to this central role of disseminating information locally and coordinating the action deployed, each regional health agency also had the task of gathering information from care homes daily (through questionnaires to identify the number of people infected, the number of deaths, and any equipment and staff accommodation requirements) and accompanying directors in making choices to apply health protocols.

Crucial inter-sectoral cooperation

At the territorial level, the objective of the ARSs was to develop care channels between care homes, general practitioners, and hospitals to create 'on-call healthcare for older people' to respond to requests from care homes. Indeed, the insufficient medicalisation of residential care homes was very apparent during the health crisis and required significant external support (Saison, 2021). As a result, numerous organisational innovations associating different actors emerged, overcoming the traditional divisions between health care and social care sectors, tackling different local situations, characterised by the determining role of geriatric networks, the intervention of *mobile geriatric teams* from hospitals at residential care homes to provide support for complex cases when hospitals were saturated, and the creation of geriatric hotlines. These organisational adaptations included more flexible conditions for implementing home hospitalisation (no medical prescription needed). This entailed increasing the number of home hospitalisation services within residential care homes. During the pandemic, the conditions for implementing the home hospitalisation (HAD) system in residential care homes were relaxed (decree of 1 April 2020), which contributed to a considerable increase in the number of admissions in 2020 (+69 per cent in 2020). Feedback on the mobilisation of HAD during the health crisis linked to COVID-19 highlighted the undeniable role of HAD in supporting residential care homes.[8] This significant evolution appears to have been one of the major responses to the problem of insufficient medicalisation in residential care homes in France.

Health and social care professionals in residential care homes were in high demand, with 'coordinating doctors' playing a significant role. The order of 25 March 2020 thus underlined their role in providing treatment for COVID cases. They were also the contact people for doctors from the Health Surveillance and Security unit at the ARS to provide updates on the situation. Although they could not visit their patients, general practitioners were present through telemedicine, which expanded considerably during the epidemic (care homes equipped with digital tablets). The network of support centres played another key role *in preventing healthcare-related infections* (Cpias): hosted in university hospitals (*Centre Hospitalier Universitaire* – CHU), which provided expertise and support to healthcare professionals and medico-social workers.

Assessment of these measures

The highly centralised state management of the crisis initially led to top-down governance, characterised by its rigidity and low capacity to take local specificities into account. While this top-down approach fostered the standardisation of measures implemented at the regional level, it did not facilitate feedback from local territories. This balance between the national and local levels was particularly crucial in the early stages of the crisis, 'where everything depends on the capacity of health systems to detect weak signals and on the capacity of political systems to move from alert to mobilisation' (Bauquet, 2020). However, reflecting the traditional conception of centralised power in the French administration, this approach showed its limits. It could be described as 'disorganised management' (Gay & Steffen, 2020), leading to an 'organisational crisis' (Bergeron et al, 2020).[9]

Beyond the centralised management, this organisational disruption also led to confusion about the role and scope of action of the different institutional actors, resulting in coordination problems between the national and local levels and within the local territories. It was, for instance, difficult to identify the respective roles of the ARS and that of the prefectures (regional administration of the ministry of the interior) or, at the level of the *départements*, the respective roles between the territorial delegations of the ARS, and the local councils. The lack of coordination between these institutional partners and different levels of public action shed light on 'the incoherence of the territorial organisation of health in France' (Giraud & Tietze, 2022).

Finally, the crisis also revealed the hospital-centric nature of the French healthcare system (Pierru, 2020b), with a large place given to the hospital sector in allocating resources and decisions. For example, unlike the hospital sector, the medico-social sector did not have an appropriate monitoring and alert system. For several weeks, monitoring the epidemic in residential care homes was very unsatisfactory, obliging the ARS teams to carry out a great deal of work to collect reliable information on contaminations and deaths in residential care homes.[10] This lack of a monitoring tool was the first source of weakness in understanding the consequences of the crisis in the medico-social sector and the inadequate public response. More broadly, the crisis highlighted how this sector remained on the fringes of national crisis management through the lack of relations between ARSs and the residential care homes and the public distribution of personal protective equipment.

This situation led the directors of residential care homes to play a significant role in managing the pandemic. Despite the crisis's highly centralised, top-down governance (from the ministry of health to the territories), directors needed to apply more than just apply government decisions in practice. They anticipated them and adjusted them according to the specific situation at their residential care home (work organisation, health status of residents). They took advantage of the margin for manoeuvre left to directors, which allowed them to be flexible. Nevertheless, this position gave them a strong sense of personal involvement (engaging their legal responsibility), which sometimes entailed high psychological pressure to make 'the right decisions at the right moment' in an uncertain context.

The health crisis as a window of opportunity for renewed management of the residential care home sector in France?

The health and regulatory situation evolved significantly during the following phases of the epidemic, partly thanks to recognising the potential of innovations and partly due to the solidarity of local actors. Based on the experience of the first wave, management of the crisis became more relaxed and more adapted to the specific situations experienced at individual care homes. Care protocols were operational, and personal protective equipment and tests were available. The measures and protocols that had been hurriedly put in place during the first wave were now fully functional (presence of doctors in care homes, organisation of hospitalisation in the home to avoid overcrowding hospitals). Moreover, they had been adjusted (the presence of families in care homes is now possible, on certain conditions). In addition, while preserving national standardisation of regulations, the responsibility to decide on which measures to apply locally, following concertation with the various institutional partners, was explicitly left to residential care home managers. Although some managers had already acted freely during the first wave, this role was now officially recognised in the organisation of health crisis management. As a result, visits from friends and family, which had been prohibited during the first wave of the epidemic, were decided on within each care home by the managers since it had become evident that isolating people from their families had negative impacts, known as 'give-up-itis'. Different solutions were thus proposed, such as creating specific visiting times, organising visits outside, and end-of-life support from loved ones, depending on the care home, to avoid isolation for all residents, whether ill or not. Similarly, the everyday life of residents was reconsidered within each residential care home to reconcile the objectives of protecting people not infected by COVID-19 with a social and community life, which is indispensable to providing quality support and ensuring well-being. The policy of confining residents to their rooms imposed in the spring of 2020 was also called into question, as was the suppression of activities, events, and common meals at residential care homes.

More generally, local actors were put at the heart of the crisis management setup and could decide on a specific organisation depending on their area's situation. ARSs could no longer only apply national recommendations but could make local recommendations depending on the *département*. For example, the Occitanie ARS in southwest France suggested ranking the 13 *départements* in the region into three zones (green, orange, and red) corresponding to the intensity of the pandemic.

The vaccination programme, which kicked off in late 2020 in residential care homes, marked the start of another phase of the pandemic in France from January 2021 (Cour des comptes, 2022). According to data from Santé public France, at the start of February, 57 per cent of care home residents had received the first dose of the vaccine, and 72 per cent in early March. In June 2021, 80 per cent of residents had received two doses of the vaccine. This inoculation campaign enabled residential care homes to escape most of the third and fourth phases of the pandemic.

In addition to this experience of crisis management, which had immediate consequences on how public authorities managed the crisis in France after the first wave of the pandemic, comes the question of how this crisis impacted the more general organisation of the sector involving care for older people in institutions. Although the high death rate due to the epidemic in residential care homes can partly be put down to the complexity of comorbidities affecting many older people, another factor is the more structural difficulties endured by the sector, brought to light by the health crisis but previously identified, such as in the Libault report (Le Bihan & Sopadzhiyan, 2019) published just before the pandemic.

The question of staffing in residential care homes is a crucial factor in the reorganisation of the residential healthcare sector. The lack of personnel qualified to care for increasingly elderly and vulnerable residents is notable. As identified in the report by the Cour des Comptes (2022), of the 377,000 FTEs working in residential care homes, doctors make up less than 1 per cent, nurses 11 per cent, and nursing assistants 33 per cent. In addition, high levels of absenteeism and turnover lead to particularly unstable teams. As a result, the staff confronted with the health crisis in 2020 was already fragile. Furthermore, some premises' unsuitability and poor condition are another dimension of the structural difficulties facing the residential care home sector (Cour des comptes, 2022). Lastly, the connection between interventions from professionals and families within care homes has also been called into question.

Managing the COVID-19 crisis generated new responses in terms of both finances and organisation. Public authorities made a considerable financial effort involving additional funding granted at the start of the first wave of the pandemic and as part of the 'Ségur de la santé' health plan signed in July 2020 involving a salary increase for all staff (carers and non-carers) in hospitals, public care homes, private, not-for-profit care homes (+€183 net per month) and private for-profit care homes (+€160 net per month). In addition to these salary increases, financial packages were set up to renovate residential care homes and develop digital capacities within care homes and medico-social services. These investments total €2.1 billion from 2021 to 2025 (Cour des comptes, 2022).

Although these long-term changes have been decided on, they are not accompanied by the necessary wide scale structural reforms. The reform of working conditions for staff in residential care homes – training, career development, prevention of occupational accidents – is still awaited, as are solutions to avoid isolation situations in some care homes, which can lead to great vulnerability, as shown by the crisis. According to the different reports and research studies produced on the need to renovate the residential care sector, the responses made to date are insufficient (Cour des comptes, 2022), and the very model of care in residential homes in France has been called into question (Gonthier et al, 2022). The management of the first wave of the epidemic highlighted the key role played by families in providing support for residents and the need to reconsider their presence within residential care homes.

The promise and announcement of a major sector reform, known as the 'old age and autonomy Act' (*loi grand âge et autonomie*), which has been repeatedly postponed for several years, may provide solutions to these particular points.

Notes

1 In France, residential care homes generally concern three types of establishment: *établissements d'hébergement pour personnes âgées dépendantes* – EHPADs, which include medical care, unlike the two other types: *logements-foyers* renamed *résidences autonomie* and *maisons de retraite*. In this paper we focus on EHPADs, which host 80 per cent of elderly residents.

2 EHPADs (with medical care), *logements-foyers* and *maisons de retraite* (without medical care).

3 And all the more so since the reorganisation of the hospital supply since the end of the 1970s has reduced accommodation capacity (Juven et al, 2019), thus contributing to the risk of hospitals being saturated following exceptional events.

4 The number of critical care beds (intensive care, intensive care and continuous monitoring), which were in great demand during the COVID-19 epidemic, increased by 3.6 per cent from the end of 2019 to the end of 2020. In particular, resuscitation capacity increased by 14.5 per cent (Brunel & Eideliman, 2022).

5 In addition to a chairperson, this council included three infectious disease specialists, a virologist, a general practitioner, a resuscitator, a modeller, a sociologist, and an anthropologist. In 2020, the council issued 22 opinions and notes, totalling 375 pages.

6 At the end of 2015, 32 per cent of residential homes declared the absence of a coordinating doctor (Grangier, 2018).

7 For example, while 57 per cent of residential care home residents had received a first dose of the vaccine in early February 2021, 72 per cent had been vaccinated in early March and, by 16 June, 80 per cent had received two doses. However, the vaccination process was slower among care professionals, since by the end of June 2021, only 50 per cent had been vaccinated (Cour des Comptes 2022).

8 Measure 28 of the 'Ségur de la santé' reinforces this partnership, encouraging the provision of integrated town-hospital-medical-social care for the elderly and supporting increased cooperation between HADs and EHPADs (Ministry of Health and Solidarity, 2021).

9 Thus, and in line with a criticism made previously (Pierru, 2020a), central authorities and ARSs were both openly blamed for their abstract and impersonal management, far removed from the needs of professionals and the expectations of individuals. For this reason, some elected representatives (Deroche et al, 2020) called to reopen the debate on 'decentralisation of the health system' in view of the adoption of the 'decentralisation, differentiation and devolvement' Act (No. 2022-217 of 21 February 2022 on differentiation, decentralisation, devolvement, and various measures to simplify local public action).

10 At the request of the DGS, Santé Publique France developed the first national surveillance system of COVID-19 situations in EHPADs. Called Voozanoo, this system was not operational until the end of March 2020, by which time the number of deaths was already in the thousands. It was also criticised for being inaccurate and unsuitable.

References

Bauquet, N. (2020) *L'Action Publique Face à la Crise du COVID-19*, Institut Montaigne, Paris.

Bazin, M. and Muller, M. (2018) Les difficultés de recrutement en EHPAD, *Etudes et Résultats*, 1067, DREES.

Boisguérin, B., Delaporte, A., and Vacher, T. (2021) Entre fin 2019 et fin 2020, la capacité d'accueil hospitalière a progressé de 3,6 % en soins critiques et de 10,8 % en hospitalisation à domicile, *Etudes et Résultats*, 1008, DREES.

Bontemps, A. (2020) Accompagner la structuration des soins primaires après la COVID-19: un nécessaire renversement du fonctionnement des institutions publiques de la santé, *Regards*, 57, 225–41.

Brunel, M. and Carrère, A. (2017) Les personnes âgées dépendantes vivant à domicile en 2015. Premiers résultats de l'enquête CARE 'ménages, *Etudes et Résultats*, 1029, DREES.

Brunel, M., and Eideliman, J. (2022) La sociabilité et l'isolement social des seniors, *Les Dossiers de la DREES*, n°98, Drees, juillet, Available from : https://drees.solidarites-sante.gouv.fr/publications/les-dossiers-de-la-drees/la-sociabilite-et-lisolement-social-des-seniors

Brunel, M, Latournelle, J., and Zakri, M. (2019) Un senior à domicile sur cinq aidé régulièrement pour les tâches du quotidien, *Etudes et Résultats*, 1103, DREES.

Clause-Verdreau, A. C., and Weil-Dubuc, P. L. (2022) Vécus et analyses de professionnels du soin et de l'accompagnement. Une enquête sur la première vague de la Covid-19, Espace Éthique d'Ille-de-France, Paris, Available from: https://www.espace-ethique.org/ressources/etuderapport/vecus-et-analyses-de-professionnels-du-soin-et-de-laccompagnement

Cour des Comptes (2022) *Les Personnes Âgées Hébergées dans les EHPAD*, Rapport public annuel, Cour des Comptes, Paris.

Deroche, C., Jomier, B., and Vermeillet, S. (2020) *Rapport du Sénat, Fait au Nom de la Commission d'Enquête pour l'Évaluation des Politiques Publiques Face aux Grandes Pandémies à la Lumière de la Crise Sanitaire de la COVID-19 et de sa Gestion*, 199, December, Sénat, Paris.

Ferras, B. (2020) Cinquième 'risque', cinquième 'branche'? Vers une politique rénovée de prise en charge de la perte d'autonomie des personnes âgées?, Regards, No. 57,195-211, Available from: https://shs.cairn.info/revue-regards-2020-1-page-195?lang=fr

Gay, R. and Steffen, M. (2020) Une gestion étatique centralisée et désordonnée, *Chronique Internationale de l'IRES*, 171: 122–38.

Giraud, O. and Tietze, N. (2022) L'organisation de l'action publique face au défi de la COVID-19 en France: Une gouvernance centralisée, politisée et parallèle, in L. Cappelletti (ed) *Crise de la Connaissance et Connaissance de la Crise: Les Points de Vue du Conservatoire National des Arts et Métiers*, Caen: EMS Editions, pp 345–63.

Gonthier, R., Adolphe, M., Michel J.P., Bringer, J., Dubois, B., Lecomte, D., Milliez, J., and Vellas, B. (2022) Après la crise COVID, quelles solutions pour l'EHPAD de demain? Au nom de la commission XIII (autonomie-dépendance-vieillissement) de l'Académie nationale de médecine, *Académie Nationale de Médecine*, Paris.

Grangier, J. (2018) Le vieillissement de la population entraîne une hausse des dépenses de santé liées aux affections de longue durée, DREES Études et Résultats 1077, Available from: https://drees.solidarites-sante.gouv.fr/publications/etudes-et-resultats/le-vieillissement-de-la-population-entraine-une-hausse-des

Halpern, C., Lascoumes, P., and Le Galès, P. (2019) Instrument, in L. Boussaguet (ed) *Dictionnaire des Politiques Publiques* (5th edn), Paris: Presses de Sciences Po, pp 321–30.

Juven, P.A., Pierru, F., and Vincent, F. (2019) *La Casse du Siècle. A Propos des Réformes de l'Hôpital Public*, Raison d'Agir, Paris.

Le Bihan, B., and Martin, C. (2010) Reforming long-term care policy in France: private–public complementarities, *Social Policy and Administration*, 44(4), 392–410, Available from: https://www.issa.int/sites/default/files/external-references/files/reforming_long_term_care_policy_in_france-56304.pdf

Le Bihan, B., and Sopadzhiyan, A. (2019) Future trends in French long-term care policy: The Libault Report. ESPN Flash Report 2019/25, European Social Policy Network (ESPN), Brussels: European Commission, Available from: https://ehesp.hal.science/hal-02180946v1

Ministry of Health and Solidarity (2021) *HAD, Feuille de Route 2021–2026*, December, Paris, Available from: https://sante.gouv.fr/soins-et-maladies/prises-en-charge-specialisees/had-10951/article/la-feuille-de-route-2021-2026

Miron de l'Espinay, A. and Pinel, L. (2021) La vaccination contre la COVID-19 en Ehpad et son effet sur la contamination des residents, *Les Dossiers de la DREES*, 86.

Miron de l'Espinay, A. and Richroch, L. (2021) En 2020, trois Ehpad sur quatre ont eu au moins un resident infecté par la COVID-19, *Etudes et Résultats*, 1196, DREES.

Muller, M. (2017) 728000 résidents en établissements d'hébergement pour personnes âgées en 2015. Premiers résultats de l'enquête EHPA 2015, Etudes et Résultats, n°1015 DREES, Available from : https://drees.solidarites-sante. gouv.fr/IMG/pdf/er1015.pdf

Olivier, C., Brunet, J. B., Bouvet, E., Abiteboul, D., Lolom, I., Pellissier, G., et al (2020) Contexte de contamination des soignants par le SARS-CoV-2 pendant la première vague de l'épidémie en France, *Bulletin Epidémiologique Hebdomadaire*, 35: 690–5.

Pierru, F. (2020a) Introduction: L'administration hospitalière, entre pandémie virale et épidémie de réformes, *Revue Française d'Administration Publique*, 174, 301–15.

Pierru, F. (2020b) Agences régionales de santé: mission impossible, *Revue Française d'Administration Publique*, 174, 385–403.

Pittet, D., Boone, L., Raoul Briet, A. M., and Parneix, P. (2021) *Rapport d'étape de la Mission Indépendante Nationale sur l'évaluation de la Gestion de la Crise COVID-19 et sur l'anticipation des Risques Pandémiques*, 13 October, Présidence de la République, Paris, Available from : https://www.vie-publique.fr/rapport/279851-gestion-crise-covid-et-anticipation-de-risques-pandemiques-rapport-final

Plateforme de Recherche sur la Fin de Vie (2021) *COVIDEHPAD, Étude des Questions Relatives aux Confinement, aux Fins de Vie et à la Mort dans les EHPAD Pendant la Première Vague de l'Épidémie de COVID-19 en France*, CNSA, Available from: https://www.plateforme-recherche-findevie.fr/sites/default/files/inline-content/PNRFV/COVIDEHPAD/rapport-covidehpad-final.pdf

Ramel, V. and Autès-Tréand, E. (2021) Gérer la crise de la première vague de COVID-19: retour d'expérience d'une agence régionale de santé, *Santé Publique*, 33: 1011–21.

Saison, J. (2021) L'organisation territoriale des soins de premier recours à l'épreuve de la COVID-19: les enseignements d'une crise sanitaire, *Droit et Ville*, 91, 11–23.

Starck, L. (2020) Science, expertises et décisions politiques, *Civitas Europa*, 45, 9–41.

Torny, D. (2012) De la gestion des risques à la production de la sécurité: l'exemple de la préparation à la pandémie grippale, *Réseaux*, 171, 45–66.

World Health Organisation (WHO) (1999) *Influenza Pandemic Preparedness Plan: The Role of WHO and Guidelines for National and Regional Planning*, Geneva: WHO.

7

Large capacities in health care: insufficient protection of vulnerable groups in Germany

Caspar Lückenbach, Eduard Klukas, Phillip Florian Schmidt, and Thomas Gerlinger

Introduction

Despite the news and experiences from Italy and Austria, the COVID-19 pandemic surprised Germany. Especially during the first wave, which according to the Robert Koch Institute (RKI), lasted from January to mid-June 2020, the healthcare system faced immense challenges. The first confirmed infection with COVID-19 occurred on 28 January 2020, the first significant outbreak about 1 month after a carnival celebration. By mid-March the virus had spread to all 16 of Germany's federal states (*Länder*). By the end of the first wave of the pandemic in mid-June 2020, 190,816 cases of COVID-19 had been reported, of which 25,697 (13.5 per cent) occurred in institutions, as defined in section 33 of the Infection Protection Act (*Infektionsschutzgesetz* – IfSG). These include residential homes, shelters for the homeless, shared accommodation for asylum seekers, and youth detention centres.

As a result of many cases, there were shortages of protective masks and other personal protective equipment (PPE), as well as problems in adequately separating infected or ill persons and maintaining the ongoing provision of healthcare services. Policymakers responded with a wide variety of short-term measures to alleviate immediate pressures on the healthcare system, gain control of the epidemic and ensure adequate treatment. Actions taken at the federal level to relieve the stress on the outpatient sector, which was the first point of contact for suspected COVID-19 infections (KBV, 2020a), included the possibility of taking sick leave without seeing a GP in person and the funding of unlimited video consultation hours. Further measures taken at regional level included, among others, mobile services for home visits, home visits by specialist COVID-19 care physicians, home visit duty schedules on demand, two daily calls to patients, video and telephone consultation hours, and a digital network with the health authorities. Nonetheless, practices suffered from economic losses and a great PPE shortage, leading to temporary closures. However, even when infections reached their peak in April 2020, about 85 per cent of COVID-19 patients were being treated in an outpatient setting, with only 11 per cent being treated in hospital (KBV, 2020b). Outpatient care was still functioning and without that many more patients would have had to be admitted to the hospital (KBV, 2020c).

The number of intensive care beds and ventilators in the inpatient sector increased due to the pandemic. Moreover, it was expected to continue to rise, according to a hospital emergency plan drawn up by the federal government and the *Länder* (Deutsches Ärzteblatt, 2020a). As a result, all scheduled admissions and operations had to be postponed as far as medically justifiable to expand ventilation and intensive care capacities (Bundesregierung, 2020a). Nonetheless, the pandemic sometimes led to isolation of patients and staff and even to the closure of wards and additional bureaucracy due to the high time and personnel requirements. Other problems included a lack of consideration of existing hospital differences, higher costs for longer treatments, coordination problems between the *Länder*, and personnel problems (Blum et al, 2020). Emergency services were also severely affected, with forecasts indicating that the capacity limits had been reached or even exceeded due, among other things, to the rising number of emergency patients and staff sickness (BAND, 2020).

Financial support packages were also put together to partially compensate for financial shortfalls and additional costs, especially in hospitals, and in the outpatient sector. For example, the number of consultations with specialists fell by up to 80 per cent (Löwenstein & Heinzle, 2020), and hospitals came under severe pressure due to the loss of revenue and rising costs (Deutsches Ärzteblatt, 2020b) and increasing levels of staff sickness (Berndt & Kunkel, 2020). Furthermore, the federal government purchased PPE and tried to organise its distribution. The same applied to rapid tests and vaccines as the pandemic progressed.

In all areas of the health care system, existing problems and shortcomings were exposed by the pandemic. It was especially so in primary care and the nursing home sector, where the consequences of many years of inadequate funding became obvious. According to an online survey conducted during the initial phase of the pandemic, 60 per cent of all deceased persons who had been in need of care came from residential or nursing homes. However, their share of the total number of people infected was only 8.5 per cent. Half of all deaths occurred in residential homes, constituting the most critical location for COVID-19 deaths (Götz, 2020).

Furthermore, claims data from the AOK nursing and health insurance funds show that, from March to May 2020, every fifth COVID-19 hospitalisation and nearly every third COVID-19 related death in a hospital concerned a nursing home resident (Kohl et al, 2021). Early on, a ban on visiting residential homes was introduced to protect residents/patients, and staff. As a result, Long Term Care (LTC) staff – in both residential homes and hospitals – had to cope with a severe lack of PPE (Langendorf, 2020), as well as other protective materials (Rattenhuber, 2020). The consequences ranged from staff absences to the isolation of entire residential homes. The loss of staff due to COVID-19 infections further exacerbated the existing shortage of personnel (Wolf-Ostermann & Rothgang, 2020: p 22), worsened working conditions (Drupp et al, 2021), and led to high overall psychological stress among them (Hower et al, 2020). Nursing home residents suffered from massive effects on social participation and, thus, well-being due to the protective measures (DGP, 2020; Kessler et al, 2020; Räker et al, 2021). Due to the improved availability of FFP2 masks and rapid tests later in 2020, obligatory testing for staff and visitors, and with the start of the vaccination programme in early 2021, working and living in nursing homes has returned to some normality. Nonetheless, the impact of COVID-19 on nursing homes is still visible daily in 2022.

In Germany, responsibility for financing and regulating the health care system, as well as the specific organisation of care in the various sectors, is distributed among numerous different actors at the federal level, in the *Länder*, and the municipalities, leading to numerous intersectoral problems. The public health service (*Öffentlicher Gesundheitsdienst* – ÖGD) showed considerable technical and staffing shortcomings in its ability to combat the pandemic. In addition, the federal structure and the decentralised responsibilities led to problems in coordinating and enforcing measures to combat the pandemic. It was reflected in a temporary overburdening of municipal administrative structures, numerous negotiations between the federal and *Länder* governments, and sometimes considerable differences in handling the pandemic between regions. Nevertheless, the measures taken during the first months can be considered relatively successful, as the numbers of infections and COVID-19 related deaths were kept reasonably low compared to other developed countries.

Politically, there was a broad consensus among the parties in the German Parliament (*Bundestag*) during the first wave of the pandemic, with only small minorities warning of the economic damage or even rejecting the measures. Most of the population also supported the measures taken by the federal government. However, there was and still is a small but very high-profile minority of people who denied the existence of the coronavirus and who vehemently reject corresponding protective measures. Even if this group of people decreased from 15 per cent of the population in 2020 to nine per cent in 2021 (Spöri & Eichhorn, 2021), they helped to ensure that the target vaccination rates of over 80 per cent were not quickly achieved. Apart from the extreme rejection of the measures taken, discussions about the relationship between restrictions to protect vulnerable groups and individual liberties increased as the pandemic progressed. The compulsory vaccination of care personnel introduced in December 2021, and the regulations enforced between October 2022, and April 2023, were no longer supported by a broad consensus.

The following sections will describe the organisation and regulation of LCT in Germany (section 2), analyse the impact of the first wave of the pandemic on the residential care sector (section 3), and finally offer some conclusions on how the pandemic has already shaped and will potentially continue to shape the evolution of LTC in Germany.

The role of the residential care sector for the elderly in long-term care (LTC)

Long-term care in Germany is strongly structured by laws and regulations passed by federal government and the *Länder*. It is highly institutionalised due to the existence of long-term care insurance. Even though care services in the outpatient sector are provided to a considerable extent by relatives and family members, LTC is characterised by a high degree of professionalisation and a comprehensive range of services. It holds especially true for the inpatient sector, where private or non-profit providers predominantly run residential homes. LTC was particularly affected by the pandemic, as recipients of LTC are significantly more vulnerable to COVID-19. Residents of nursing homes and the care workers employed there were identified as particularly vulnerable groups quite early on.

The trajectory of LTC to the current model

LTC was introduced in 1995 and is organised as a mandatory insurance system (Gerlinger & Rosenbrock, 2023). Benefits are funded by the contributions-based long-term care insurance scheme (LTCI). LTCI covers only parts of LTC costs (Gerlinger & Rosenbrock, 2023). Until 2017, the characteristics of LTCI were mainly left unchanged. From 1995 to 2008, LTCI benefits were not increased despite the rising costs of LTC goods and services, resulting in a significant decline in purchasing power. Outpatient benefits in kind and cash have since been increased in stages starting in 2008 and dynamically adjusted to price trends every 3 years, starting from 2015. However, this has only partly compensated for the initial decline. Recent reforms adopted since 2017 – especially the payment of a monthly contribution to relieving the burden on caring relatives – were intended to create financial incentives for providing informal care at home by family members or volunteers to avoid some of the cost of more expensive residential care. In 2017, the regulations governing entitlement to LTCI benefits were fundamentally reformed. Before this, there were three levels of care based on the severity of only the physical health condition and the expected care time required to help with daily living activities. Now, patients are allocated to one of five care grades depending on their physical, mental, and psychological disabilities and placed into one of six categories according to the extent to which their independence is restricted. The assessment is carried out by the independent Medical Review Board (*Medizinischer Dienst* – MD). The reform has considerably increased the number of benefit recipients, but predominantly in home care settings.

Current arrangements in LTC

The provision of LTC in Germany is based on the insurance principle. LTCI is mandatory via the social long-term care insurance (LTCI) scheme or a private equivalent. In general, all members of the statutory health insurance scheme (SHI) are automatically members of the social LTCI scheme, and all members of a private health insurance scheme (PHI) are members of a private LTCI. At the end of 2021, 73.51 million people (around 89 per cent of the population) were insured under the social LTCI scheme, while at the end of 2020, 9.19 million (around 11 per cent) held a private LTCI policy (BMG, 2022a: p 1). Social LTCI is almost exclusively financed through contributions paid equally by employers and employees. In 2022, the federal government, for the first time, paid an annual tax-financed subsidy of €1 billion to the social LTCI scheme (out of a total annual expenditure of around €54 billion in 2021). In 2023, the contribution rate of gross wages was 3.05 per cent (3.40 per cent for childless people). Children and spouses with an income of less than €520 per month are co-insured at no extra cost.

In contrast to the SHI, the LTCI covers only part of LTC costs, with benefits depending on the care grade and the type of benefit provided. As benefits do not fully cover the costs, recipients must make substantial co-payments. If the individual recipient cannot afford the co-payments, the shortfall must be paid out of social welfare grants provided by the municipalities. The reform passed in 2021 reduced private co-payments, but the reform was widely criticised as insufficient and private co-payments are still very high (Gerlinger, 2022). Regarding benefits, there are no differences between social and private LTCI. People are eligible for long-term care if they require frequent or substantial assistance due to a certain degree of restriction of their independence on a long-term basis because of a physical, mental, or psychological illness or disability, irrespective of their age. The benefits of LTCI do not differ between regions and are not time limited. They are granted on the basis of a care grade and the care arrangements in place (either at home or in a residential home for the elderly). Assistance may be provided for prevention and rehabilitation, for instance measures to overcome, reduce or prevent an increase in the need for long-term care.

These measures are given priority over care. Home care is also given priority over residential care.

In general, claimants can choose between three different arrangements: care allowance, home care (in kind), and residential care:

- Care allowance refers to informal care, that is, care provided at home by close relatives or volunteers, for which the LTCI pays a certain amount of money that is lower than the costs of home care in kind.
- Home care (in kind) means that a professional care provider (for example, a social services agency or home care service) visits the recipient regularly at home. The provider is under contract with the LTCI fund and is paid directly by the LTCI scheme.
- Residential care is provided in a residential home. The LTCI scheme bears the costs of primary care, social support, and treatment according to the individual care level. In addition, recipients pay for food and board.

Additional benefits are provided under LTCI, such as holiday stand-ins, part-time institutional day and night care, short-term care, nursing aids, and nursing care courses for relatives. At the end of 2020, around 4.6 million people required long-term care (BMG, 2022a: pp 1–3). Of these, around 0.76 million people lived in residential homes (BMG, 2022a: pp 1–3). Residential homes constitute the most expensive form of care, accounting for 27.3 per cent (2021) of total expenditure (BMG, 2022b). Residential care is dominated by private providers, both for-profit and non-profit. In December 2019, there were 15,380 residential homes (Statistisches Bundesamt, 2020: p 33), 43 per cent of which were private for-profit establishments, 53 per cent private, not-for-profit establishments and 5 per cent publicly owned and run (Statistisches Bundesamt, 2020, p 33). It is mainly because under the Long-Term Care Insurance Act, non-profit and private providers have priority over public providers when concluding LTC contracts (Social Code Book XI: section 11, para 2)[1]. Around 796,500 (also mostly qualified) persons are employed in residential homes (Social Code Book XI: section 11, para 2). More than two-thirds of the employees (around 85 per cent of women) work part-time (Social Code Book XI: section 11, para 2).

Every LTC facility that meets the legal requirements (especially regarding personnel structure and quality assurance) is generally entitled to conclude a care contract with the LTCI funds and remuneration for their services. The federal legislature draws up the basic regulations on the remuneration of care services. The *Länder* are responsible for the legal supervision of the LTCI funds, which in turn conclude the care contracts with the individual facilities (Gerlinger & Rosenbrock, 2023). In contrast to inpatient and outpatient medical care, the number and location of LTC facilities are not subject to need assessment or planning. The legislators assumed that the law of supply and demand would lead to an adequate supply of care facilities and good access to care. However, particularly in disadvantaged regions, there are complaints about an insufficient number of care facilities. As a result, people needing care cannot always be cared for close to their residence or obtain the type of care they prefer. Despite several reforms, LTC in Germany faces serious problems. Firstly, it suffers from a serious lack of qualified staff due to relatively low wages and poor working conditions (Schmucker, 2020). Secondly, the quality of care needs to be improved, a problem exacerbated by staff shortages. Furthermore, the private co-payments are too high for many recipients of care benefits and their relatives to be paid entirely by themselves, leaving for instance around 30 per cent of nursing home residents dependent on social grants (Rothgang et al, 2020: p 15).

Analysis of the measures adopted to address the impact of the pandemic on the residential care sector for the elderly

Preparedness

The Robert Koch-Institute (RKI) is the central federal institution in Germany for disease detection and health reporting. It draws up nationwide pandemic plans and collects nationwide data on notifiable diseases. In addition to the RKI, the Federal Office for Civil Protection and Disaster Assistance (*Bundesamt für Bevölkerungsschutz und Katastrophenhilfe* – BBK) is responsible for risk prevention in the field of public health. As early as January 2013, a risk analysis paper on civil protection presented to the Bundestag warned of the possibility of a great epidemic with a hypothetical viral pathogen from the Coronaviridae virus family (Deutscher Bundestag, 2013).

The Federal Government initiated the first concrete steps toward developing a National Influenza Pandemic Plan in the early 2000s (RKI, 2017). The RKI was commissioned to develop a National Pandemic Plan based on the recommendations of the WHO. The plan has regularly been revised and updated, for example, to implement the findings from the H1N1 influenza pandemic in 2009. Its main objectives are to reduce pandemic-related morbidity and mortality, to ensure care for ill people, to maintain essential public services, and to provide the public with reliable information during a pandemic.

The *Länder* implements the federal pandemic plan in individual plans, which are based on the federal baselines but take regional specifics (such as population density) into account. The *Länder* play a key role in combating the pandemic due to their prime responsibility in the area of infection control. The public health service of the *Länder* and their local authorities, together with other local administrative bodies, are responsible for the containment of pandemic situations. Furthermore, the *Länder* are a central link in the system of Federal Health Monitoring (*Gesundheitsberichterstattung des Bundes*).

The National Pandemic Plan contains explicit planning aids for inpatient LTC (RKI, 2017: p 55). The recommended measures aim to protect staff and residents and ensure continuing care. In the event of a pandemic, organisations need to establish appropriate spatial separation of sick and non-sick persons. In the event of illness, parenteral nutrition and oxygen administration may be necessary, especially for persons with existing care needs. The RKI requires residential homes to prepare themselves accordingly. Stockpiling of PPE is recommended. LTC staff displaying influenza-associated symptoms should be removed from the workplace. If this leads to staff shortages, consideration should be given to drafting in other workers, such as trainees (RKI, 2017: p 55). Generally, the RKI recommends vaccination of personnel in inter-pandemic and acute pandemic phases, provided that a vaccine is available (RKI, 2017: p 55). Retirement and residential homes should train their staff regularly, especially regarding the procedures and stricter hygiene measures required in a pandemic. The RKI published its recommended hygiene measures during an influenza pandemic (RKI, 2010).

In March 2020, the RKI amended the National Pandemic Plan by adding specific recommendations and measures to cope with the COVID-19 pandemic (RKI 2020). Besides the recommendations on surveillance of the pandemic, most of the recommendations concern infection hygiene. They also refer explicitly to providers of inpatient LTC (RKI, 2020: p 11). Infection-preventing and contact-reducing measures are listed first. In case of an infection, these include using single-bed rooms, reducing community activities, and, if necessary, cohort isolation measures. For the staff, training courses are recommended. In possible danger, a ban on activities under the Infection Protection Act should also be considered (RKI, 2020: p 11). Furthermore, the RKI points out that individual institutions are responsible for maintaining stocks of PPE.

Additionally, there are several recommendations for LTC staff on behavioural measures such as hand hygiene and cough etiquette, as well as specific rules of conduct for intersectoral contact, for example, with members of the emergency services during patient transport. Nursing staff should wear gloves and a face mask during care measures (RKI, 2020: p 11). If possible, the patient should also wear a face mask during transportation. Comprehensive disinfection measures and the safe handling of dishes, laundry, and waste are also detailed.

LTC facilities are legally obliged to document internal procedures for infection hygiene in so-called hygiene plans (*Hygienepläne*) to protect residents and staff (RKI, 2005). Furthermore, both the Infection Protection Act and the Home Act (*Heimgesetz*) require comprehensive measures to ensure infection protection, as does Social Code Book V (*Sozialgesetzbuch V*) as a part of quality assurance (RKI, 2005: p 1063).

The following aspects must be considered in these internal hygiene plans (Bales & Baumann, 2003; RKI, 2005):

- risk analysis of the institution's specific infection hazards,
- comparison of individual risks and corresponding risk-minimising measures,
- determination of the concrete risk-minimising measures,
- methods for the appropriate monitoring of compliance with the risk-minimising measures,
- determination of the intervals at which the institution's internal hygiene plan is reviewed and updated, and
- determination of the documentation method for the hygiene plan and staff training.

The hygiene plan is to be drawn up by an internal team of employees, the so-called Hygiene Committee, and, if necessary, in consultation with the respective local health authority (RKI, 2005: p 1064).

Management capacity

Despite the existence of these pandemic plans, the COVID-19 pandemic caught inpatient LTC 'off guard' (Keller, 2020). Due to the lockdown measures taken, including closures, visiting bans, access restrictions, and the cancellation of social activities, residential homes were forced to compensate for the lost care and service structures. Based on the RKI recommendations, all residential homes took measures to contain the incidence of infection. Thus in almost all homes, measures were taken to reduce contact within the facility (98.7 per cent), a crisis team was set up (96.1 per cent), and absence regulations were implemented for symptomatic nursing home staff (97.0 per cent). In addition, many homes stopped admissions (49.1 per cent) or closed individual areas (30.7 per cent) (Wolf-Ostermann et al, 2022). However, many facilities were not sufficiently stocked with PPE for a pandemic of this size (Wolf-Ostermann et al, 2022). The isolation of infected persons was also often complicated by the spatial conditions. Increased sick leave combined with additional workload due to the pandemic further complicated the working conditions of nursing staff in the first wave (Drupp et al, 2021). This situation led to high psychological stress overall (Hower et al, 2020). Regardless of the health consequences of a COVID-19 infection, residents had massive effects on social participation and, thus, well-being because of the protective measures (DGP, 2020; Kessler et al, 2020; Räker et al, 2021).

Furthermore, there was considerable divergence between facilities handling and applying hygiene plans. Although many facilities were well prepared, quite a few experienced considerable difficulties dealing with the pandemic. Despite the legal obligation to maintain institution-specific hygiene plans, problems arose because the plans either did not exist or were available only in rudimentary form. These differences cannot be explained by types of ownership, funding, or region. Rather, the differences were due to the commitment of individual managers on the ground. Moreover, deficiencies were aggravated by the fact that staff was too seldom trained in these cases. Finally, it should be noted that LTC in Germany is, to a considerable extent, provided by auxiliary staff with little or no training in dealing with infectious diseases.

In addition to these shortcomings in quality, the supply of PPE was also inadequate in quantitative terms. Inpatient LTC facilities were experienced in dealing with minor incidents of infection, which, like norovirus, were often limited to the institutions themselves. A pandemic situation with a veritable external threat of infection was beyond their experience. This circumstance, coupled with the economic pressure to increase efficiency, led to an undersupply of PPE in the long-term care system, quickly becoming a nationwide problem. It was not only the PPE stocks that were quantitatively insufficient, but also the staffing itself. Across Germany there is a shortage of skilled workers in nursing care for the elderly (Bundesagentur für Arbeit, 2020: p 16), which has not yet been effectively defused despite many countermeasures taken in recent years. The pandemic hit an LTC system that was partly under-equipped in terms of structural quality and was not always able to provide the necessary human and material resources to cope with the COVID-19 pandemic.

The lack of equipment, especially the inadequate stockpiling of PPE, is also an epiphenomenon of an overarching restrictive budgetary policy. About 10 years ago, the Federal Republic of Germany and its constituent states committed themselves to reducing budget deficits and extensively limiting the incurring of new debts. Although this 'austerity culture' only indirectly affects long-term nursing care, in conjunction with the increasing importance of economic efficiency criteria it has led to comprehensive cost avoidance strategies, especially for storage costs.

Governance

It should first be noted that the *Länder* are responsible for protecting public health. Although the competence to adopt some legal framework provisions lies with the federal government, these provisions (for example, the Infection Protection Act) require the approval of the *Bundesrat*, the chamber of the *Länder*. It opens up a variety of independent options for the *Länder*. The federal government saw this division of competency as an obstacle to rapid nationwide interventions to fight the pandemic and therefore tried to expand the scope of its competency. Accordingly, at the end of March 2020, the *Bundestag* passed the Act for the Protection of the Population in the Event of an Epidemic Situation of National Significance (*Gesetz zum Schutz der Bevölkerung bei einer epidemischen Lage von nationaler Tragweite*), which amends the Infection Protection Act (BGBl, 2020: I: p 587[2]). It gives the Federal Minister of Health, for a limited period, the authority to take measures to protect the population and to guarantee the provision of health care to the population by statutory order. The prerequisite is that the *Bundestag* should previously have declared an epidemic situation of national importance (IfSG: section 5)[3]. The resulting Federal Minister competency (IfSG: section 5, para 2) covers a wide range of actions, for instance, provisions on cross-border travel, on reporting and examination obligations, on ensuring the supply of medicines. Furthermore, it explicitly includes the right to adapt, restrict or suspend provisions applicable to residential homes (IfSG: section 5, para 2, no 8a–c). To this extent, this law strengthens the federal government's powers vis-a-vis the *Länder*, and the self-administration of the nursing care insurance scheme. Overall, one can speak of a moderate centralisation of competency to contain an 'epidemic emergency'.

Until 2006, the operation of residential homes and the quality of the care services provided were subject to statutory framework regulations enacted by the federal government (Lückenbach et al, 2021). However, they were transferred to the *Länder* in September 2006. The *Länder* are also responsible for monitoring compliance with these regulations. In addition, the legal provisions of the Long-Term Care Insurance Act, which constitute Social Code Book XI, which also gives the *Länder* various options for structuring the system, apply throughout Germany. Monitoring compliance with provisions under the Long-Term Care Insurance Act is the responsibility of the MDK, which is organised at the *Länder* level. Due to the COVID-19 pandemic, measures under the Infection Protection Act have gained considerably in importance. In this respect, the *Länder* have the competence to independently shape the federal legal framework, a competence they have made extensive use of during the COVID-19 crisis. The local health authorities are responsible for monitoring compliance with these regulations. However, the legal bases mentioned, and the resulting powers of control, apply to all residential home operators, irrespective of whether the residential home operators are public, non-profit, or private organisations. To that extent, the COVID-19 crisis has not led to significant shifts in the distribution of responsibilities between the public and private sectors. However, one can speak of an increase in the importance of public regulation since the *Länder*, based on the Infection Protection Act, issued a large number of detailed regulations specific to residential homes, which also apply to private residential homes, which account for the vast majority of residential homes and residential home places. The extent to which this was also accompanied by an increase in the incidence of checks on (private) residential homes by (public) institutions cannot be determined based on the available data.

Furthermore, an amendment to the Occupational Health and Safety Act (*Arbeitsschutzgesetz* – ArbSchG) enabled the individual *Länder* to temporarily increase the maximum daily working hours to up to 12 hours in order to reduce changeovers of personnel and thus the risk of infection. Additionally, quality checks on residential homes were suspended. All physical assessments by the Medical Review Board of the Statutory Health Insurance Funds were suspended and replaced by document- and telephone-based assessments (MDK, 2020).

Other general measures are also largely the responsibility of the individual *Länder*. For example, the Bavarian State Ministry of Health and Nursing established a committee of experts on long-term care, including representatives of the nursing profession, to identify the problems from a nursing perspective and to develop joint solutions (StmGP Bayern, 2020). Individual nursing councils, and their respective *Länder* have also launched a call for nursing professionals to volunteer their services to improve staffing levels in the short term. In addition, the *Länder* concerned have found solutions to enable foreign medical and paramedical personnel to commute from neighbouring countries. Notwithstanding the legal regulations and recommendations by the federal government and the Länder, individual residential homes were required to take their initiatives to deal with the pandemic in the best possible way. For example, residential homes had to provide sufficient room capacities to be able to comply with quarantine regulations in case of infection (Lückenbach et al, 2021). Furthermore, they had to try to make room to store PPE, as many homes did not have enough storage space available (Lückenbach et al, 2021).

From the beginning to mid-May, the visiting bans were relaxed individually under certain conditions set by the respective *Länder* (Bundesregierung, 2020b). The lack of protective equipment and the mandatory preparation and implementation of visiting arrangements were enormous challenges for residential homes. The *Länder* and home nursing bodies drew up measures and recommendations for developing the visiting arrangements. However, the responsibility for implementation lies with the individual residential homes. As a result, even residential homes in the same community used different measures. Thus, the different solutions devised by individual residential homes led to injustice for those needing care. These differences between individual residential homes and between regions were also intensively discussed by the media and the public. Just as the moral and ethical conflicts between protecting people by isolating them and thus restricting their freedom of movement (and that of others), and causing other social and health-related problems.

Since lifting the bans on visits increased the risk of infection, individual *Länder* conducted random tests in residential homes. At the end of March

2020, for example, an initiative launched by members of the Paderborn Practice Network (*Praxisnetz Paderborn* e.V.) identified positive cases through extensive testing (RKI, 2020). The federal government was therefore called upon to increase testing for the risk groups and reacted shortly afterwards with a new test regulation. The new directive aimed to provide comprehensive testing for asymptomatic individuals for whom COVID-19 infection would be a great risk because of the potential danger to themselves or others (BMG, 2020). Thus with backdated effect from May 2020, residential homes and nursing services were refunded for testing individuals even in the absence of symptoms. Before this measure was adopted testing costs were covered by the statutory health insurance scheme only when symptoms occurred.

Intersectoral coordination

Residential homes were subjected to contact restrictions by legislation at Land level. The residential homes themselves were responsible for applying these provisions with the effects described previously. Although residential homes may employ doctors, medical care is mostly not provided by employed doctors in the residential homes but rather by doctors in private practice or medical care centres (*Medizinische Versorgungszentren* – MVZ). Bans or restrictions on visits imposed following infection surges also applied to external service providers to residential homes, including doctors. In a nationwide online survey of residential homes, only 5.7 per cent of the responding institutions stated that they granted unrestricted access to external service providers.

In comparison 27.7 per cent did not allow access, and 66.6 per cent only in exceptional cases (Wolf-Ostermann & Rothgang, 2020: p 24). Among the residential homes hit hardest by the pandemic, the proportion of homes that did not grant access rose to 38.5 per cent (Wolf-Ostermann & Rothgang, 2020: p 24). The case of the city, the district, and the Würzburg health authority caused a furore: to limit the number of contacts between doctors and residential home residents; they made provision for one doctor, who had previously treated the majority of patients in a home, to be responsible for the entire home, while at the same time excluding all other doctors from providing care in this home. This limited the individual's right to free choice of doctor on the one hand and the doctor's right to free exercise of his profession on the other and was sharply criticised by the umbrella organisation of doctors working in outpatient care for the statutory health insurance scheme, the National Association of Statutory Health Insurance Accredited Physicians (KBV). Some *Länder* (for example, Lower Saxony) provided residential homes with tablets to enable residents to have tele consultations with doctors. The intersection between residential homes and medical care was barely addressed in the pandemic plans. The online survey just mentioned shows that only a few facilities purchased special software to enable residents to have a video or online consultation (Wolf-Ostermann & Rothgang, 2020: p 28). However, a good three-quarters of all facilities procured additional software to counteract the isolation of home residents and enable contact with relatives or friends (Wolf-Ostermann & Rothgang, 2020: p 28).

Assessment of these measures

The measures taken by the federal government and the other actors at the federal and *Länder* level cannot be described as proactive as looking at the development of the pandemic over time in a European context. Despite the developments in Italy, Spain, and France, the potential extent of the crisis for Germany was initially underestimated. However, when the pandemic became a reality in Germany as well, all relevant actors, under the leadership of the BMG, responded in anticipation and at an early stage by adopting relatively far-reaching and strict measures that enabled Germany to contain the spread of the virus relatively well. The existence of well-equipped intensive care units and good laboratory capacities was undoubtedly helpful. In addition, the ad-hoc measures taken (contact restrictions, procurement of PPE, containment scouts, creation of additional intensive care capacities, and others) can be considered very effective. Furthermore, initial measures have also been initiated to address the structural deficits in the public health service and long-term care revealed by the crisis.

Problems arose with the information flows from federal and *Länder* level to local authorities and residential homes. For example, there were some exceptions to the visit ban, for example, to enable relatives to be with a dying family member. However, these were often not applied due to the lack of information given to individual residential homes (Lückenbach et al, 2021). The fact that individual residential homes were ultimately responsible for applying the regulations often led to cautious behaviour on the part of managers. Preventing infection was the highest priority for many managers, and the resulting negative consequences for residents and relatives were sometimes serious (Interview BMG 2: 28:04).

Several aspects are relevant concerning the role and importance of relevant actors in developing and implementing policies. First of all, the BMG included the LTC insurance funds and LTC associations in the political discussion rounds at the federal level right from the start, for instance, in order to decide on the financing of additional protective measures (protective clothing, masks, gloves, and so on) and contact reduction measures as early as the beginning of March 2020. These were then incorporated into legislation (Hospital Relief Act – *Krankenhausentlastungsgesetz*). The Federal Ministry of Health, in close coordination with the Länder via the Conference of Health

Ministers, can be regarded as a central actor in this regard. There was also broad agreement among the associations of non-statutory social welfare and other providers of retirement and residential homes on the necessity of the measures taken to protect against infection, and corresponding decisions were taken at joint conferences at federal level. However, at the municipal level, where the measures were implemented, information on current regulations and possible exemptions varied greatly (for instance, on terminal care). The fact that the professional nursing associations were not represented in the municipal crisis committees – in contrast to doctors and representatives of residential home operators – was criticised both by the associations and by the Federal Commissioner for Nursing (Interview BMG, 2: 16:44). Overall, the membership of such bodies at the municipal level was very heterogeneous (Interview BMG, 2: 16:44). The individual house rules of each home operator also permitted deviations. Accordingly, the actual design of the visiting regulations varied within the nationally uniform framework. It ranged from strict closure of the facility to outsiders to the provision of protective measures and equipment that enabled relatives to visit the residents regularly (Interview BMG, 2: 23:54). Particularly at the beginning of the pandemic, the lack of PPE and the preparation and implementation of visiting arrangements were perceived as challenges by the providers' associations. However, legal uncertainties and unwanted media interest may have played a role in the sometimes very restrictive interpretation of visiting regulations by individual facilities (Interview BMG 2: 28:04 / 32:53).

The measures' efficacy remains challenging to assess, even in retrospect. All in all, the residential homes were very differently affected by the first wave. According to a cross-sectional study from April to May 2020, no infections occurred in 80 per cent of the facilities. In contrast, 75 per cent of residents who died from COVID-19 were in residential homes, with more than five deaths, and 81 per cent of infected residents lived in more than ten infected ones. In addition, smaller facilities were significantly more affected than large ones, and most infections were concentrated in a few facilities with more significant outbreaks (Wolf-Ostermann et al, 2022). It suggests that the measures taken were insufficient to prevent larger outbreaks in residential homes effectively. Furthermore, according to claims data from the AOK nursing and health insurance funds, mortality in nursing homes was comparable to that in the general population (Kohl et al, 2021). Also, among residential home residents with greater care needs and persons with dementia, mortality was higher than among residents with lower care needs and without dementia (Kohl et al, 2021). Therefore, it seems that, even within the facilities, it was impossible to protect particularly vulnerable groups adequately.

According to data from the ECDC Public Health Emergency Team (2020) on infections and deaths in LTCF in selected European countries, Germany came through the first wave comparatively well. However, whether and to what extent this was due to the measures taken cannot be assessed.

Further evolution of the situation in the care home sector and challenges for the future of LTC

In LTC during the first wave of the pandemic, there was a lack of protective equipment, a high level of psychological stress for staff, and significant effects on the social well-being of patients and their relatives due to the lockdown measures. In contrast, during the second and third waves at the end of 2020 and in the course of 2021, basic contacts and (social) care structures could be maintained. It was achieved through mandatory testing for staff (several times per week) and visitors, sufficient availability of FFP2 masks, and extensive vaccination coverage of residents in the first quarter of 2021. However, significant restrictions and the associated burdens remained for all involved. In addition, the number of outbreaks in elderly care and nursing facilities increased substantially compared with the first wave (RKI, 2022). With the emergence and rapid spread of the Omicron variant(s) starting in November 2021, infection numbers also skyrocketed in Germany. The nationwide 7-day incidence rose to nearly 2,000 in March 2022. The number of outbreaks in elderly care and nursing homes also rose considerably again but remained just as significantly below the numbers of the second wave. In February 2022, the federal government and the *Länder* decided to gradually abolish most protective measures, such as testing or vaccination certificates and the obligatory use of masks, starting in April 2022 (Bundesregierung, 2022). Only particularly vulnerable groups will continue to be protected. For example, since March 2022, employees in residential healthcare facilities must prove that they have either been vaccinated or recovered from COVID-19 to protect patients and/or residents. The local health authorities must monitor this and impose sanctions if necessary (Bundesregierung, 2022). However, given the shortage of nursing staff and health authorities' high workload, strict enforcement is unlikely.

Regardless of the further evolution of the pandemic, institutional LTC will continue to gain importance in Germany. The demographic development, or more precisely, the ageing of the population, continues. Especially from the mid-2030s onwards, large cohorts of baby boomers will significantly raise the number of people in need of LTC. The numbers will grow from the current 3.7 million recipients of social LTC insurance benefits to over 5 million in 2050 Jacobs et al, 2018: p 11). The number of people receiving inpatient long-term care will almost double (Jacobs et al, 2018: p 11). In addition to the foreseeable increase in LTC recipients, the socio-structural and socio-cultural changes associated with increasing individualisation continue to progress. This fact does not suggest that a disproportionate increase in the use of domiciliary long-term care is to be expected.

On the contrary, due to the flexibility and mobility requirements of the modern labour market and especially due to women's labour market participation, family members' ability and willingness to provide care for their parents or grandparents themselves are dwindling throughout the population. These demographic and social developments will increasingly direct long-term nursing care into the inpatient (residential) sector, even though domiciliary care provided by relatives and nursing services will continue to play a major role. The COVID-19 pandemic has revealed structural weaknesses in residential long-term care in Germany. Among the most striking crisis phenomena, the causes of which can be traced back to the time before the pandemic, are staff shortages and the inadequate provision of PPE for staff. The pandemic acted as a catalyst for these two problems, making it evident to large parts of the public that these problems have taken on serious proportions. This applies above all to the lack of professionally trained nursing staff in residential long-term care, which to some extent, calls the system's resilience into question.

In recent years, the government has introduced various measures to make the nursing profession more attractive and alleviate the shortage of skilled personnel. For example, the Nursing Staff Strengthening Act (*Pflegepersonal-Stärkungsgesetz*), passed in January 2019, provided funding for 13,000 additional jobs in nursing care for the elderly. The recruitment of skilled workers from abroad has also been intensified. In addition, the content of vocational training has been reformed. Regularly uprated minimum wages for the nursing professions and an obligation on nursing facilities to comply with collective wage agreements, which came into force in September 2022, is also intended to raise the profession's profile significantly in financial terms. Nevertheless, these measures will presumably not be enough to solve the nursing shortage.

Regarding other epidemiological and infectiological experiences as well as lessons from the organisation of health and care provision during the coronavirus, such as the inadequate stockpiling of PPE, antiquated reporting chains and so on, it can be assumed that these aspects will be incorporated into a revised version of the National Pandemic Plan. Similar to the situation after the H1N1 pandemic, aspects will be supplemented and identified omissions addressed in an amendment. Thus, the plan can be expected to include concrete specifications for the quantity and quality of PPE to be stockpiled. Overall, the revised plans are likely to focus more strongly on long-term care facilities. This is likely to manifest itself, among other things, in an expansion and strengthening of infectiological guidelines. In such a nationwide amendment of the pandemic plan and its regional-specific details, particular consideration should be given to the problems caused by inadequate or insufficiently developed hygiene plans and to the training required to implement them.

The lack of PPE, its scarcity, and high cost in the free market may lead to the development of national or Europe-wide production capacities to replace the previous strategy of outsourcing production to East Asian countries.

Strengthening local public health services will supposedly be one of Germany's most far-reaching long-term changes that can be directly linked to the COVID-19 pandemic. During the peak phase of the pandemic, the local health authorities were provided with additional personnel resources to monitor and contain infections. Therefore, it can be assumed that Germany's public health service, which has been neglected for decades, will see its personnel substantially increased and its technical infrastructure modernised.

Furthermore, several smaller developments outside the standard pandemic control instruments are expected. On the one hand, the use of telemedicine for people in need of long-term care in residential facilities is likely to become more important. On the other hand, the controversies around the long-term reorganisation of medical care for people in retirement and residential homes will be fuelled again.

At this point, it should be noted that no fundamental changes in the institutional setting are expected in the long-term care regime. Individual actors, such as the public health service, will be upgraded and strengthened, and necessary amendments will be made to the pandemic plans. However, from the current point of view, there are no substantial reforms in restructuring responsibilities in the long-term care system. The German LTC system could be more convenient, where segmented responsibilities and conflicting interests have prevented substantial reforms. Moreover, for decades, there has been a need for more political consensus to raise funding and service delivery to a new level.

Notes

1. https://www.bundesgesundheitsministerium.de/service/begriffe-von-a-z/p/pflegestaerkungsgesetz-zweites-psg-ii.html
2. Bundesgesetzblatt Jahrgang (2020) Teil I Nr. 14, ausgegeben zu Bonn am 27. März 2020.
3. https://dip.bundestag.de/vorgang/gesetz-zum-schutz-der-bev%C3%B6lkerung-bei-einer-epidemischen-lage-von/260577

References

Bales, S., Baumann, H. G., Schnitzler, N. (2003) §36 Einhaltung der infektionshygiene, in S. Bales, H. G. Baumann and N. Schnitzler (eds) *Infektionsschutzgesetz Kommentar und Vorschriftensammlung* (2nd edn), Stuttgart: Kohlhammer, pp 247–9.

BAND –Bundesvereinigung der Arbeitsgemeinschaften Notärzte Deutschlands e.V. (2020) Leitplanken für notärztinnen und notärzte bei der zuteilung von behandlungsressourcen im kontext der COVID-10-pandemie, *BAND*, 30 March [online], Available from: http://www.band-online.de/download/8468.pdf

Bernd, C. and Kunkel, C. (2020) Ich bekomme nur einen Mund-Nasen-Schutz pro Tag, *Süddeutsche Zeitung*, 19 May [online], Available from: https://www.sueddeutsche.de/gesundheit/ coronavirus-krankenhaeuser-ansteckung-1.4911294

Blum, K., Heber, R., Löffert, S., Offermanns, M., and Steffen, P. (2020) Auswirkungen der COVID-19-pandemie und des krankenhausentlastungsgesetzes auf die krankenhäuser. Krankenhausbefragung des Deutschen krankenhausinstituts für die Deutsche krankenhausgesellschaft, *Deutsches Krankenhausinstitut* [online], Available from: https://www.dkgev.de/fileadmin/default/ Mediapool/0_Home/2020-05-29_Anlage_Corona-Befragung.pdf

BMG – Bundesministerium für Gesundheit (2020) Verordnung zum anspruch auf bestimmte testungen für den nachweis des vorliegens einer infektion mit dem Coronavirus SARS-CoV-2, *BMG* [online], Available from: https://www.bundesgesundheitsministerium.de/fileadmin/Dateien/3_Downloads/C/Coronavirus/Corona-Test-VO_20i_SGB_V_mit_Begruendung.pdf

BMG (2022a) *Zahlen und Fakten zur Pflegeversicherung* [online], Available from: https://www.bundesgesundheitsministerium.de/fileadmin/Dateien/3_Downloads/Statistiken/Pflegeversicherung/Zahlen_und_Fakten/Zahlen_und_Fakten_Stand_April_2022_bf.pdf

BMG (2022b) Die finanzentwicklung der sozialen pflegeversicherung. Ist-ergebnisse ohne rechnungsabgrenzung, *BMG* [online], Available from: https://www.bundesgesundheitsministerium.de/fileadmin/Dateien/3_Downloads/Statistiken/Pflegeversicherung/Finanzentwicklung/03-Finanzentwicklung-der-sozialen-Pflegeversicherung__2021_bf.pdf

Bundesagentur für Arbeit (2020) *Statistik der Bundesagentur für Arbeit. Berichte: Blickpunkt Arbeitsmarkt–Arbeitsmarktsituation im Pflegebereich*, Nürnberg: Bundesagentur für Arbeit.

Bundesregierung (2020a) Besprechung der bundeskanzlerin mit den regierungschefinnen und regierungschefs der Länder (Press release), 12 March [online], Available from: https://www.bundesregierung.de/breg-de/themen/ coronavirus/beschluss-zu-corona-1730292

Bundesregierung (2020b) Telefonschaltkonferenz der bundeskanzlerin mit den regierungschefinnen und regierungschefs der Länder (Press release), 6 May [online], Available from: https://www.bundesregierung.de/resource/blob/975226/1750986/ fc61b6eb1fc1d398d66cfea79b565129/ 2020-05-06-mpk-beschluss-data.pdf

Bundesregierung (2022) Videoschaltkonferenz des bundeskanzlers mit den regierungschefinnen und regierungschefs der Länder (Press release), 16 February, [online], Available from: https://www.bundesregierung.de/resource/ blob/974430/2005140/c4b34f495b329f74f43616dd7ccd7d7c/ 2022-02-16-mpk-beschluss-data.pdf

Deutscher Bundestag (2013) Unterrichtung durch die bundesregierung: bericht zur risikoanalyse im bevölkerungsschutz 2012, Drucksache 17/12051, 3 January, Berlin: Bundesanzeiger [online], Available from: https://dserver.bundestag.de/btd/17/120/1712051.pdf

Deutsches Ärzteblatt (2020a) Bund und Länder beschließen krankenhausnotfallplan, *Deutsches Ärzteblatt*, 17 March [online], Available from: https://www.aerzteblatt.de/nachrichten/111125/Bund-und-Laender-beschliessen-Krankenhaus-Notfallplan

Deutsches Ärzteblatt (2020b) Krankenhausgesellschaft in bayern sorgt sich um finanzen der kliniken, *Deutsches Ärzteblatt*, 27 April [online], Available from: https://www.aerzteblatt.de/nachrichten/112328/Krankenhausgesellschaft-in-Bayern-sorgt-sich-um-Finanzen-der-Kliniken

DGP – Deutsche Gesellschaft für Pflegewissenschaft e.V. (eds) (2020) *S1-Leitlinie – Soziale Teilhabe und Lebensqualität in der Stationären Altenhilfe unter den Bedingungen der COVID-19-Pandemie*, Langfassung – AWMF-Registernummer 184–001 [online], Available from: https://www.awmf.org/leitlinien/detail/ll/184-001.html

Drupp, M., Meyer, M., and Winter, W. (2021) Betriebliches gesundheitsmanagement (BGM) für pflegeeinrichtungen und krankenhäuser unter pandemiebedingungen, in K. Jacobs, A. Kuhlmey, S. Greß, J. Klauber, and A. Schwinger (eds) *Pflege-Report 2021 Sicherstellung der Pflege: Bedarfslagen und Angebotsstrukturen*, Berlin: Springer, pp 71–89.

ECDC – Public Health Emergency Team, Danis, K., Fonteneau, L., Georges, S., Daniau, C., Bernard-Stoecklin, S., et al (2020) High impact of COVID-19 in long-term care facilities, suggestion for monitoring in the EU/EEA, *Euro Surveill*, 25(22), pii=2000956.

Gerlinger, T. (2022) *Financial Reform of German Long-term Care Insurance*, ESPN Flash Report 2022/05, Brussels: European Commission [online], Available from: https://ec.europa.eu/social/BlobServlet?docId=25253&langId=en.

Gerlinger, T. and Rosenbrock, R. (2023) *Gesundheitspolitik. Eine Systematische Einführung* (4th edn), Bern: Hogrefe.

Götz, K. (2020) Ambulante versorgung pflegebedürftiger destabilisiert, *BIQuaM – Bremer Initiative für Qualitative Methoden*, 10 June [online], Available from: https://www.uni-bremen.de/biquam/news/detailansicht/ambulante-versorgung-pflegebeduerftiger-in-corona-krise-destabilisiert

Hower, K. I., Pfaff, H., and Pförtner, T. -K. (2020) Pflege in zeiten von COVID-19: onlinebefragung von leitungskräften zu herausforderungen, belastungen und bewältigungsstrategien, *Pflege*, 33(4): 207–18.

Jacobs, K., Kuhlmey, A., Greß, S., Klauber. J., and Schwinger, A. (2018) Pflege-Report 2018 Qualität in der Pflege, Springer Open, Berlin, Available from: chrome-extension://efaidnbmnnnibpcajpcglclefindmkaj/https://link.springer.com/content/pdf/10.1007/978-3-662-56822-4.pdf

KBV – Kassenärztliche Bundesvereinigung (2020a) Bericht von Dr. Andreas Gassen an die Vertreterversammlung. Rede des KBV-Vorstandsvorsitzenden, *KBV*, 12 June [online], Available from: https://www.kbv.de/html/46544.php

KBV (2020b) Aktueller stand derambulanten versorgung während der Coronavirus-pandemie, *KBV*, 16 April [online], Available from: https://www.kbv.de/html/45889.php

KBV (2020c) Bericht von Dr. Andreas Gassen an die vertreterversammlung. Rede des KBV-vorstandsvorsitzenden, *KBV*, 12 June [online], Available from: https://www.kbv.de/html/46544.php

Keller, M. (2020) Corona in alten- und pflegeheimen: Die pandemie hat uns kalt erwischt, *Der Tagesspiegel*, 24 April [online], Available from: https://www.tagesspiegel.de/wissen/corona-in-alten-und-pflegeheimendie-angehoerigen-reagieren-zu-95-prozent-mitverstaendnis/25756662-2.html

Kessler, E-M., Strumpen, S., Kricheldorff, C., Franke, A., Pantel, J., and Gellert, P. (2020) Partizipation und soziale teilhabe älterer menschen trotz Corona-pandemie ermöglichen, Gemeinsames Statement der Sektionen für Geriatrische Medizin (II), Sozial- und verhaltenswissenschaftliche Gerontologie (III), Soziale Gerontologie und Altenhilfe (IV) der Deutschen Gesellschaft für Gerontologie und Geriatrie (DGGG e.V.), 24 April [online] Available from: https://www.dggg-online.de/files/dggg/downloads/COVID-19/20200424_DGGG_Statement_Sektionen_II_III_IV_Soziale_Teilhabe_und_Partizipation.pdf

Kohl, R., Jürchott, K., Hering, C., Gangus, A., Kuhlmey, A., and Schwinger, A. (2021) COVID-19-betroffenheit in der vollstationären langzeitpflege, in K. Jacobs, A. Kuhlmey, S. Greß, J. Klauber, and A. Schwinger (eds) *Pflege-Report 2021 Sicherstellung der Pflege: Bedarfslagen und Angebotsstrukturen*, Berlin: Springer, pp 3–20.

Langendorf, M. (2020) Pflege- und altenheime zu festungen machen, *Caritas Deutschland*, 7 April [online], Available from: https://www.caritas.de/magazin/schwerpunkt/corona/pflege-und-altenheime-zu-festungen-mache

Löwenstein, M. and Heinzle, C. (2020) Fachärzte: erst leere wartezimmer, jetzt termin-stau, *NDR*, 26 May [online], Available from: https://www.ndr.de/nachrichten/info/Drastischer-Rueckgang-von-Facharztbesuchen,facharzt124.html

Lückenbach, C., Klukas, E., Schmidt, P. H. and Gerlinger, T. (2021) Governmental response to the COVID-19 pandemic in Long-Term Care residences for older people: preparedness, responses and challenges for the future: Germany, MC COVID-19 working paper 06/2021, CSIC, Available from: chrome-extension://efaidnbmnnnibpcajpcglclefindmkaj/https://digital.csic.es/bitstream/10261/227268/3/210204_CSIC_covid_ALEMANIA.pdf

MDK – Medizinischer Dienst der Krankenversicherung (2020) Fragen und antworten zur Corona-pandemie, *MDK* [online], Available from: https://www.mdk.de/fileadmin/MDK-zentraler-Ordner/Downloads/19_Corona/FIN_Fragen_und_Antworten_zur_Corona.pdf

Räker, M., Klauber, J., and Schwinger, A. (2021) Pflegerische versorgung in der ersten welle der COVID-19-pandemie, in K. Jacobs, A. Kuhlmey, S. Greß, J. Klauber, and A. Schwinger (eds) *Pflege-Report 2021 Sicherstellung der Pflege: Bedarfslagen und Angebotsstrukturen*, Berlin: Springer, pp 33–58.

Rattenhuber, E. (2020) Coronavirus: altenheime sind dem virus ausgeliefert, *Süddeutsche Zeitung*, 27 March [online], Available from: https://www.sueddeutsche.de/politik/coronavirus-pflege-altenheime-atemschutzmasken-1.4858231

RKI – Robert Koch-Institut (2005) Infektionsprävention in heimen: empfehlung der Kommission für Krankenhaushygiene und Infektionsprävention beim Robert Koch-Institut (RKI), *Bundesgesundheitsblatt – Gesundheitsforschung – Gesundheitsschutz*, 48(9): 1061–80.

RKI – Robert Koch-Institut (2010) Empfehlungen des Robert Koch-Institutes zu präventions: und kontrollmaßnahmen bei bewohnern mit verdacht auf bzw. Nachgewiesener influenza in heimen, *RKI* [online], Available from: https://www. rki.de/DE/Content/Infekt/Krankenhaushygiene/Erreger_ausgewaehlt/Influenza/Influenza_Heim_pdf.pdf?blob=publicationFile

RKI – Robert Koch-Institut (2017) *Nationaler Pandemieplan Teil I. Strukturen und Maßnahmen*, Berlin: Robert Koch-Institut.

RKI – Robert Koch-Institut (2020) *Ergänzung zum Nationalen Pandemieplan: COVID-19 – Neuartige Coronaviruserkrankung*, Berlin: Robert Koch-Institut, Available from: https://www.rki.de/DE/Content/InfAZ/N/Neuartiges_Coronavirus/Ergaenzung_Pandemieplan_COVID.pdf?__blob=publicationFile

RKI – Robert Koch-Institut (2022) Wöchentlicher lagebericht des RKI zur Coronavirus-Krankheit-2019 (COVID-19) – aktualisierter stand für Deutschland, *RKI*, 31 March [online], Available from: https://www.rki.de/DE/Content/InfAZ/N/Neuartiges_Coronavirus/Situationsberichte/Wochenbericht/Wochenbericht_2022-03-31.pdf

Rothgang, H., Müller, R., and Preuß, B. (2020) *BARMER Pflegereport 2020*, Berlin: BARMER, Available from: https://www.socium.uni-bremen.de/uploads/News/2020/20201201_BARMER_Pflegereport_2020.pdf

Schmucker, R. (2020) Arbeitsbedingungen in pflegeberufen. Ergebnisse einer sonderauswertung der beschäftigtenbefragung zum DGB-Index Gute Arbeit, in K. Jacobs et al (eds) *Pflege-Report 2019: Mehr Personal in der Langzeitpflege – Aber Woher?*, Berlin: Springer, pp 49–60.

Spöri, T., and Eichhorn, J. (2021) Wer Glaubt an Corona-verschwörungsmythen? Der Einfluss von Soziodemographie, politischen Einstellungen und Wertehaltungen in Deutschland, d|part, Berlin, Available from: chrome-extension://efaidnbmnnnibpcajpcglclefindmkaj/http://wordpress.dpart.org/wp-content/uploads/2024/05/Corona-Verschworungsmythen-und-Wertevorstellungen-in-Deutschland.pdf

StBA – Statistisches Bundesamt (2020) *Pflegestatistik 2019: Pflege im Rahmen der Pflegeversicherung. Deutschlandergebnisse*, 15 December [online], Available from: https://www.destatis.de/DE/Themen/Gesellschaft-Umwelt/Gesundheit/Pflege/Publikationen/Downloads-Pflege/pflege-deutschlandergebnisse-5224001199004.pdf;jsessionid=4DCFDF88FB7FBEDB6D3E6C0B9296BDD6.live722?__blob=publicationFile

StmGP Bayern – Bayerisches Staatsministerium für Gesundheit und Pflege (2020) Huml hat expertengremium zur eindämmung der Corona-pandemie in der langzeitpflege einberufen – bayerns gesundheits- und pflegeministerin: kampf gegen infektionen konsequent fortsetzen, Press release, 3 May [online], Available from: https://www.stmgp.bayern.de/presse/huml-hat-expertengremium-zur-eindaemmung-der-corona-pandemie-in-der-langzeitpflege/

Wolf-Ostermann, K. and Rothgang, H. (2020) *Zur Situation der Langzeitpflege in Deutschland während der Corona-Pandemie. Ergebnisse einer Online-Befragung in Einrichtungen der (teil)stationären und ambulanten Langzeitpflege*, Bremen: Universität Bremen [online], Available from: https://www.uni-bremen.de/fb11/corona-fb11/zur-situation-der-langzeitpflege-in-deutschland-waehrend-der-corona-pandemie

Wolf-Ostermann, K., Rothgang, H., Domhoff, D., Friedrich, A. C., Heinze, F., Hess, M., Preuss, B., Ratz, K., Schmidt, A., Seibert, K., Stolle, C., and Wiegelmann, H. (2022) Die erste welle – auswirkungen der COVID-19-pandemie auf die versorgung von menschen mit pflegebedarf in Deutschland, in V. Breitbach and H. Brandenburg (eds) *Corona und die Pflege Denkanstöße – die Corona-Krise und Danach*, Wiesbaden: Springer.

8

The Greek long-term care sector against COVID-19: an effort for excellence

Costis Prouskas and Michael Goudoumas

Introduction

The coronavirus pandemic COVID-19 appeared and spread in Greece from 26 February 2020 onwards. Most cases in the early days were related to people who had travelled to Italy for business, and to a group of pilgrims who had visited Israel and Egypt and, subsequently, to their contacts.[1]

Table 8.1 refers to the general population data as presented in the NHPO's official report of 31 May 2020. The highest level of mortality occurred in the over-65s and especially in men, who made up 51.4 per cent of COVID-19 deaths. In contrast, women over 65 appeared to be less diseased in the general population and over-65s, with the mortality rate almost half that of men, at 24.6 per cent.

From 27 February 2020, to 31 May 2020, confirmed cases and deaths due to COVID-19 were very low. Greece was among the countries with the lowest mortality rate due to COVID-19, with only 175 deaths despite the 2,915 confirmed cases (6 per cent of confirmed cases). Following the opening of the borders at the end of June, the daily number of confirmed cases reported included those detected following checks at the country's entry gates. In addition, a total of 3,562 recoveries had been announced by 26 July (Prouskas, 2020a).

In Greece, the overall COVID-19 death rate in the elderly care units was minimal, almost zero per cent for the semester of 2020 (February to July 2020). The Greek long-term care (LTC) sector exceeded expectations during the outbreak of the COVID-19 pandemic. The Greek elderly care units managed to work together and overcome obstacles and bureaucratic impediments. With 97.5 per cent occupancy (13,613 residents), until the end of the Greek 2020 lockdown, only two deaths were recorded due to COVID-19, whereas there were only 13 (less than 0.001 per cent) cases in two of the 300 units of the country.

Table 8.1: Cases by sex and age until 31 May 2020, Greece

Classification		Cases		Fatal cases		Cases treated in ICU	
		Number	(%)	Number	(%)	Number	(%)
All		**2,719**	**100**	**175**	**100**	**13**	**100**
Sex	**Male**	1,499	55.1	123	70.3	9	69.2
	Female	1,220	44.9	52	29.7	4	30.8
Age	**≥65**	576	21.2	133	76.0	8	61.5
	40–64	1,139	41.9	39	22.3	5	38.5
	18–39	844	31.0	3	1.7	0	0.0
	0–17	160	5.9	0	0.0	0	0.0

In this chapter, we will describe the situation during the first wave of COVID-19 as it played out in Greece. Mainly we will discuss how the whole situation and the pandemic affected the LTC sector and how the care units responded. The first part is a brief review of the modern reforms in the LTC sector. Moreover, the importance of the family in the care of the elderly is given. It then presents a case study of the Greek LTC sector, the measures taken to prevent the transmission of COVID-19, and the impact of the pandemic on the sector and on the elderly residents in the elderly care units. In the concluding section, an attempt is made to present the reality of the LTC sector after the end of the pandemic wave.

The LTC sector in Greece

Current arrangements in LTC and social welfare

According to the Ministry of Labor report, in 2020, approximately 300 long-term care units (LTCUs) were licensed in Greece, with an average of 45 beds each. Of these, 53 per cent were private (for profit), and the rest of them (not for profit) are operated by NGOs and the Church (Ministry of Labour, 2020). Of the total 14,571 beds in LTCUs, almost 50 per cent were located in the Attica Region (Athens, Piraeus, and the suburbs). The country has only one characterised as Public Entity, but actually, it is an ecclesiastic foundation without operational authorisation. In addition, there are 30 unauthorised units in the private and third sectors. The reasons for non-registration are bureaucratic, due to the fact that they have to wait for the regional administrative bureaus to publish the operating authorisation. Or church institutions that started as humanitarian institutions or asylums, elder care charities with an initial authorisation that has never been renewed since then.

Registered units provide nursing and medical care, hospitality services, and some recreational activities. Elderly care units operate under the supervision of the Social and Welfare Services of the Regions. The older adult or their family pays the fees. The current legal framework does not include any quality indicators or standards except spatial and personnel standards (Government Gazette, 2018).

The Greek State is the primary mechanism for ensuring social well-being and redistributing economic resources (Prouskas, 2000). It is also the exclusive insurance institution, and through three mechanisms: i) social security, ii) social care, and iii) health care, it supports the social security system.

The average pension is €882 per month (€713 main pension, €169 for supplementary). According to the Ministry of Labour, Social Security & Social Solidarity's display of pension benefits, about 1.5 million older adults aged 71 to over 90 years old receive a pension of no more than €880. Those aged 85 to over 90 do not receive more than €650 on average, and 34 per cent of pensioners receive over €1000 but at most €1150 on average.

The benefits policy cannot meet the needs of destitute older people since the benefit amount is usually relatively small. At the same time, ineffective bureaucratic procedures have made the process more difficult, unsurprisingly. Material benefits related to providing clothing, medicines, and food to helpless or destitute older adults are administered through their local church, or NGOs.

In Greece, there are no 'intermediate institutions' such as medical or convalescent homes, to complete treatment after a hospital so that there can be a full recovery. Concerning LTC, the State is just an observer and a regulator for LTC providers. Except for the local day centres and community or home care programmes, mentioned previously, the State is absent in the provision of LTCUs.

Greek LTC is based on a mixed 'quasi-system' of services, comprising formal (public, private, and non-governmental providers) and informal elderly care. Formal care providers include primary (local) health centres, secondary and university hospitals, day care centres, counselling centres, rehabilitation centres, private clinics, private hospitals, elderly care units, services from non-governmental/non-profit organisations (such as Alzheimer centres), and home care services.

As far as informal care is concerned, the primary responsibility for the financial and practical support of a family's dependents rests squarely and legally on the family and plays the dominant role in providing LTC for older people. Therefore, it constitutes the main determining feature of the Greek LTC system (Kagialaris et al, 2010; Ziomas et al, 2018).

There is no specific model for organising LTC: there are combinations that are relevant to the 'Ever Care' model (a personalised and holistic approach) and the 'Guided Care' model – but this is not a central management policy choice. A common point of the two models is the importance of nurse caregivers, cooperation with the treating physician, and connections with the local community and the National Health System (Pierakos, 2013; Ziomas et al, 2018; Prouskas, 2020).

The issue lies in the non-coverage of LTC by state insurers. Thus, regarding the LTC of the elderly, day hospitalisation expenditure is not justified, nor has it been costed. In contrast, the costs of medical care, medicine, and other therapeutic costs (such as physiotherapy, occupational therapy) is justified by state insurance funds and private insurance companies operating in Greece. Furthermore, non-coverage applies to other LTCUs, such as psychiatric structures and treatment centres (Prouskas et al, 2012).

The State's involvement in this policy area is limited, while governance and organisational arrangements are grossly inadequate. The state finances and controls the national health system – health centres, hospitals, and the social services mentioned previously, that is, the home care program, and the social benefits (social assistance allowances and pensions).

The rest of the state social structures for older people are funded and controlled by the Regions and the respective Municipal authorities. The regional authorities also license and control the elderly care units in their operational and health activities. Therefore, the main changes introduced into the health system have focused on the work and role of the central State.

There are actions concerning funding, with common new trends in service delivery and the emergence of hybrid systems. These trends refer to variations in the systems of public supply. The State as a direct service provider of health is parallel with a shift from hospital to primary care, where private providers traditionally play a more critical role. Finally, rearrangements in the regulation of relations between the three leading institutions of the healthcare system – the State, the health funds or associations of health care providers, and the private doctors involved in the 'health market'.

Legislation upon LTC

After the fall of the dictatorship of the colonels (Greek junta) in 1974, the normalisation of political life and the modernisation of the primary institutions began, part of a general process of achieving Greece's accession to the European Community. In this context, the State's construction that includes the law and welfare is included (Stathopoulos, 2005; Rapti, 2007).

Numerous laws were declared, and ministerial decisions were taken from 1975 onwards, with the last one taking place in 2012. They are mainly concerned with licensing conditions (surfaces/persons and buildings), human resources requirements, and changes in labour provisions. The most significant changes were those made in 1996 and 2007. The 2007 Act modernises LTCUs based on international standards by increasing support and care staff and emphasising quality care delivery and quality of life. The changes affect medical-nursing staff, paramedical specialists (such as occupational therapists, speech and language therapists), and psychosocial support specialists.

There has been a growing awareness among Greek governments of possible problems associated with the rapidly increasing number and proportion of older people in the Greek population. Thus, no national plan for developing health and social services for older adults has been made. However, some programmes were initiated by service providers such as local authorities and NGOs, and broader policy measures are currently under review by the Ministry of Labour and Social Solidarity.

General functioning of the residential care system

Although relevant official statistical data concerning the demand and supply of LTC services/facilities are not available, all the indications are that formal care is available to only a small number of beneficiaries. For example, the Eurostat data show that in 2015 (ELSTAT, 2015), for every 100,000 inhabitants, there were only 17 LTC beds in nursing and residential care facilities; this was the lowest ratio among the EU Member States.

Most LTCUs and services for older adults are located near to urban areas. However, almost 50 per cent of them can be found in Athens, leading to a geographically unequal development (Athens contains 40 per cent of the Greek population). It implies that access to LTC is heavily dependent on where the older person lives, which constitutes one of the main barriers to accessing LTC services, especially for those living on the islands and in isolated rural areas (Ziomas et al, 2016, 2018).

Several other barriers have been identified concerning access to and availability of LTC services (including home care services). For example, according to the latest available data (European Quality of Life Survey 2011 – Eurofound, 2012), more than 80 per cent of LTC service users in Greece experienced difficulties with availability (such as waiting lists and lack of services). In contrast, over 70 per cent of service users experienced difficulties with access (for example, because of distance or opening hours). One example is that the care services provided through the public day-care centres for the elderly and the 'Help at Home' programme are available only on weekdays, in the morning and early afternoon, and for up to 8 hours per day.

In addition, most of the existing public formal LTC services entail rather strict eligibility criteria that make them inaccessible to many persons in need of such care. As Tinios (2017: p 104) argues, 'those left out are probably the majority of those who need LTC; they would be excluded either *de jure* through the exclusion criteria or *de facto* through the limited places available'. It should also be underlined that, despite the fact that disability is one of the main factors driving the demand for LTC services, the capacity of such services in Greece falls far short of meeting the needs of people with disabilities, the great majority of whom are aged 65+ (Ziomas et al, 2018).

As Ziomas (Ziomas et al, 2018: p 9) argues, '552,700 people aged 65+ reported difficulty with personal care activities, while almost 2/3 of them needed assistance. Although these data are not up to date, they reveal that disability is prevalent among older age groups, and thus demand for LTC services is likely to increase'. Furthermore, the 'closed' institutions for the disabled of all ages are found to be inefficient and with serious shortcomings, to the detriment of patients.

The Greek Association of Alzheimer's Disease and Related Disorders (2017) mentions that the existing community-based LTC services for the disabled and older adults with dementia with or without Alzheimer's remain strongly limited. Overall, there is an urgent need to increase the system's capacity to meet the demand for LTC services. That constitutes the most profound challenge in this policy area. Still, and most importantly, action to increase the system's capacity should go hand in hand with efforts to ensure sufficient quality of LTC services provision.

Adopted measures and preparedness level on public health

Since 1980, many laws have endeavoured to modernise the public health system. Nowadays, the network of public health services is structured at national, regional, and prefectural level. Greek legislation on the protection of public health against communicable diseases includes a wide range of areas affecting health, such as the adoption of the International Health Regulation, legislation on the declaration of infectious diseases and epidemiological surveillance, legislation on the control of the health market and health service providers, and legislation on water, food, environmental hygiene, and standards for vaccination (Sidiropoulou, 2009).

In the 1990s and millennial Greece, outbreaks of poultry and swine influenza viruses – Influenza A(H7N9) and A(H1N1) – as well as respiratory control coronaviruses such as MERS and SARS, were treated, which did not result in epidemic situations, since the NHS, in cooperation with the HCDCP[2] and the government agencies, was able in a timely manner to inform the public of their risk and to check travellers coming from countries where the disease was on the rise.

Due to the frequent epidemics worldwide, HCDCP and the Ministry of Health cooperate in launching guidelines about preventing and treating infectious diseases. Among those guidelines, four are essential here:

1. The Guide for the 'National Action Plan to Tackle the Influenza Pandemic', first published in 2005 for the treatment of H5N1, was

renewed based on WHO and EU guidelines until 2009, when H1N1 first appeared (Prouskas, 2020a).

2. In 2007 the Hospital Infections Scientific Committee of the HCDCP issued the 'Diagnosis and Empirical Treatment of Infections Guidelines' to be shared in Hospital and Clinical Units of Greece, given the concern raised by the resistance of viruses due to the overconsumption and over-prescription of antibiotics.
3. In 2015 in the context of the implementation of the Ministerial Decision (FEK 388/18-2-2014) on the basis of which each hospital should draw up an Internal Regulation for the control of antimicrobial resistance and hospital infections, the Commission developed 'Guidelines for the drafting of the Rules of Procedure for the Prevention and Control of Infections in Health Service Areas', a standard of Rules of Procedure for Greek hospitals. This standard mainly defines the role of human resources, explains infection control surveillance indicators by which hospital practices will be assessed, and gives guidelines on control and prevention measures and the rational use of antibiotics.
4. In 2019, the Ministry of Health and the National Council for Public Health published the 'National Action Plan for Public Health' (NAP-PH), developed by the General Secretariat for Public Health (GSPH). In the context of the reconstruction of public health services, the NAP-PH adopted the main priorities of the WHO to achieve the key strategic objectives relating to reducing social inequalities, improving health for all, and participatory governance for health. It has seven main axes of action, selected using the main criteria of their mental burden, their economic consequences, and the resources of the health system, as well as the emergencies caused by international economic and political circumstances. Axis 6 describes the exact plan for health emergencies set out by the International Health Regulations (IHR) for cross-border threats and communicable diseases (Prouskas, 2020a).

A common feature of all these directives is their attention to cooperation between various governmental bureaus, ministries, health and state departments. Secondly, to the systematic use of personal protection measures (masks, gloves, protective glasses, and special suits when necessary) as well as to the working environment and equipment sterilisation. Continuous training and awareness for all of this are also essential, such as the information and awareness of the public.

The NPHO and government sources proposed similar measures to deal with COVID-19.

Due to the population they serve, LTCUs for the elderly must follow instructions and provisions relating to (a) hospital/clinical environments and (b) health regulations addressed to the community. LTCs for the elderly in Greece are open care structures, so on the one hand, they are clinical environments, and on the other, the population they serve is integrated and can act freely within the community outside the residential unit and through visiting contacts. Thus, infectious diseases, in particular, and health regulations, in general, are no different from a primary care clinic. No matter what, LTCUs are obliged to follow every public health regulation that is taken.

Many of the measures taken during the pandemic of COVID-19 are the result of the historical experiences discussed previously, good cooperation, and information sharing among the directors and managers of the LTCUs, and their staff's ethical and correct behaviour. Therefore, the lack of specialised regulations and government guidelines for the LTCUs in the treatment of epidemic infections affecting public health at both clinical and community level makes the work of LTCUs more challenging to implement and open to criticism from the public opinion and the media.

The first time the government mentioned the announcement of measures to prevent and treat the spread of infectious diseases specifically for LTCUs, was on 28 August 2020, with the statement that they will be certified by the National Public Health Organisation (NPHO) specialists. Until then, measures to deal with COVID-19 were only mentioned in ministerial decisions.

Governmental guidelines for LTC sector

The first official national guidelines for the pandemic handling were announced in March 2020, and they regulated visits to LTCU's residents. They originated within the Ministry of Health and were distributed by the regional authorities on 14 March 2020. On the same day, an Act of Legislative Content was published in the Government Gazette issue 64, under which the State could commandeer the human resources and the equipment of the private Primary and Secondary Health Units, including LTCUs.

On 24 March 2020, the NHPO announced the General Guidelines for precautionary measures against COVID-19, officially adopted by the Ministry of Health on 7 April 2020.

They were concerned, in particular, with personal protection and hygiene measures in the event of a coronavirus case. More specifically, the NPHO page (NPHO, 2020) states that medical and nursing staff, external partners, and administration officers shall be alert for possible symptoms consistent with a respiratory infection and measure their temperature daily before starting work. In addition, everybody had to wear masks during working time. Furthermore, in case they had symptoms compatible with COVID-19 infection or were contacted with a confirmed or suspected case, it was mandatory for the person to leave the workplace instantly and stay in home quarantine. Also, systematic observance of cleaning, disinfection of premises and surfaces, and safe management of infectious waste should be recorded.

The NHPO produced a table with guidelines on the exposure risk ratio and the measures to be taken. According to this table, the personal protection measures taken by the worker and the degree of exposure was a measure of whether or not the worker had to be removed from the workplace, the time period and the conditions under which this was to be done, and the self-quarantine period.

Furthermore, continuous awareness activities and training sessions on the proper use of personal protective equipment with emphasis on the application and removal process should be provided.

On 24 March 2020, visitations were prohibited for the LTCUs. The only exception referred to relatives of residents in a near-death condition. However, even in such a case, visiting was prohibited if they had any symptoms compatible with a respiratory infection. The LTCUs would have to update families regarding their admitted relative via video conferencing, SMS, phone, or other alternatives.

Regarding the LTC residents, the measures were stringent and concerned with personal hygiene and using the unit's premises. More specifically, the measures involved the all-day use of masks, personal hygiene, restrictions of movement and feeding only in their rooms, and restriction of activities and social contacts, even if these involved specific treatments such as physiotherapy, occupational therapy, or psychological support sessions. These measures even included older people with dementia or other neurological conditions who may not have been able to perceive the condition under which their daily routine was being changed. In a suspected or confirmed COVID-19 case, the resident should be immediately transferred to a health service provider. The ambulance service, the NPHO, and the reception hospital shall be instantly informed to take all necessary measures to prevent and control the spread of the infection. In the case of a resident's death who was suspected or confirmed as COVID-19 infected, there were instructions given by NHPO on the management of dead bodies that should be followed.

The guidelines also referred to logistics management and upgrading, for example the posting of printed instructions on the five steps of hand hygiene and the correct procedures for the application and removal of personal protective equipment upon entry into the unit or isolation room, installing closets with personal protective equipment at the rooms' entrances. Even trash cans had to be of a specific type (foot operated).

LTC sector policies and impact

Prouskas and Goudoumas surveyed nursing home directors in the first 6 months of 2020 (Prouskas, 2020). A questionnaire[3] was administered to 61 managers and owners of LTCUs from all regions of Greece. The percentage of completed questionnaires (21 per cent) compared to the total number of units (n = 295) and the coverage areas of the respecting units allows a claim for it being a representative sample.

According to this survey, 44 per cent of the LTCUs that did not already have them developed health risk protocols following the measures just discussed. Fifty-two per cent had protocols or internal regulations, which were readjusted with additions regarding the threats from COVID-19. The remaining 3 per cent had no protocols and did not form any. Nevertheless, it is likely to have been corrected due to the situation's development and frequent checks by the health authorities. In addition, in the case of a COVID-19 outbreak, isolation rooms were increased in 54 per cent of the units.

As to what procedures they would follow if there were a COVID-19 outbreak, 72 per cent replied that they would follow the standard treatment procedure as defined by the EODY and take additional measures. Finally, 28 per cent said they would only follow the EODY procedure.

LTC sector measures

The overall results of that survey indicated that government agencies need to take action on COVID-19 in LTC faster. According to the survey's results, 60 per cent of the elderly care units in Greece had already started to take emergency precautions earlier. Twenty-four per cent of them took the measures before the virus appeared in Greece. However, only 7 per cent took action after government instructions or during the lockdown.

Most LTCUs (44 per cent) received the first updates on the risks of COVID-19 in February 2020. Only 8 per cent started to be updated in December 2019, and 28 per cent in January 2020. However, 3 per cent were updated about the measures in April, 2 months after the first cases in Greece, but this was when the Ministry of Health decided to adopt the General Precautionary Measures for LTCUs.

When asked about the information source regarding the measures to be taken for COVID-19, 82 per cent answered that the media and the Internet mainly informed them. On the other hand, the percentage of information coming from government sources, that is, the central government, the regional authorities, and the NPHO, reached 90 per cent. Another 21 per cent included GCHA as a source of information.

Most of the measures proposed by the Ministry of Health and the NHPO were already being followed in the LTCUs due to the vulnerability of their residents. Masks, gloves, disinfectant liquids, soaps, and various methods of disinfection of the premises were essential for living within the units even before COVID-19. Therefore, the answers by all the units were 100 per cent for adopting these measures and single-use handkerchiefs in rooms and bathrooms. The vast majority of these measures will continue after the COVID-19 outreach. Moreover, more than 50 per cent of the units were supplied with shoe covers, face shields, and single-use suits, but less than 20 per cent stated that they were likely to use them after the pandemic. Most of these materials were not in use before. Nearly 40 per cent of the units had yet to have a contract with a disinfection company, but they decided to cooperate with one due to the situation. More than 65 per cent of the units were disinfecting the units using their resources.

In order to better control the situation, the LTCUs took additional protection and precaution measures not mentioned in the official state briefings. The Government, through the intervention of the Greek Care Home Association and after discussions with relevant authorities such as the Directorates of Public Health of the Regions and the Competent Committee of the Ministry of Health took a diversity of measures: the prohibition of group eating in the dining room, maintenance of air conditioning, and an increase in doctors' visits and frequency of temperature measuring both for the staff and the residents.

Impact of the epidemic on the residents and relatives

Greek LTCUs are small- to medium-sized enterprises with an average capacity of 60 beds. Only 9 per cent exceed 100 beds, and just 2 per cent of them can host more than 200. A quarter of the units have a capacity of at most 80 beds. The situation emerging due to COVID-19 was harmful to their occupancy rates. Most units stated that admissions for 2020 were reduced compared to the same period (January to May) of the previous year. More than 45 per cent of the units reported a significant reduction in occupancy. An almost similar proportion (43 per cent) mentioned that their occupancy remained the same. Ten per cent of the participants stated that they saw an increase in the occupancy rate from January to May 2020.

Departures of residents for reasons related to COVID-19 occurred in 11 per cent of units, and not for more than five residents per unit. Mostly, this was decided by the relatives mainly for financial reasons, arising from the pandemic and the lockdown situation, and less because of their concern about staying in a LTCU.

Except for the personal protection directives and the visitation prohibition, the Government did not take any other severe measures to protect LTCUs in the first semester of 2020, and the LTCUs had to face COVID-19 alone.

By the answers of the LTCUs managers, the level of adjustment difficulty was divided almost 50 per cent among the residents. Eventually, more than 75 per cent of the residents accepted the lack of visitations, which affected the excellent performance of the units in terms of precaution and service provision.

However, a difficulty emerged within the units. Given that within most elderly care units are many people with dementia, Alzheimer's disease, or other neurodegenerative diseases that affect their cognitive functionality and behaviour, less than 25 per cent were able to follow 'easily' the implementation of personal protection and prevention measures. A third of the managers state that the residents found it difficult (30 per cent) or very difficult (21 per cent).

Another factor that must be considered is the psychological effects of all the measures on the psycho-emotional state of recipients of LTC services. Especially those for whom the expression of emotions is difficult due to cognitive decline or limited functionality. The unit managers were also asked to respond to this through their impressions or information from the unit professionals.

Forty-six per cent of the LTC managers reported that the most commonly occurring impact was psycho-emotional instability followed by sadness and feelings of loneliness. Also, due to the managers' reports, a large number – almost a third of tenants (30–33 per cent) – experienced stressful feelings and felt excluded. However, psychosomatic or behavioural disorders and other purely psychiatric indications remain low (from 5 to 10 per cent).

The majority of the relatives (62 per cent), despite their fears – caused by high mortality levels and unpleasant developments in other European countries – accepted the ban on visitation. All of them considered that the suspension of their rights to visit was of 'high necessity', but it 'lasted too long' (50 per cent). They deemed the measure necessary even though a large proportion of them (36 per cent) did not completely understand the urgency and the long duration of the visitation ban (27 per cent). Just 22 per cent disagreed with the measure's continuation. Their level of cooperation demonstrated the general agreement and acceptance of the measure. On a five point scale, from 'non-cooperative' to 'very cooperative', 80 per cent of the relatives were reported as 'sufficiently' or 'very cooperative' in the opinion of the units' directors or managers. Only 3 per cent of the relatives were found to give 'little' cooperation (Figure 8.1).

LTCU managers stated that although relatives largely trust the place of hospitality and care of their loved one, they do not cease to feel guilt (67 per cent) and sadness (55 per cent). Usually, they think they have left the older adult alone. In addition, stress, caused by the feeling of abandonment, affects 65 per cent of relatives.

Good cooperation also comes from the alternative means of communication the units offer. Managers also reported that due to new technologies, almost

Figure 8.1: Relatives' cooperation rate

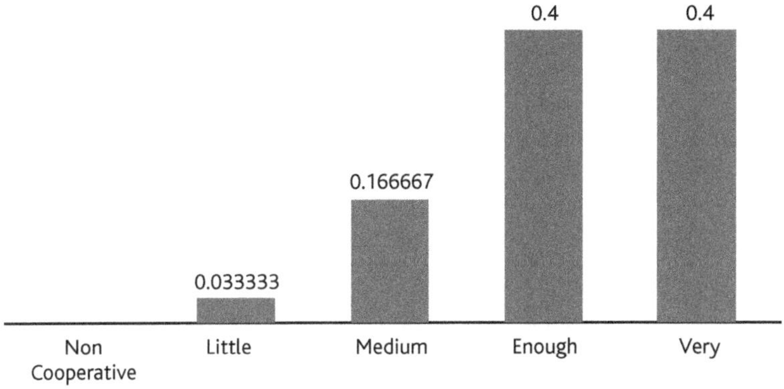

Source: Prouskas (2020); NHPO (2020)

75 per cent of the residents could communicate with their loved ones via videoconferencing applications.

Impact upon LTCUs

Over 90 per cent of the units participating in the survey employ the specialties required by law (doctors, nurses, nursing assistants, administration officers). Very few employ additional specialist therapists, for example speech or occupational therapists (5 per cent and 15 per cent, respectively). It is essential to mention that fewer than 60 per cent of the units employ psychologists, and fewer employ social workers (48 per cent).

In 84 per cent of the units in the survey, their employees were tested for COVID-19 at least once. Most of the tests (47 per cent) were conducted after the lockdown. Just one third of the participants stated that the testing occurred during the quarantine. The tests were mainly conducted by the units of NHPO (62 per cent) and private laboratories or hospitals (29 per cent).

Concerning personnel, 65 per cent of the units replied that their human resources remained the same, while 25 per cent noted an increase in numbers for reasons related to COVID-19. The results showed that 97 per cent of the employed staff and the external partners accepted 'to a large extent' or 'fully' the measures taken for precaution against and treatment of COVID-19. About a tenth of the nursing staff left to be employed in the public sector.

All units seem burdened by the increase in the price of products, medical services, laboratory tests related to COVID-19, and the inability to find sanitary and personal protective equipment. At the same time, occupancy reduction was reported by 66 per cent of the units and reduced demand by 62 per cent.

Furthermore, there was an increased expenditure on sanitary and personal protection materials: 97 per cent of the units increased their expenditure for masks, gloves, nurse suits, single-use suits, diapers, incontinence bed pads, disinfection, and personal hygiene materials. During the period that drugstores did not have materials or increased their prices, Attica Regional Authority's initiative with the Greek Care Homes Association (GCHA/PEMFI), a small number of masks (200 pieces) and sanitisers (8 litres) were distributed to local units as a donation. However, there were no government initiatives to overcome the lack of protective equipment and materials in case of virus spread within the units. On the other hand, in case of an increased spread of COVID-19 cases, LTC facilities would have been very useful in supporting NHS and covering its needs for beds for chronic or even asymptomatic COVID patients.

The pandemic and its consequences financially damaged the LTC sector in Greece. Not only were they not supported by the Government (lack of grants, increased taxation, continuous state controls, and increased safety conditions), but they faced a sharp increase in their costs due to reduced outflows (reduced occupancy, checkouts). The average loss was 25 per cent, while some unit managers reported a 40–50 per cent profit loss. Only 10 per cent reported the same income as for the previous year in the same period.

The future of the LTC sector in Greece

The LTC sector in Greece is still developing, both in terms of market and internal operations. Factors such as aggressive competition, or lack of any central plan for healthy development to adequately meet the needs of local populations, have led to 'scissors scale' phenomena, such as the evident inequality between very large or small units in the same area. The State plays the supervisor role and does not consider the sector as an area working under special conditions and capabilities but integrates it into the more comprehensive health and welfare sector.

However, the Greek LTCUs for elderly people are not included in national lists of state funding, making them inaccessible to the broader population, thus creating market distortions and forcing them to remain in the private or Third sectors initiative. Furthermore, pricing is determined by the owners or managers of the units, depending on the customer audience to which they want to refer. It means that an older person whose pension is, on average, €750–800 will have to be helped to meet out-of-pocket expenses from their children, relatives, or even friends. This reduces the options for a unit of their choice. Alternatively, an older person is forced to stay home, assisted, and cared for by their family or a paid caregiver.

During the COVID-19 outreach period, the LTCUs were not subsidised by the Government to overcome their needs and difficulties, and only a few of the governmental measures (remote workability, the prohibition of redundancies at the time of the virus's intense outbreak) applied to them. Nevertheless, on the other hand, creating new protocols or upgrading existing ones offered a sense of security to residents' relatives and employees at regional and state administration levels.

The difficulty in finding skilled or unskilled caregivers continued to exist and intensified during this pandemic. Unfortunately, in Greece, as globally, nurses and caregivers do not easily choose to work in elderly care units. Even when workforce demands due to COVID-19 increased, nurses hardly ever chose to work in a unit. The mass media chose to cultivate the fear instead of highlighting the positive outcomes in the sector in Greece compared to other countries in Europe or even worldwide with its information.

The fact that the LTC market in Greece is still small gives a variety of prospects for the sector. The foundations can be laid for a more customer-oriented, well-developed sector that integrates well with other existing services and considers the needs of all the stakeholders, such as residents, employees, managers, owners, and inspectors. In that way, it can achieve the equilibrium between quality of care and quality of life (Prouskas, 2020b).

Conclusion

Watching the negative development of the pandemic in other countries closely, the instructions of the global scientific community as reflected in the guidelines of the World Health Organization, timely measures were taken, which were welcomed and then incorporated into the directives of the Region of Attica, the NHPO and the Ministry of Health.

The outstanding outcome is the result of their timely reaction, the initiatives and early measures they introduced, and the government's early reaction and measures that kept rates of COVID-19 infections in the community low. Also, it results from their managers working together within the GCHA and cooperating with regional authorities and the government.

The decisions made by the units' owners or managers to isolate the units, regularly check employees and residents, increase protection measures, and closely observe employees' and residents' temperatures and possible symptoms were also correct. Many units took these precautions even before the national bodies adopted them. Time has been earned to design a better, common, solid strategy and make the necessary adjustments to 'heal wounds' and effectively deal with COVID-19 in the future.

Notes

1 Reuters (2020); www.eody.gov.gr (2020)

2 Hellenic Centre for Diseases Control and Prevention (KEELPNO/HCDCP). The Hellenic Centre for Diseases Control and Prevention, HCDCP (Greek: Κέντρο Ελέγχου και Πρόληψης Νοσημάτων, ΚΕΕΛΠΝΟ) was Greece's public health organisation until 2019. It was based in Athens, Greece, and was named 'HCIDC' (Hellenic Centre for

Infectious Diseases Control) up to 2005. HCDCP was replaced in 2019 and its full successor is the National Public Health Organization (NPHO/EODY).

3 The questionnaire consisted of 165 questions divided into seven Sections and 34 sub-sections. Questions related to operational issues, pandemic handling, measures and incidents, residents and family reaction, personnel attitudes towards the disease, company finances, and inspections by authorities. The analysis of the questionnaire shows the general impact of the pandemic on the residential care sector.

References

Arkouli, M. (2013) Nursing homes emptying during crisis, Greek Reporter, 19 August [online], Available from: https://greece.greekreporter.com/2013/08/19/nursing-homes-emptying-during-crisis/

Civil Protection (2020) Urgent briefing of the Deputy Minister of Civil Protection and Crisis Management Nikos Chardalias on additional measures to limit the spread of the new coronavirus, General Secretariat for Civil Protection, 31 July [online], Available from: https://www.civilprotection.gr/el/simantika-themata/ektakti-enimerosi-toy-yfypoyrgoy-politikis-prostasias-kai-diaheirisis-kriseon

COVID19.Gov (2020) Daily monitoring – COVID-19 live analytics, 4 August [online], Available from: https://COVID19.gov.gr/COVID19-live-analytics/

ELSTAT – Hellenic Statistical Authority (2015) *Survey on Social Care Units* [online], Available from: https://www.statistics.gr/el/statistics/-/publication/SHE27/-

Eurofound (2012) *Third European Quality of Life Survey – Quality of life in Europe: Impacts of the crisis*, Luxembourg: Publications Office of the European Union [online], Available from: https://www.eurofound.europa.eu/sites/default/files/ef_publication/field_ef_document/ef1264en_0.pdf

Greek Association of Alzheimer's Disease and Related Disorders (2017) A Note for Alzheimer's Disease, Quarterly Edition, 71(December) [online], Available from: http://www.alzheimer-hellas.gr/periodiko/dec17.pdf (in Greek)

Government Gazette (2018) Amendment and supplementation of the decision A3a/876 / 16.5.2000 (B 661) of the Ministers of Finance and of Health and Welfare of Law 2716/1999 'Determining the manner of organisation and operation of the Psychosocial Rehabilitation Units (Boarding Schools, Hostels) and the Programs of Protected Apartments of article 9 of law 2716/1999', *Government Gazette*, Issue B 1157 / 29 March.

IMF (2020) Policy responses to COVID-19, 4 August [online], Available from: https://www.imf.org/en/Topics/imf-and-COVID19/Policy-Responses-to-COVID-19#G

Kagialaris, G., Mastroyiannakis, T., and Triantafillou, J. (2010) *The Role of Informal Care in Long-Term Care – National Report: Greece*, Athens: Work Package 5, Interlinks, April.

Kyriopoulos, G. (2008) *Public Health and Social Policy: Eleftherios Venizelos and His Era*, Athens: Papazisis.
Lyberaki, A. and Tinios, P. (2018) Long-term care, ageing and gender in the Greek crisis, *GreeSE*, Paper No.128, Hellenic Observatory Papers on Greece and Southeast Europe, London: LSE.
NHPO (2020) *Risk Assessment and Management of Health Care Personnel with Possible Exposure in a Confirmed Case of COVID-19 Infection in Service Areas Health* [online], Available from: https://eody.gov.gr/wp-content/uploads/2020/03/COVID-19-eppag-ygeias-ektimisi-kindinou.pdf
Petmezidou, M., Papanastasiou, S., Pempetzoglou, M., Papatheodorou, C., and Polizoidis, P. (2015) *Health and Long-term Care in Greece*, INE GSEE, Athens, Available from: https://www.researchgate.net/profile/Ioannis-Apostolakis/publication/355192829_The_existence_of_welfare_states_in_the_front_of_Long-Term_Care_in_Greece/links/616692bd3851f95994f76bcb/The-existence-of-welfare-states-in-the-front-of-Long-Term-Care-in-Greece.pdf
Pierakos G. (2013) *Long Term Care Management models in the Local Community*, Athens: Papazisis.
Prouskas, C. (2000) *Investigating aspects of health among older Greeks: The development and utilisation of an hellenic version of a multidimensional and functional assessment questionnaire*, PhD Thesis, London: King's College London, School of Health – Age Concern Institute of Gerontology [online], Available from: doi: 10.12681/eadd/22724
Prouskas, C. (2012) Home care or assignment to a care unit, MedicalNews.gr, 25 September [online], Available from: https://medicalnews.gr/frontida-sto-spiti-i-anathesh-se-monada/
Prouskas, C. (2019) Choosing of an elderly care unit: an important decision, Amarysia, 25 October [online], Available from: https://amarysia.gr/ygeia-news
Prouskas, C. (2020a) Long term care units during the COVID-19 era, Amarysia, 18 July [online], Available from: https://amarysia.gr/ygeia-news/
Prouskas, C. (2020b) COVID-19 and elderly care units in Greece: initiatives, protocols, procedures, and developments, 7th Pancretan Interdisciplinary Conference on Alzheimer's Disease and the 3rd Panhellenic Conference on Active and Healthy Ageing, Herakleion, Greece: 'Solidarity' Association of Alzheimer's Disease of Herakleion.
Prouskas, C., Theleriti, M., Vougiouka, A., and Vassou, V. (2012) *Guide for the Inclusion of Gender Mainstreaming in Greek Municipalities Focusing on Socially Disadvantaged Women Budgeting*, Athens: General Secretariat for Gender Equality.
Rapti, V. (2007) The postwar Greek welfare model within the context of southern European welfare, in G. Hagemann *Reciprocity and Redistribution. Work and Welfare Reconsidered*, Pisa: Pisa University Press, pp 43–60.

Reuters (2020) Greece confirms first coronavirus case, a woman back from Milan, 26 February [online], Available from: https://www.reuters.com/article/us-china-health-greece-idUSKCN20K1IA

Sakellariou, E. (2015) *National Report For Young Caregivers Who Belong to Special National and Ethnic Groups*, Family and Child Care Center.

Sextant (1998) *COPE – Country Report for Greece*, Athens: Sextant.

Sidiropoulou, M. (2009) Medicine today: prevention as a measure to protect public health, *Medical Issues*, 56, Thessaloniki: Medical Association of Thessaloniki.

Tinios, P. (2017) Greece: forced transformation in a deep crisis, in B. Greve (ed), *Long-term Care for the Elderly in Europe: Development and Prospects*, London: Taylor & Francis, pp 93–106.

Ziomas, D., Sakellis, I., Spyropoulou, N., and Bouzas, N. (2016) *ESPN Thematic Report on Work-Life Balance Measures for Persons of Working Age with Dependent Relatives – Greece*, Brussels: European Social Policy Network [online], Available from: http://ec.europa.eu/social/BlobServlet?docId=15825&langId=en

9

Long-term care of older people in residential care settings in Ireland during waves 1 and 2 of the COVID-19 pandemic: lessons (still to be) learned

Sara Burke, Katharine Schulmann, Virpi Timonen, and Eimir Hurley

Introduction

The arrival of COVID-19 was a major shock to health systems globally, and had immediate and major effects on the Irish health system (Government of Ireland, 2020; WHO, 2020). COVID-19 highlighted pre-existing deficiencies and inequalities in the health care system and broader society and resulted in many agile health system responses (Burke et al, 2020; Department of Health, 2020a; Murray, 2020). The pandemic hit during the second year of implementation of a major Irish health reform programme, known as Sláintecare – a 10-year plan to deliver universal access to timely, integrated care (Houses of the Oireachtas Committee on the Future of Healthcare, 2017; Department of Health, 2018b; Department of Health, 2019).

As part of Ireland's whole-of-Government coordinated approach, the National Public Health Emergency Team (NPHET), and HSE National Crisis Management Teams for COVID-19 were convened and commenced their work at the end of January 2020 within days of confirmation of Europe's first cases (Department of Health, 2020b). NPHET was chaired by the Chief Medical Officer and advised by a Coronavirus Expert Advisory Group (CEAG) (Department of Health, 2020c). Its remit was to oversee and provide national direction, guidance, support, and expert advice on the development and implementation of a strategy to contain COVID-19 in Ireland (Department of Health, 2020c).

On 12 March 2020, the government announced immediate closure of schools, colleges and childcare facilities, cancelling of indoor mass gatherings of 100 people or more and outdoor mass gatherings of more than 500 people and a strong encouragement for people to work remotely (Department of the Taoiseach, 2020a; (Pierce, 2020; Nolan et al, 2021). On 16 March 2020, the government published 'Ireland's National Action Plan in response to COVID-19' (Department of the Taoiseach, 2020b). The Plan set out a whole-of-society response and the mobilisation of resources across Government and society to fight the spread of the virus (Department of the Taoiseach, 2020b). Delay phase measures were intensified on 27 March and Ireland moved into a mitigation phase through what are referred to as 'stay at home' measures, whereby people were advised to stay at home except for specific reasons including to shop for food, essential household goods, collect medical supplies or attend medical appointments, take care of essential family needs, and exercise within 2 kilometres of home. Only workers providing essential services could travel to work. People over 70 years of age and those at very high risk of severe illness from COVID-19 were advised to 'cocoon', advice that many older adults understood as a government directive to confine themselves to living indoors (Department of the Taoiseach, 2020a; Pierce, 2020).

While it is not feasible to give a detailed account of the pandemic measures that followed during the rest of 2020 and in 2021, it is useful to note that the lockdowns in Ireland were more severe and lasted longer than in most other EU countries (Nolan et al, 2021). A particularly noteworthy feature of the lockdowns in Ireland were the long-lasting and severe restrictions on freedom of movement which many older adults and their families interpreted as extending even to situations where there was a great need for care and support (Casey, 2021). Nursing homes experienced lockdowns for even longer stretches with the result that residents (and in some instances staff) were unable to see family members in person for extended periods of time.

In part due to public pushback following the protracted and severe restrictions in 2020, the government decided in December 2020 to provide the people of Ireland with a so-called 'meaningful Christmas' (in other words, to ease restrictions for the festive season), with the result that COVID-19 cases increased rapidly in the early months of 2021, leading to many deaths, predominantly among the older population and in congregated settings. By February 2021, 1,543 COVID-19 deaths were recorded in care homes, comprising 40 per cent of all COVID-19 deaths (CSO, 2022). Of the total deaths recorded in care homes, 369 occurred in January 2021 at the height of the Delta wave (CSO, 2022). Ireland effectively went from having one of the lowest rates of cases in Europe in autumn 2020, to among the highest in January 2021. The surge in early 2021 led to further severe restrictions that lasted until summer 2021, by which time the vaccination programme had resulted in a very high proportion of the adult population being vaccinated.

The pandemic brought into sharp focus existing deficiencies and inequalities in the Irish health and social care system. These include (a) a failure to implement policies on the delivery of universal access to integrated healthcare; (b) the lack of coordination between levels and institutions of governance; (c) lack of State regulatory oversight of majority private/voluntary sector long-term care providers; (d) the inadequacies of the long-term care system, in particular the still strong emphasis on residential care and shortcoming within that sector; (e) the paternalistic discourses and practices that frame older adults as vulnerable to the point of erasing their personhood and existence as persons with social needs.

The first and second features – failure to implement reform and the lack of coordination – in turn reflect the broader problem of policy non-implementation and sectoral (mis)alignment in health and social care in Ireland whereby the lack of structured coordination between levels and sectors marks the healthcare system as a whole (Barry et al, 2021; Thomas et al, 2021). The residential care (nursing homes) sector in Ireland suffers from inadequacies in staffing and infrastructure – features that the pandemic accentuated (Pierce, 2020). The paternalistic management of the COVID-19 crisis in Irish residential care settings evinces the ongoing predominance of the 'medical model' in the care of older people. These features will be elaborated after a short overview of the residential care sector.

Residential care for older adults in Ireland

Most older people in Ireland live independently at home and care for themselves. As the role of the family has changed with increasing numbers of women in the workforce, families in Ireland increasingly rely on the formal care sector (Timonen & Doyle, 2008). Similar to many welfare states across Europe, there has been a move since the 1980s to deinstitutionalise and to facilitate people to live in the community (Timonen & Doyle, 2008). However, this intent of deinstitutionalisation has not been properly implemented due to failure to invest in home and community care services that could enable more people to live in their own homes (Timonen et al, 2012). State-funded homecare is limited and hard to access, and many people pay private home care agencies out of pocket for formal care at home (McDonald et al 2019). The bulk of public investment for formal care for older people is directed to residential (nursing home) care.

The delivery of residential long-term care (LTC) in Ireland has been marred with controversy, from underfunding, to poor State provision historically supplemented by voluntary sector (often religious) providers, to more recent privatisation of nursing home care (Burke, 2009). The Nursing Home Support Scheme (NHSS) was introduced in 2009 in response to outcry about illegal fee charging practices, with the aim of providing consistency in how nursing home care is funded by the State and individuals (Department of Health and Children, 2009). While major improvements were achieved through the introduction of the NHSS and a statutory body tasked with monitoring standards (the Health Information and Quality Authority, HIQA), the stated ambition of moving away from emphasis on residential care (towards more home and community care) has not been achieved despite multiple political commitments over several decades (Timonen et al, 2012).

The introduction of the NHSS made residential care a statutory entitlement. There is no comparable entitlement to home care, despite political consensus on the need for the same since at least 2017 when the State's 10-year health and social care programme (Sláintecare) was published (Houses of the Oireachtas Committee on the Future of Healthcare, 2017). Universal home care is one of the programme's recommendations. Amidst health officials' preoccupation with the pandemic, the implementation of the Sláintecare programme has slowed. It has also been marked by interdepartmental conflicts, resulting in the resignation of the director of the programme and several members of the board in the second half of 2021, leading the Minister for Health to establish a new governance structure to oversee the quasi-governmental body. As a result, 5 years and halfway into the reform programme, State funding for home and community care continues to be subject to political will and annual availability rather than being needs-driven. Furthermore, the home care model being pursued by the current government (in 2022) deviates from Sláintecare's recommendation of publicly funded universal access to home care, mimicking instead the NHSS's contributory model.

The executive arm of the health and social care systems, the Health Service Executive (HSE) administers the NHSS but the contract is between the older person and the nursing home. HIQA sets the standards, but has no role in setting the price and has no powers to investigate complaints. The price of private nursing home care is negotiated on a case-by-case basis by the National Treatment Purchase Fund, which was established in 2002 (Burke, 2019). Public nursing home care is delivered through HSE-run public LTC facilities, which are funded out of the exchequer through the overall HSE budget. These different funders, providers, and regulators of care result in a complicated system that is hard for (prospective) residents and their families to navigate and also poses challenges for providers to deliver high quality care.

Current nursing home fees do not take into account dependency levels, which has implications for care of residents with greater needs. Public nursing home costs are set out by the HSE and are largely determined by historic running costs (Department of Health, 2018a) whereas rates paid by the State to private nursing homes are negotiated by the National Treatment Purchase Fund (NTPF) without proper consideration of the range of needs. Private nursing homes are paid less than public ones, and residents in private nursing homes can find it difficult to access public services such as public health nursing, occupational therapy, and physiotherapy – residents often have to pay additional fees for such services.

In 2016, HIQA's National Residential Care Standards for Older People gave until 2021 to refurbish, upgrade, or replace public facilities in order to reach compliance with the standards (HIQA, 2012, 2016). In 2019, there were plans for 400 new publicly provided beds in long stay, dementia and rehabilitation facilities, with €265 million earmarked to spend on this by 2021 in Phase 1 of Project Ireland 2040 (Government of Ireland, 2018). This included the upgrade or replacement of over 58 Community Nursing Units (HSE, 2019). More public nursing home facilities have been promised, but refurbishment and replacement has not kept up with standards (HIQA, 2019). In 2019, a HIQA report detailed the reasons for the closure of nursing homes including 'the sustainability of the financial model underpinning smaller centres, financial implications of achieving regulatory compliance – particularly the requirement to provide improved living space for residents from 2021' (HIQA, 2019).

In 2020, there were 576 registered nursing homes in Ireland, with approximately 32,000 residential places; private entities have become, over time, by far the largest providers in the sector, managing eight out of ten beds nationally (HIQA, 2020b). While the average number of beds in nursing homes nationally in 2020 was 56, they ranged in size from as small as nine beds to the largest centre which had 184 beds. There is considerable variation in the type of nursing home accommodation available across the country. Many of the newer nursing homes provide single en suite bedrooms and have ample communal and outdoor spaces for residents. Some of the older facilities – many operated by the HSE and voluntary providers – are reliant on multi-occupancy rooms (where residents share bedrooms and bathrooms). It is easy to see how these features proved problematic during a pandemic that necessitated physical distancing and infection control measures (HIQA, 2020c).

Nursing Homes Ireland (NHI), the representative body of private and voluntary nursing homes, has requested annually that the Government should lead in establishing a forum on LTC, in light of the requirement for a better and more integrated working relationship between the State and the entire nursing home sector (Houses of the Oireachtas Special Committee on COVID-19 Response, 2020c). This lack of consistent coordination between sectors and levels of governance and provision is another feature of the Irish LTC system that proved problematic during the pandemic. The next section provides a summary of pandemic management in Ireland with a specific reference to the residential care sector.

Residential care in Ireland during the pandemic

The pandemic exposed how reliant the Irish public health system is on the acute hospital system to deliver care. In 2017, occupancy rates for acute beds in Ireland were at 94.5 per cent, the highest of all OECD-28 countries reporting the metric (OECD-28 average = 75.2 per cent) (Organisation for Economic Cooperation and Development, 2019a). Despite increasing since 2012, the number of hospital beds remains low, at 2.9 per 1,000 population (compared to an EU average of 5.1) (Organisation for Economic Cooperation and Development, 2019b).

In anticipation of the expected surge in hospitalisations, efforts in February and March 2020, focused on increasing bed capacity in the acute hospital sector. This involved freeing up capacity in public hospitals and reaching an agreement that made all private hospitals available to the public health system, at the cost of over €100 million a month (WHO Regional Office for Europe European Commission and European Observatory on Health Systems and Policies, 2020). Another initiative designed to free up hospital beds was the transfer of patients from the acute hospital system to nursing homes in March 2020. Approximately 800 people in hospital were discharged to nursing homes during this period without having been tested for COVID-19 unless they were symptomatic (Houses of the Oireachtas Special Committee on COVID-19 Response, 2020b, 2020c). The large scale discharge of patients from the acute system to the nursing home sector, which does not have the clinical resources of the acute hospital system, was later heavily criticised (Houses of the Oireachtas Special Committee on COVID-19 Response, 2020b). The Department of Health and the HSE stated that older people were discharged in adherence to guidelines published by the HSE on 10 March 2020, in which the testing of asymptomatic patients was not yet advised (Houses of the Oireachtas Special Committee on COVID-19 Response, 2020b). Although follow-up data on each individual person who was transferred was never collected, there is consensus among experts that inadequate risk assessment protocols contributed to the subsequent proliferation of outbreaks in nursing homes.

Coordination in health and social care is important at a number of different levels, and across sectors: among relevant government departments, between the policymakers and executive agency tasked with provision (the Health Services Executive), and between public and private actors involved in the provision of services. Responsibility for Ireland's public health policy lies with the Office of the Chief Medical Officer in the Department of Health and the HSE's public health departments. While the HSE runs public nursing homes and largely funds private and voluntary homes, it does not have authority or a legislative basis for oversight of private and voluntary residential centres. The legal responsibility for care rests with the nursing home provider. Considering that 77 per cent of nursing homes (and 79 per cent of nursing home beds) are operated by private/voluntary providers, this lack of public sector oversight perpetuates a significant regulatory 'black box' at the heart of the State's system of care for older people (Houses of the Oireheactas Special Committee on COVID-19 Response, 2020c). The disjointed structure of powers and responsibilities gave rise to great difficulties, especially in the early stages of responding to the pandemic in residential care settings.

There is a lack of a specific national structure or clinical oversight of the care of residents in nursing homes with differences between types of provider (public, private, and voluntary) and place of provider (for example, some community geriatricians, who are often hospital based, have made links with local nursing homes, but this is neither consistent nor nationwide). Individual homes have a system where they have GPs or medical officers assigned who take responsibility for clinical governance. The lack of statutory clinical oversight of care for residents in private nursing homes was one of the biggest weaknesses highlighted by COVID-19. The current model of private residential care for older persons has no formal clinical governance links with the HSE, that is, there is no national clinical oversight of nursing home care (Houses of the Oireachtas Special Committee on COVID-19 Response, 2020d). As a consequence, the infrastructure required by the HSE to support the private sector was under-resourced and became increasingly challenged at the start of the pandemic (Houses of the Oireachtas Special Committee on COVID-19 Response, 2020c).

Nursing Homes Ireland reported a lack of engagement and poor communication on the part of the HSE and the Department of Health in the crucial first weeks of the pandemic (Houses of the Oireachtas Special Committee on COVID-19 Response, 2020b). Private nursing home providers responded to public criticism and lack of direction from health officials by asserting their own proactive stance in infection control and other measures. For instance, on 6 March 2020, Nursing Homes Ireland advised a blanket ban on visitors in its member nursing homes. Despite Nursing Homes Ireland's evident concerns about transmission of the virus in nursing homes, the NPHET delayed recommending visitor restrictions in all nursing homes in the State (public, private, and voluntary) for another week, and not before first directly contradicting Nursing Homes Ireland's advisory (Department of Health, 2020b).

Following initial stumbles, the HSE in coordination with Nursing Homes Ireland and the network of regional healthcare authorities (Community Healthcare Organisations) set up Crisis Management Teams to support nursing homes, especially those dealing with outbreaks of the virus. The Crisis Management Teams provided management support, procurement of personal protective equipment (PPE) and other supplies, support with staffing, including in some cases the deployment of HSE staff (Department of Health, 2020b).

At the level of the management of residents with COVID-19 and the protection of residents exposed to the virus, the inadequacy of physical infrastructure and staffing featured prominently. The current design and layout of many facilities acted as a barrier to ensuring adequate infection prevention and control (COVID-19 Nursing Homes Expert Panel, 2020). The public health emergency threw into sharp relief the need for nursing homes to meet new physical environment regulations aimed at providing residents with more living space, dignity, comfort, and safety (HIQA, 2020b).

Most nursing homes have limited or inequitable access to the expertise of consultant geriatricians, old age psychiatrists, gerontological nursing, and allied health professional expertise (Houses of the Oireachtas Special Committee on COVID-19 Response, 2020c). End-of-life care/palliative care and expertise is not universally available in care settings. There is long-standing unanimity on the need for adequate staffing/minimum staffing requirements, contingency plans and training of staff, and the persistent failure to address these was showcased during the pandemic. The Department of Health-commissioned COVID-19 Nursing Homes Expert Panel, which consulted stakeholders as part of its review of the national and international response to the first wave of the pandemic in nursing homes, highlighted the need to support healthcare assistants at work and in their living standards. It also highlighted the importance of utilising qualified nursing staff to their full potential and optimising their scope of practice and role of the nurse in the care of the older person (COVID-19 Nursing Homes Expert Panel, 2020).

Despite the Expert Panel's exhortations to improve practice across these and other domains, the management of COVID-19 in nursing homes was strongly marked by inadequacy of staff, lack of training for some, not to mention periodic shortages of PPE in the earlier stages of the pandemic. The Expert Panel's findings reinforced prior independent and government-commissioned reports citing inadequate numbers and skill mix of staff in nursing homes (Browne, 2016; Houses of the Oireachtas Committee on the Future of Healthcare, 2017). The Expert Panel's report called on government actors to use the lessons of the pandemic as an opportunity to address long-standing staffing issues.

The major difficulties in obtaining adequate PPE and testing capacity reflect the general weaknesses of health sector procurement processes and inadequate infrastructural investment. In many cases the solutions were short-termist and relied on outsourcing, for instance, sending COVID-19 tests to foreign companies, with the result that at several stages (especially in 2020), obtaining test results took over 10 days (effectively negating any rationale for testing). While waiting for their (often negative) test results, nursing home residents were kept in maximum feasible isolation, an arrangement that especially those with cognitive impairments found impossible to understand and hard to bear (Hennelly & Cahill, 2020). There is consensus that a more comprehensive and rapid testing strategy should have been in place in nursing homes and particularly for the transfer of patients from the acute hospital system (Houses of the Oireachtas Special Committee on COVID-19 Response, 2020d).

The pandemic exposed shortages in staff and staff skills mix in Ireland's nursing homes. Many nursing homes were significantly challenged in maintaining safe staffing levels and managing enhanced infection prevention measures (HIQA, 2020a). This was especially problematic in terms of enabling staffing to be organised to care for residents in separate, self-contained groups; and maintaining staffing levels in the event of sudden and unplanned absences. Many nursing homes were hampered in their response to the virus due to the impact of senior staff and management falling ill with COVID-19 (HIQA, 2020b). Tensions arose early between Nursing Homes Ireland and the HSE at what was seen as the poaching of staff from the nursing home sector to work in the acute hospital sector during the HSE recruitment campaign 'Be on Call for Ireland', launched on 17 March 2020 (Houses of the Oireachtas Special Committee on COVID-19 Response, 2020c). Nursing Homes Ireland followed by launching a separate recruitment campaign for private and voluntary nursing homes (Nursing Homes Ireland, 2020).

The impact of the pandemic and the pandemic response on the Irish care workforce has been heavily gendered (Wickhan, 2022). As in most countries, women make up the majority of care staff, and while no official national data is available on the subject, research by advocacy groups points to a significant percentage of the workforce in the private sector coming from migrant backgrounds (MRCI, 2012; MRCI, 2015). Care staff with families and with young children in particular found themselves under profound strain for many reasons. These included having to self-isolate away from family members in order to comply with nursing homes' infection control guidelines, trying to arrange childcare while crèches across the country were closed and alternatives were slow to be provided by the State, and coping with often inadequate sick leave benefits and overwork due to colleagues' absences (Houses of the Oireheactas Special Committee on COVID-19 Response, 2020a). Despite their alacrity in imposing many rigid restrictions, the NPHET were slow to recommend mandatory face masks and there were high numbers of cases and deaths in nursing homes as the early focus of the crisis was on public health measures and freeing up beds in the acute sector in anticipation of the health system being overwhelmed by COVID-19 cases. The advice to over 70-year-olds and vulnerable groups to 'cocoon' resulted in increased fragility, decreased mobility, feelings of isolation and loneliness, and poor quality of life (Costello et al, 2021; Ward et al, 2021). The paternalism of the cocooning measures and the failure to address the crisis in nursing homes reflect broader societal ageism.

Ireland's preparation for the pandemic between January and March 2020 was heavily criticised as being too focused on public health measures and acute hospitals, with little emphasis placed on the nursing home sector. As a response to the high number of deaths in nursing homes in the early months of the pandemic, between May and June 2020, there were three sittings of the Irish government's Special Committee on COVID-19 focused on nursing homes. The Committee set out to examine the response to the pandemic in the nursing home sector and whether nursing home residents were adequately protected. An interim report summarising the oral testimonials of representatives of the HSE, HIQA, Department of Health, among other stakeholders, as well as written submissions to the Committee, was published in July 2020 (Houses of the Oireachtas Special Committee on COVID-19 Response, 2020d), followed by the committee's final report and recommendations in October 2020 (Houses of the Oireachtas Special Committee on COVID-19 Response, 2020a). It found that at the start of the pandemic, there was a lack of substantial engagement, guidance, and two-way dialogue between nursing homes, the HSE and the Department of Health. It also found that the guidance issued to nursing homes from January was inadequate, lacking a coherent overarching response. Specifically, it found that visitation protocols were incoherent, contradictory, and initially lagging behind the sector's own sentiments and recommendations, which led to further confusion. The work of the Special Committee on COVID-19 Response, which sat between May and October 2020, was the only State-sanctioned effort to date to investigate and assess the success of the government's response to the pandemic. To some extent, the parliamentary Joint Committee on Health, which held its first session on 1 October 2020, continued the work of the Special Committee, holding hearings on the evolving situation in nursing homes, on testing/tracing capacity, vaccine rollout, workforce planning, progress on implementation of Sláintecare, and so on, but its mandate has not been explicitly to examine the government's response to the pandemic but rather to hold hearings on issues affecting the healthcare sector more generally (Houses of the Oireachtas Committee on Health, 2020e, 2020f, 2020g). So, while the crisis in nursing homes in the first months of the pandemic contributed to the formation of the Special Committee and a degree of introspection among officials and members of parliament, the State's handling of (later stages of) the pandemic has not been subject to any official, comprehensive critical analysis since.

Very early in the pandemic, on 13 March 2020, NPHET recommended visitor restrictions in LTC settings. One of the immediate concerns following the announcement of these restrictions was the impact of social isolation and separation from their families on residents. The HIQA report on the impact of COVID-19 on nursing homes, together with the Alliance of Age Sector NGOs report 'Telling It Like It Is' provided a comprehensive account of the human impact of the virus and of the restrictions on residents, relatives and staff of nursing homes (HIQA, 2020b; Gilbert, 2021). Many residents spoke about missing the human touch of a family member or staff. While some limited visits were permitted in some nursing homes on 'compassionate grounds', such as for families of those residents who were facing the end of their lives, there were strict controls around physical distancing, the use of screens and the number of people that were permitted to visit. The facilitation of such visits was also often constrained by staff shortages. This was extremely challenging for residents who may have been accustomed to seeing people every day and who looked forward to these social occasions. During the summer of 2020, there was much media and public attention on those whose loved ones died in nursing homes during the height of the COVID-19 pandemic in spring/summer 2020 and the impact this had on those dying as well as on their family and friends. There was innovation in trying to ameliorate the impact of isolation measures, such as the use of tablet computers to talk to family and friends, not to mention the exceptional efforts by care home staff and carers to provide comfort, but nothing could replace the time spent with loved ones in person during their last hours. There was a very public depiction in the media of people visiting and seeing their loved ones for the last time through nursing home windows.

The HIQA report also highlighted that heightened measures around infection prevention and control meant that nursing homes became more clinical in nature, with significant changes to the overall environment (HIQA, 2020b). For example, bright yellow signage warned people of infection risks, staff had to wear PPE, and clinical waste bins were much more prevalent throughout centres. After years of moving towards a more homely, social model of care, the pandemic measures brought strong reinforcement of the medical model of care. These infection controls involved many residents being largely confined to their own bedrooms, which meant that in addition to being externally cut off from family and loved ones, they were also internally restricted and cut off from their friends in the nursing home.

The Oireachtas Special Committee set up to examine the government response to COVID-19 heard witness testimony and received written submissions from those in the nursing home sector in relation to the profound impact the virus and the restrictions put in place in the homes had on residents and relatives. The CEO of Nursing Homes Ireland told the Special Committee that the impact of an outbreak was frightening for many residents, and that for those with dementia, the arrival of people in full PPE was terrifying. Serious shortages of staff meant that there was little, if any, time to provide psychological support to residents in facilities where many had died. For families with relatives who were extremely ill or dying, the inability to visit or even to talk to their loved ones by phone was a source of considerable distress and frustration. The Irish Hospice Foundation told the Oireachtas Committee that many of the experiences of dying, death, and bereavement during the COVID-19 pandemic fell short of people's expressed wishes in relation to what they want for themselves or their loved ones at end-of-life (Houses of the Oireachtas Special Committee on COVID-19 Response, 2020d).

Despite the failings of pandemic management in residential care, it is important to acknowledge the evident drive by many actors and institutions to respond quickly, attempts at thoroughness and 'learnings' from mistakes. For example, Ireland is one of the few countries that undertook a mass testing programme in LTC. Following a recommendation of the NPHET on 17 April 2020, all staff in long-term residential facilities was tested; 95,900 tests were completed with a positivity rate of 5.5 per cent (Department of Health, 2020c). This was followed by a mass testing strategy which commenced 21 April 2020, with testing in all LTC facilities completed by 15 May 2020. The HSE introduced a weekly rolling programme of testing staff in nursing homes for a 4-week period to track and target any emerging infection which continued into Autumn 2020 (WHO Regional Office for Europe European Commission and European Observatory on Health Systems and Policies, 2020). Such measures speak to attempts to follow good practices, albeit they were hampered by various inefficiencies and deficits in testing capacity.

Comparative data on COVID-19 related deaths are fraught with difficulties due to differences in testing and categorisation of what is included in a 'COVID-19 death', as well as in the timeliness of reporting (Unruh et al, 2021). For example, did the person die of or with COVID-19? How does one know if testing was not in place? Data from the Central Statistics Offices show that by February 2021 there were 1,543 COVID-19 deaths recorded in care homes (40 per cent of all COVID-19 deaths), 369 of which, nearly one quarter, occurred in January 2021 at the height of the Delta wave (Central Statistics Office, 2022). HIQA reported a huge spike in unexpected deaths in nursing homes compared to previous years (HIQA, 2020c). Despite the challenges of reporting comparative data, multiple sources compiling mortality data show Ireland with a relatively modest excess mortality rate due to COVID-19, with the result that average life expectancy did not decline greatly compared to some other European countries. Overall, these data indicate that the relatively strict and lengthy social distancing measures enacted in Ireland succeeded to a great extent in protecting people from dying from the virus, in keeping people alive. The question that remains is, at what cost? Older people, particularly those living in nursing homes, were stripped of their autonomy and did not have a say in how they wished to live out the months and years of the pandemic (a period of time that constitutes a very large share of their likely remaining lifespan). Arguably, there is a particularly strong moral imperative to allow older persons in their very final years and months much greater latitude in autonomous decision making than was granted during the pandemic in Ireland. As it was, older persons were not allowed any such latitude in an environment of medically imposed restrictions that always put 'safety' (against the virus) first vis-à-vis any other priority, even if it was the last wish of a person to be allowed a degree of 'risk' in how they spent their remaining time.

Although the response of the regulator (HIQA) to the pandemic was delayed, HIQA wrote to the providers and asked them to review the contingency plans they had in place to manage an outbreak. It then acted quite quickly undertaking a programme of inspections to assess the preparedness and contingency planning for outbreaks in those nursing homes that had not yet had a suspected or confirmed case of the disease. This was followed by a separate targeted programme of risk-based inspections focusing on those nursing homes that were most impacted by COVID-19. As part of its response, a quality assurance process was set up, whereby all nursing homes were phoned on a fortnightly basis by an inspector of social services. These calls were to assess the welfare of the residents, how nursing homes were coping, any concerns they had, and any deficiencies identified in their ability to sustain a safe, high-quality service. It was through these interactions that inspectors were able to determine where nursing homes were struggling, for example, in relation to access to equipment such as PPE or advice. HIQA escalated all risks to the HSE for their support. The Infection Prevention and Control Hub, also established by HIQA, provided a direct line for staff to offer guidance on infection control and the frequent revisions to the HSPC guidance, as well as escalating high-risk centres to the HSE (HIQA, 2020b). In short, although greatly hampered by broader structural problems, several examples can be identified of actors and agencies who 'tried their best' in the midst of an unprecedented crisis within what is generally acknowledged to be a health and social care system with many challenges.

Lessons and challenges for the future

A failure to implement long-promised health system reforms including timely, universal access to care in the community pre-COVID-19 contributed to many of the difficulties encountered during the pandemic. The fragmented nature of the structural relationship between key State actors and the residential care sector also led to delays in response to the crisis in nursing homes. A key learning from the response to the crisis is that nursing homes should be prioritised early on in public health emergency planning, and that clearer lines of communication between the different organisations are needed.

The pandemic highlighted key weaknesses in the nursing home setting, especially in terms of deficits in clinical governance. Private nursing homes are generally clinically supported by local GPs and therefore do not have a formalised clinical governance relationship in place with the HSE. Other weaknesses exposed include the lack of skilled staffing, the lack of minimum staffing requirements, and inadequate premises especially in terms of ability to isolate suspected cases. The State's responsibility to respond to the public health emergency created the need for the HSE to set up a structured support system in line with NPHET recommendations to build sector resilience. From the end of March 2020, the HSE agreed to provide substantial support for the private nursing home sector. Supports provided included new HSE national and regional governance structures, the setting up of a variety of systems to provide immediate practical support such as PPE and oxygen logistics, and the deployment of crisis management teams to oversee the response where outbreaks occurred (Department of Health, 2020c).

Against this backdrop of decision-making and structures of provision, it is perhaps not surprising that the management of COVID-19 in nursing homes became distinctly paternalistic and medicalised in character. The overwhelming prerogative was protection of residents' physical health against the virus, to the point where all other needs of older persons were negated. This led to scenes such as people spending the last days of their lives in isolation, and 'interacting' with relatives through windows and screens.

While there appears to have been a degree of 'learnings' and adaptation in some regards, question marks remain about the degree of reform and meaningful improvements for older persons and for people working in residential care settings. In the absence of universal access to a statutory scheme for homecare, it remains the case that there is no formal legislative basis for support and care in the community, despite several decades of policy commitments and recommendations to remove perverse incentives that de facto incentivise entry into residential care. The NHSS means that the State continues to provide more support to older people who live in residential care than those who want to live in the community where infection control would be more feasible and more humane in the event of similar future pandemics.

Current financing arrangements continue to 'push' people into nursing home care as there is an absence of an adequate state funded home care scheme and the continuum of integrated care required to care for older people towards the end of their live. Sláintecare, Ireland's 10-year plan for health reform – which outlines a path to universal access to timely, quality care with a very strong emphasis on prevention, public health, and providing as much care as possible in the home or close to the home – is yet to be implemented (Houses of the Oireachtas Committee on the Future of Healthcare, 2017; Department of Health, 2019; Thomas et al, 2021). The implementation of a high-quality continuum of care for older people which prioritises enabling people to live at home requires political will and significant public resources to deliver changes in how care for older people is provided. Despite some lessons learned, many of the challenges in the care of the older population experienced during COVID-19 are likely to be repeated during future crises due to the persistent problems in the structure and organisation of health and social services provision in Ireland, including the failure to resource properly alternatives to residential care in the form of home and community care.

References

Barry, S., Stach, M., Thomas, S., and Burke, S. (2021) Understanding service reorganisation in the Irish health & social care system from 1998 to 2020: lessons for reform and transformation, *HRB Open Research*, 4 [online], Available from: https://hrbopenresearch.org/articles/4-106

Browne, M. (2016) *Responding to the Support & Care Needs of our Older Population: Shaping an Agenda for Future Action*, Dublin: Sage Advocacy [online], Available from: https://www.sageadvocacy.ie/media/1124/report_of_forum_on_ltc_for_older_people.pdf

Burke, S. (2009) *Irish Apartheid: Healthcare Inequality in Ireland*, Dublin: New Island.

Burke, S., Brugha, R., and Thomas, S. (2019) The National Treatment Purchase Fund – a success for some patients yet a public policy failure? *Administration*, 67, 47–69.

Burke, S., Thomas, S., Stach, M., Kavanagh, P., Magahy, L., Johnston, B., and Barry, S. (2020) Health system foundations for Sláintecare implementation in 2020 and beyond – co-producing a Sláintecare living implementation framework with evaluation: learning from the Irish health system's response to COVID-19. A mixed-methods study protocol, *HRB Open Research*, 3, 70 [online], Available from: https://pubmed.ncbi.nlm.nih.gov/33728398/

Casey, O., Doyle, O., Kenny, D., and Lyons, D. (2021) *Ireland's Emergency Powers During the COVID-19 Pandemic: Report prepared for The Irish Human Rights and Equality Commission by The COVID-19 Law and Human Rights Observatory*, Dublin: The Irish Human Rights and Equality Commission.

Central Statistics Office (2022) COVID-19 Deaths and Cases Series 38, Dublin: CSO, Table 2.2A.

Costello, N., Ward, M., O'Mahoney, P., and Kenny, R. (2021) In their own words: The Voices of Older Irish People in the COVID-19 Pandemic, The Irish Longitudinal Study on Ageing, Dublin, Available from: https://tilda.tcd.ie/publications/reports/pdf/Report_C19ParticipantVoices.pdf

COVID-19 Nursing Homes Expert Panel (2020) *Examination of Measures to 2021. Report to the Minister for Health (August 2020)* [online], Available from: https://www.gov.ie/en/publication/3af5a-COVID-19-nursing-homes-expert-panel-final-report/

Department of Health (2018a) *Long stay Activity Statistics 2017, Ireland*, Dublin: Department of Health.

Department of Health (2018b) *Sláintecare Implementation Strategy*, Dublin: Department of Health.

Department of Health (2019) *Sláintecare Action Plan 2019*, Dublin: Department of Health.

Department of Health (2020a) *Briefing to the Minister June 2020*, Dublin: Department of Health.

Department of Health (2020b) *Overview of the Health System Response to Date: Long-Term Residential Healthcare Settings*, NPHET Meeting Paper, 22 May [online], Available from: https://www.lenus.ie/handle/10147/627723

Department of Health (2020c) *Summary Paper Provided to Special Committee on COVID-19 Response*, 15 June [online] Available from: https://www.gov.ie/en/collection/8d7df-department-of-health-nursing-homes-papers-special-COVID-19-committee-june-2020/

Department of Health and Children (2009) *Nursing Home Support Scheme* [online], Available from: http://www.dohc.ie/issues/fair_deal/

Department of the Taoiseach (2020a) Briefing on the government's response to COVID-19, 28 March [online], Available from: https://www.gov.ie/en/publication/cfc502-daily-briefing-on-the-governments-response-to-COVID-19-saturday-28-m/

Department of the Taoiseach (2020b) Government publishes national action plan on COVID-19, 16 March [online], Available from: https://www.gov.ie/en/publication/47b727-government-publishes-national-action-plan-on-COVID-19

Gilbert, M. (2021) *'Telling It Like It Is': What Older People Told Us About Their Experience of COVID-19, and What Ireland Should Do About It*, Dublin: Alliance of Age Sector NGOs.

Government of Ireland (2018) *Project Ireland 2040 National Planning Framework*, Dublin: Government of Ireland.

Government of Ireland (2020) *National Action Plan in Response to COVID-19*, Dublin: Government of Ireland.

Hennelly, N. and Cahill, S. (2020) The impact of COVID-19 on people living with dementia in Ireland, International Long-Term Care Policy Network, CPEC-LSE [online], Available from: https://ltcCOVID.org/wp-content/uploads/2020/06/COVID-19-and-Dementia-Ireland.pdf

HIQA – Health Information and Quality Authority (2012) *National Standards for Safer and Better Healthcare*, Ireland: Health Information and Quality Authority.

HIQA (2016) *Statutory Notifications. Guidance for Registered Providers and Persons in Charge of Designated Centres*, Ireland: Health Information and Quality Authority.

HIQA (2019) *Overview Report on the Regulation of Designated Centres for Older Persons – 2018*, Ireland: Health Information and Quality Authority.

HIQA (2020a) *The Impact of COVID-19 on Nursing Homes in Ireland*, Ireland: Health Information and Quality Authority [online], Available from: https://www.hiqa.ie/sites/default/files/2020-07/The-impact-of-COVID-19-on-nursing-homes-in-Ireland_0.pdf

HIQA (2020b) The impact of COVID-19 on nursing homes in Ireland (July 2020), Ireland: Health Information and Quality Authority. Available: https://www.hiqa.ie/sites/default/files/2020-07/The-impact-of-COVID-19-on-nursing-homes-in-Ireland_0.pdf

HIQA (2020c) The impact of COVID-19 on nursing homes in Ireland. https://www.hiqa.ie/sites/default/files/2020-07/The-impact-of-COVID-19-on-nursing-homes-in-Ireland_0.pdf:HIQA

Houses of the Oireachtas Committee on Health (2020) *Committee on Health*, Dublin: Houses of the Oireachtas [online], Available from: https://www.oireachtas.ie/en/committees/33/health/

Houses of the Oireachtas Committee on the Future of Healthcare (2017) *Houses of the Oireachtas Committee on the Future of Healthcare Sláintecare Report*, May, Dublin: Houses of the Oireachtas.

Houses of the Oireachtas Special Committee on COVID-19 Response (2020a) *Special Committee on COVID-19 Response: Final Report*, 9 October, Dublin: Houses of the Oireachtas [online], Available from: https://data.oireachtas.ie/ie/oireachtas/committee/dail/33/special_committee_on_COVID_19_response/reports/2020/2020-10-09_final-report-of-the-special-committee-on-COVID-19-response-sccr004_en.pdf

Houses of the Oireachtas Special Committee on COVID-19 Response (2020b) *Special Committee on COVID-19 Response: Debate Record*, 18 June, Dublin: Houses of the Oireachtas [online], Available from: https://data.oireachtas.ie/ie/oireachtas/debateRecord/special_committee_on_COVID-19_response/2020-06-18/debate/mul@/main.pdf

Houses of the Oireachtas Special Committee on COVID-19 Response (2020c) *Special Committee on COVID-19 Response: Debate Record*, 26 May, Dublin: Houses of the Oireachtas [online], Available from: https://data.oireachtas.ie/ie/oireachtas/debateRecord/special_committee_on_COVID-19_response/2020-05-26/debate/mul@/main.pdf

Houses of the Oireachtas Special Committee on COVID-19 Response (2020d) *Special Committee on COVID-19 Response: Interim Report on COVID-19 in Nursing Homes*, 31 July, Dublin: Houses of the Oireachtas [online], Available from: https://data.oireachtas.ie/ie/oireachtas/committee/dail/33/special_committee_on_COVID-19_response/reports/2020/2020-07-31_interim-report-on-COVID-19-in-nursing-homes_en.pdf

Houses of the Oireachtas Special Committee on COVID-19 Response (2020e) *Special Committee on COVID-19 Response: Debate Record*, 25 June, Dublin: Houses of the Oireachtas [online], Available from: https://www.oireachtas.ie/en/debates/debate/special_committee_on_COVID-19_response/2020-06-25/2/

Houses of the Oireachtas Special Committee on COVID-19 Response (2020f) *Special Committee on COVID-19 Response: Debate Record*, 26 May, Dublin: Houses of the Oireachtas [online], Available from: https://data.oireachtas.ie/ie/oireachtas/debateRecord/special_committee_on_COVID-19_response/2020-05-26/debate/mul@/main.pdf

Houses of the Oireachtas Special Committee on COVID-19 Response (2020g) *Special Committee on COVID-19 Response: Interim Report on COVID-19 in Nursing Homes*, 31 July, Dublin: Houses of the Oireachtas [online], Available from: https://data.oireachtas.ie/ie/oireachtas/committee/dail/33/special_committee_on_COVID-19_response/reports/2020/2020-07-31_interim-report-on-COVID-19-in-nursing-homes_en.pdf

HSE (2019) *Health Service Executive National Service Plan 2020*, Dublin: Health Service Executive (HSE).

Mcdonald, A., Lolich, L., Virpi, T., and Warters, A. (2019) Time is more important than anything else: tensions of time in the home care of older adults in Ireland, *International Journal of Care and Caring*, 3(4): 501–15, Available from: https://bristoluniversitypressdigital.com/view/journals/ijcc/3/4/article-p501.xml

MRCI (2012) *Who Cares? The Experience of Migrant Care Workers in Ireland*, Dublin: Migrant Rights Centre Ireland [online], Available from: https://www.mrci.ie/app/uploads/2020/02/Who-Cares-The-experience-of-Migrant-Care-Workers-in-Ireland-Nov-2012.pdf

MRCI (2015) *Migrant Workers in the Home Care Sector: Preparing for the Elder Boom in Ireland*, Dublin: Migrant Rights Centre Ireland [online], Available from: https://www.mrci.ie/app/uploads/2020/01/Migrant-Workers-in-the-Home-Care-Sector-Preparing-for-the-Elder-Boom-in-Ireland.pdf

Murray, D. (2020) Experience of dealing with the COVID-19 crisis will speed up systemic reforms in healthcare, says HSE chief, Interview with HSE chief Paul Reid, *Sunday Business Post*, 9 August 2020, Available from: https://www.businesspost.ie/health/experience-of-dealing-with-the-covid-19-crisis-will-speed-up-systemic-reforms-in-healthcare-says-hs/

Nolan, A., Burke, S., Burke, E., Darker, C., Barry, J., O'Connell, N., Zgaga, L., Mather, L., Nicolson, G., Dempster, M., Graham, C., Crowley, P., O'Connor, C., Tobin, K., and Scally, G. (2021) Obstacles to public health that even pandemics cannot overcome: the politics of COVID-19 on the Island of Ireland, *Irish Studies in International Affairs*, 32: 225–46.

Nursing Homes Ireland (2020) Recruitment drive launched by Nursing Homes Ireland, 17 March [online], Available from: https://nhi.ie/recruitment-drive-launched-by-nursing-homes-ireland/

Organisation for Economic Cooperation and Development (2019a) *Health at a Glance 2019: OECD Indicators* [online], Available from: https://www.oecd.org/en/publications/2019/11/health-at-a-glance-2019_f58fa178.html

Organisation for Economic Cooperation and Development (2019b) *Ireland: Country Health Profile 2019* [online], Available from: https://www.oecd-ilibrary.org/social-issues-migration-health/ireland-country-health-profile-2019_2393fd0a-en;jsessionid=VijZVaub_WbDQQBLyW0FudqJ.ip-10-240-5-120

Pierce, M., Keogh, F., and O'Shea, E. (2020) *The Impact of COVID-19 on People who Use and Provide Long-term Care in Ireland and Mitigating Measures*, 13 May, International Long-Term Care Policy Network [online], Available from: https://ltccovid.org/wp-content/uploads/2020/05/Ireland-COVID-LTC-report-updated-13-May-2020.pdf

Thomas, S., Johnston, B., Barry, S., Siersbaek, R. and Burke, S. (2021) Sláintecare implementation status in 2020: Limited progress with entitlement expansion. *Health Policy*, 125(3), 277–83.

Timonen, V. and Doyle, M. (2008) From the workhouse to the home: evolution of care policy for older people in Ireland, *International Journal of Sociology and Social Policy*, 28, 76–89.

Timonen, V., Doyle, M., and O'Dwyer, C. (2012) Expanded, but not regulated: ambiguity in home-care policy in Ireland, *Health & Social Care in the Community*, 20(3), 310–18.

Unruh, L., Allin, S., Marchildon, G., Burke, S., Barry, S., Siersbaek, R., Thomas, S., Selina, R., Andriy, K., Alexander, M., Merkur, S., Webb, E., and Williams, G. A. (2021) A comparison of health policy responses to the COVID-19 pandemic in Canada, Ireland, the United Kingdom and the United States of America, *Health Policy*, 126(5), 427–37.

Ward, M., O'Mahoney, P., and Kenny, R. (2021) Altered lives in a time of crisis: The impact of the COVID-19 pandemic on the lives of older adults in Ireland Findings from the Irish Longitudinal Study on Ageing. Dublin: TILDA, Available from: https://tilda.tcd.ie/publications/reports/C19ReportKeyFindings/index.php

WHO (2020) *Strengthening the Health System Response to COVID-19: Recommendations for the WHO European Region*, Policy brief, 1 April [online], Available from: http://www.euro.who.int/__data/assets/pdf_file/0003/436350/strengthening-health-system-response-COVID-19.pdf?ua=1

WHO Regional Office for Europe European Commission and European Observatory on Health Systems and Policies (2020) *WHO COVID-19 Health System Response Monitor* [online], Available from: https://eurohealthobservatory.who.int/monitors/hsrm/hsrm-countries/hsrm/ireland

Wickhan, J. (2022) Revaluation of working conditions and wages for essential workers. Country study on Ireland (Annex 3.3.), in Scientific and Quality of Life Policies, European Parliament, Luxembourg (eds) *Publication for the Committee on Employment and Social Affairs, P.D.F.E.*, European Parliament [online], Available from: https://www.europarl.europa.eu/RegData/etudes/STUD/2021/695491/IPOL_STU(2021)695491(ANN03)_EN.pdf

10

Neglecting nursing homes: the management of the pandemic crisis in Italy

Costanzo Ranci, Marco Arlotti, and Stefania Cerea

Introduction

Italy was the first western country to be strongly hit by the COVID-19 outbreak. The first relevant clusters of infection were officially registered in two northern Italian regions (Codogno in Lombardy, and Vo' in Veneto) on 21 February 2020. At that time, scientific information about COVID-19 and its potential dangers was still very scarce. The WHO did not proclaim COVID-19 as a 'high global risk' until 28 February 2020: on that same day, Italy already had 888 officially infected persons, 345 hospitalised COVID-19 patients, 105 patients in intensive therapy units (ICUs), and 21 deaths (open data from Protezione Civile).[1]

Considering the total number of COVID-19 infections during the first phase of the pandemic, the cases counted at the end of May 2020 were 232,639. However, the peak was reached in March 2020, with 113,351, while in the following months, the trend decreased, reaching 'only' 22,893 cases in May 2020 (ISTAT - ISS, 2020).

According to available data, more than 70 per cent of positive cases reported between February and May 2020 were concentrated in a limited number of Northern Italian provinces in which the circulation of the infection was exceptionally high (that is, COVID-19 infection higher than 450 cases per 1000 residents) (ISTAT - ISS, 2020).

The rate of excess deaths provides a more fine-grained analysis of the substantial social impact of the COVID-19 pandemic. Data from the previous years (2015–19), show that a relevant deviation took place in March 2020 (+49.4 per cent) and April 2020 (+36.6 per cent), particularly in Northern Italy (+96.4 per cent in March and +71.7 per cent in April) and among those provinces affected by high circulation of the virus (+122.2 per cent in March and +85.3 per cent in April) (ISTAT - ISS, 2020).

Lombardy was the main Italian region affected by the pandemic (Arlotti et al, 2021). In March 2020, the rate of excess deaths was +190.1 per cent, and +111.9 per cent in April 2020. This deviation was also persistent in May 2020 (+8.6 per cent). It is, therefore, in Lombardy that the pandemic showed its most dramatic consequences. For example, in the province of Bergamo (where in March 2020 the photographs of the army transporting 65 coffins of COVID-19 deaths from the hospital to other cities for overnight burial travelled the world in all media), the mortality excess was +573.6 per cent in March 2020, and +125.7 per cent in April 2020 (ISTAT - ISS, 2020).

The spread of infections in Northern Italy, and especially in Lombardy during the first wave of the pandemic, was presumably due to a variety of factors, including the global economic integration of the area, climate and morphological characteristics favouring a high exposure to environmental risks, high population density and intra-regional mobility, and weak development of territorial health services in Lombardy (Casti et al, 2022).

This evolution of the pandemic had a dramatic impact on the healthcare sector. Since the end of February 2020, the National Health Ministry stated that healthcare facilities (with no further specifications) were required to strictly and systematically comply with standard precautions. Confirmed cases of COVID-19 were hospitalised wherever possible in single isolation rooms. Healthcare professionals in contact with a suspected or confirmed case of COVID-19 were required to wear appropriate PPE (face protection, waterproof gown, gloves). Visits to the patient in hospitals were suspended. However, the massive increase in the number of infected patients in the following weeks made the pressure on hospitals unsustainable. At the beginning of March 2020, for instance, in the Lombardy region, there was a considerable deficiency in ICU beds despite the supply of these beds in this region already being higher than the national average (8.98 per 100,000 inhabitants vs. 8.40 per 100,000 inhabitants at the national level) (Altems, 2020). Also, the availability of ventilators and healthcare staff was inadequate in coping with the strong effects of the epidemic. The pressure on the healthcare system was so intense that the Italian Association of Anesthesiologists (SIAARTI) developed specific ethics recommendations for admission to intensive treatments, and their suspension in exceptional conditions of imbalance between needs and available resources (SIAARTI, 2020).

In the residential care sector, the pandemic's impact was also dramatic. It has been estimated that deaths in nursing homes during the first phase of the pandemic represented 32 per cent of the total number of COVID-19 deaths in the country (Pesaresi, 2020). According to a national survey carried out in April–May 2020 by Istituto Superiore di Sanità (ISS) (ISS, 2020b), a national scientific institution responsible for providing data and consultancy on public health, the mortality rate due to COVID-19 was calculated to be 3.8 per cent at the national level, but rose to 7.5 per cent in Lombardy. Southern regions were only partially affected by the pandemic, with mortality rates lower than the national average (ISS, 2020b). According to a study of the International

Long-term Care Policy Network (based at the London School of Economics) (Comas-Herrera et al, 2020), the only source for comparative data on the impact of COVID-19 on LTC systems,[2] mortality rates due to COVID-19 in nursing homes ranged between 0.5 per cent in Germany, to 6.2 per cent in Spain (France: 2.5 per cent, Sweden: 3.3 per cent, UK: 5.1 per cent).

While these figures show that mortality in nursing homes was very high in Italy, the relative incidence of COVID-19 mortality in nursing homes was not exceptionally high in Lombardy once we weigh it by the incidence of COVID-19 mortality over the total population (our estimation based on 2020 excess mortality data of ISTAT).

Against this background, this chapter presents the impact of the pandemic on the residential care sector in Italy, with a specific focus on Lombardy, the region most seriously hit by COVID-19 in the first wave. After a short description of the sector in the next section, the primary regulation to manage the emergency is discussed: the use of preventive plans, lockdown measures, testing and reporting, management of human and financial resources, and coordination with health services. Finally, in the last section, we investigate the room for future change in the sector's regulation.

The role of residential care within the long-term care system

Italy's long-term care (LTC) policy field is characterised by entrenched, long-standing inertia. Compared to other European countries, Italy has been traditionally characterised by a scarcity of measures to support the needs of frail older people. In such a context, care needs have traditionally been covered by families and informal means (Saraceno et al, 2010; Saraceno, 2016).

Public LTC benefits are organised along two main lines of intervention, with low coordination. The first is a national cash-for-care benefit called Indennità di accompagnamento (IdA). IdA constitutes the mainstay of the Italian LTC system. In 2019, 46 per cent of the total public LTC expenditure was estimated to go through IdA (Gori et al, 2021). It is a national, universalistic, non-means-tested cash allowance (€530 per month in 2022), accessed by people with certified 100 per cent disability and needing permanent help to perform their daily activities (as stated by Law n. 18/1980). The central state funds this scheme through fiscal resources. Introduced in 1980 to support adults with disability, IdA was extended to the elderly only in 1988. Over the last 25 years, its use for dependent older adults has grown exponentially: it covered less than 3 per cent of the population over 65 in 1989, rising to 11.8 per cent in 2018 (Gori et al, 2021). While the elderly (aged 64 years and more) accounted for 20 per cent of all beneficiaries in 1989, this figure rose to 70 per cent in 2018 (ISTAT, 2020a, 2020b).

The support provided by IdA is an unconditional cash transfer that beneficiaries can freely spend as they wish (Da Roit et al, 2016). Given the unconditional character and absence of controls, the IdA has been extensively used to pay migrant care workers (MCWs) employed directly by Italian families, very often on an informal, non contractual basis (Da Roit, 2007; van Hooren, 2014; Pavolini et al, 2017). The number of MCWs has recently been estimated at around 1 million, with only 40 per cent having a regular contract (Pasquinelli et al, 2021).

The existence of a large, unregulated care market, broadly tolerated at the social and political level, has kept the costs of private care arrangements low while guaranteeing a high degree of flexibility in terms of working hours and care tasks. Italian families appreciate the economic benefits and round-the-clock coverage of such arrangements (24/7 care in the case of live-in MCWs), which are also in keeping with dominant cultural attitudes which attach high value to 'ageing-in-place' strategies (as opposed to the institutionalisation of the elderly in nursing homes).

In the context of growing care pressure, the shift to a 'migrant-in-the-family' care regime (Bettio et al, 2006) has been strongly stimulated by a persistent marginal role of public care services (residential and home care services). These services are provided under the responsibility of local and regional governments. However, due to the lack of central regulation and inadequate financial support provided by the national government, these services are traditionally affected by marked geographical inequality (Fargion, 1997; Ascoli et al, 2015).

More specifically, considering the residential care system, in 2018,[3] there were 12,857 residential structures in Italy, with 312,565 beds for patients over 64. The distance between Italy from other countries is considerable. Let us consider the coverage rate according to the number of beds in residential structures per 1,000 population aged 65 years old and over. Italy is less than half of Spain, almost one-third of Germany, and one-quarter compared to Sweden and the Netherlands. Japan, Korea, and even the United States also surpass Italy. Only Poland is behind Italy (OECD database).[4]

In Italy, a *residential structure* for dependent older people is defined as a public or private facility providing social assistance services (assisted hospitality with overnight stays) and social health services to needy people (DPR 14/01/1997). Therefore, public and private hospitals are excluded. While the classifications of such structures vary across regions, ISTAT (the National Institute for Statistics) distinguishes three types according to the level of health care:

- high-level (intensive treatments that are essential for the support of vital functions)
- medium level (extensive treatments such as daily medical and nursing care, rehabilitation treatments, and administration of therapies)
- low level (hospitality and social care services)

According to the data released by ISTAT for 2018,[5] 81 per cent of beds in such institutions are eligible for a high level of health care assistance.

In this context, residential care services are not only residually provided but face enormous difficulties due to their peculiar configuration. They are occupied by older adults (76 per cent of the older patients are aged over 80) with little or no autonomy in daily life (95 per cent of the total) (ISTAT, 2018).[6] Often these structures are mainly considered long-term health services rather than housing solutions for older people. Recent trends highlight the critical nature of this situation. In the face of the ageing process of the population, in the period 2009–18, the number of hospitalised patients in residential care services decreased by 2 per cent, equal to 6,000 people. Self-sufficient patients decreased (–16,000 users) while severely impaired patients requiring intensive care increased (+25,000 users). Such changes in the number and profile of inpatients came with an organisational change in the residential structures, which increasingly were transformed into 'high health-intensive residential facilities', that is, nursing homes providing intensive treatments that are essential for the support of the vital functions of their patients.

This shift towards high health-intensity services was not the result of an intentional reform but of growing resistance against the institutionalisation of the elderly in the population. Only when the dependent person is frail or affected by mental problems does the recourse to residential services become an obligatory choice for families. This negative attitude towards residential institutions was due not only to a general favour towards 'ageing in place' strategies but also to the high fees paid in nursing homes and the long waiting time to obtain a bed in such institutions.

The high fee for nursing homes results from strong underfunding by public authorities. Though public health funding should cover at least 50 per cent of hospitalisation costs of high health-intensive residential facilities by national law, in many regions, the amounts are significantly lower. For example, in Lombardy, the public funding per user paid is, on average, €41.3 per day, while the fee paid by users is between €60 and €69 per day (Tidoli et al, 2019). Tight in the grip between rising costs due to the progressive increase of inpatients requiring high-intensity health services and insufficient public funding, many structures have rationed the expenses through increased fees and under-staffing strategies. In the 2009–18 period, the medical staff was significantly reduced (by 10 per cent), compensated by an increase of equivalent proportions in less skilled care workers (by 6 per cent) and the nursing staff (+10 per cent). Hence as intensive health care increased, the presence of qualified medical personnel strikingly decreased. These changes were due to austerity policies intended to contrast the economic recession of 2011 and more structural disinvestment in public healthcare expenditure in the last decade (Fattore, 2019).

In addition to these trends, it should be noted that similarly to what happens in other countries (OECD, 2020), also in Italy, there are difficulties in the recruitment and retention of care workers. It is mainly due to their contractual arrangements (which are mainly temporary, with the spreading of involuntary part-time positions) and related low wages, if compared to the contractual conditions enjoyed by workers with equal qualifications employed in hospitals (Arlotti et al, 2020).

Finally, the residential care sector in Italy has been characterised for decades by high institutional fragmentation and decentralisation. Not only are services mainly provided by small-sized private organisations, but also the sector's regulation is devolved to regional governments, which have developed highly differentiated systems of NH classification and funding. This peculiarity of the Italian system has already been highlighted in recent comparative research on the reactions of LTC systems to the pandemic (Daly et al, 2021; León et al, 2021).

Managing the pandemic emergency: the regulation of the residential care sector

In this section, we reconstruct the regulation concerning nursing homes adopted to manage the COVID-19 emergency. First, we will focus on the first wave when national and regional authorities introduced most regulations. Then, we consider five aspects: the level of preparedness before the onset of the pandemic, lockdown measures, regulation concerning testing and diagnosis, rules about the management of human and financial resources, and finally, aspects concerning the coordination among nursing homes and health services (mainly hospitals). These aspects are to be considered crucial in managing the pandemic emergency.

Preparedness

The World Health Organization (WHO), following the A/H5N1 bird flu virus, recommended that all countries develop a pandemic plan and constantly update it following agreed guidelines. In Italy, in 2006, a 'National Influenza Pandemic Preparedness and Response Plan' was drawn up and approved (Ministerio della Salute, 2020). It contains an annex providing guidelines for drawing up regional pandemic plans, which were supposed to be drawn based on the National Plan.

In the Plan, care homes are mentioned twice. In Section 7.2, nursing homes are included in the number of institutions that should carry out actions to prevent and control the spread of the contagion. To limit infection, such institutions are required 'to avoid overcrowding in public spaces and provide such spaces with adequate aeration equipment'. However, only hospitals are required to provide staff with adequate PPE, separate paths inside the structure for infected patients, and plan an adequate number of beds in isolation. When considering the alert phase and the ongoing pandemic, the plan considers only infected persons to be kept at home to reduce the congestion of hospitals, and prescribes more severe recommendations only for hospitals. Nursing homes are considered here (Section 7.3) only as places to transfer infected patients from hospitals to reduce their pressure and never as places of virus transmission. Finally, while the pandemic plan is expected to be updated every three years, no updating has been done since 2006.

Following the National Plan, in the same year, the Lombardy Region approved a Regional Pandemic Plan[7] in which the national guidelines were translated, by highlighting responsibilities, actions, and implementation deadlines, and defining the institutional parties delegated to adopt the various provisions and measures for the different phases. Unfortunately, this plan was updated only in 2009 and had never been amended, although, in 2010, a Regional Government Resolution[8] noted critical issues for its 'maintenance' (Amnesty International Italia, 2020; Noli, 2020; Sparaciari, 2020).

Finally, the Regional Pandemic Plan was grounded on the activation of two players – the Regional Government and Local Health Authorities (ASL). Nevertheless, under the healthcare reform passed by the Lombardy Regional Government in 2015, ASL became agencies of mere bureaucratic and administrative control over the activity of hospitals. While their role was officially transferred to Local Social and Health Authorities (ASST), most of their operational tasks were not shifted to the new authorities (Sparaciari, 2020). These tasks include providing, storing, and distributing PPE to health and social care institutions. According to a report by Amnesty International (Amnesty International Italia, 2020), the missing implementation of the new institutional setting may have contributed to the shortage of PPE during the COVID-19 pandemic, which was one of the main problems for the residential care sector during the first wave.

Lockdown measures

As mentioned, on 21 February 2020, Italy dealt with its first certified clusters of COVID-19 infections. On the same day, the Health Ministry activated hospital prevention protocols regarding visits, testing, monitoring, and hospitalisations. Visits to patients in hospitals were discontinued. All people with symptoms or who had come into contact with a COVID-19 patient had to be tested and monitored for 14 days. All confirmed COVID-19 cases had to be hospitalised in isolation rooms. Healthcare staff working in hospitals and contacting COVID-19 patients had to wear appropriate PPE. However, care homes were not mentioned in all these initial interventions.

The following day, 23 February 2020, an agreement between the Health Ministry and the Lombardy Region suspended all public and private events. It closed all schools, museums, and cinemas, but no specific mention was made of nursing homes.[9] In similar agreements with Veneto and Emilia Romagna Regions (both hardly hit by the outbreak), external access to nursing homes was instead limited. Thus, relatives of nursing home residents in Lombardy could still access the facilities, even though immediately on 24 February 2020, the Lombardy Region clarified that this possibility was allowed, but 'not exceeding one daily visitor per patient'.[10] It implied that hundreds of people were allowed to visit large structures daily. Most of them complimented the staff's work with everyday caring routines. Moreover, since the regional government also clarified that day centres connected to care homes had to remain open, many institutions, which had already closed these centres to users or external visitors, re-opened to avoid legal action being taken against them by the Region. Finally, on 27 February 2020, the regional government ordered visitors to have their temperatures taken before entering the nursing home (with the implicit assumption that they could enter if they were not ill).

More restrictive instructions came partially only later, from the national Decree of 4 March, already 2 weeks after the total closure of hospitals. This Decree left the regulation of relatives' access to the discretion of care homes managers.[11] Then, on 8 and 9 March, the arrangement was confirmed in two following decrees through which the national government introduced a general lockdown of the country. Therefore, from this period, visits to residents in care homes were stopped and allowed only for specific circumstances under the full responsibility of care home managers.[12]

Testing and reporting

At the onset of the pandemic in Italy, testing was required for all people with symptoms,[13] including nursing home patients. In reality, testing was concentrated in hospitals, but data for the Lombardy region show that 10 per cent of COVID-19 infections were already concentrated in care homes at the end of February 2020 (Bettoni et al, 2020). Therefore, on 10 March 2020, testing in hospitals became a priority officially; in Lombardy, only hospitalised patients ('subjects with respiratory symptoms and in urgent need of hospitalisation') could be tested according to the regional protocol. Consequently, there was no way to test care home patients and workers: COVID-19 became a hidden phenomenon in care homes, although it spread quickly.

Data about Lombardy show that in mid-March 2020, only 2 per cent of the official COVID-19 infections were in care homes. However, according to a national retrospective survey carried out by the National Institute for

Public Health, the majority of COVID-19 deaths (including deaths of people with similar symptoms but not officially tested) occurred in the second half of March 2020: 42 per cent of deaths recorded during the period 1 February to 30 April 2020 occurred in Lombardy between 16 and 31 March 2020 (ISS, 2020a), at a time when the official deaths in care homes were not registered at all.

Only on 25 March 2020, following the first reports and claims about the increasing number of deaths in nursing homes and the lack of protection for their staff, the National Health Minister established the priority of testing also for healthcare staff working in nursing homes as well as specific indications about the adoption of PPE in nursing homes.[14]

However, it is essential to note that such indications were already introduced for the hospital sector at the end of February 2020, when the epidemic started. This delay in the decision taken by the national government to consider also care homes as a crucial sector in terms of intervention was presumably related both to the fact that the priority was oriented to tackle the critical conditions of the hospital sector (including the shortages of PPE, tests) and, in particular, to the fact that the national policy strategy completely neglected and primarily delegated to regional governments the definition of the interventions to be taken to protect this frontier of contagion.

A few days later, on 5 April 2020, the shockingly high number of deaths in nursing homes entered the public debate. Only a few days before, on 3 April 2020, the Minister of Health enforced the testing of care home patients and asymptomatic workers.[15] However, on 21 April 2020, there was a news report that many care homes in the Lombardy region had yet to obtain access to the testing provided by the health service (Corriere Della Sera – Milano, 2020b).

Human and material resources to contrast COVID-19

Since the onset of the COVID-19 pandemic, the national government adopted a complex set of extraordinary measures to support the healthcare system and, in particular, the hospital sector. Consequently, care homes became the target of specific policy attention only later.

On 25 March 2020, for the first time, a guideline provided by the Ministry of Health indicated the importance of 'strengthening' the staff in these facilities and implementing an extraordinary recruitment plan already in place for hospitals.[16] However, there is no indication that this plan was ever executed, even at the regional level. In many care homes, the lack and inadequacy of staff level due to the infections of care workers and the difficulty in finding new nurses and doctors constituted one of the most important critical features that undermined their capacity to cope with the new circumstances by the spreading of the virus. National newspapers reported cases of nursing homes in which the situation was so problematic that army doctors were requested as external support (Brera, 2020).

The lack of PPE for staff was a crucial difficulty in fighting infections in care homes. During the critical weeks of the outbreak, the scarcity of supply meant that priority was given to professionals working in hospitals at the expense of nursing homes. Moreover, in the Lombardy region, while a general protocol prescribed PPE for all healthcare service providers on 27 February 2020, there needed to be more clarity about whose responsibility it was to provide them.

The National Civil Protection Service was in charge of providing PPE. However, on 17 March 2020, a national decree authorised the 'requisition of medical and medical-surgical devices and movable assets' necessary 'to ensure the supply of structures and equipment to hospitals'.[17] This indication created even more difficulties in providing PPE to care homes, as most were directed or redirected towards hospitals.

Only on 25 March, a Health Ministry circular established rules to guarantee a minimum supply to protect nursing home workers (discussed earlier).[18] However, the lack of PPE continued to be persistently denounced by nursing home managers and their associations during April 2020 (Marocchi et al, 2020). According to the ISS survey, by mid-April 2020, more than 86 per cent of nursing homes declared the absence of PPE a significant difficulty (ISS, 2020a).

The coordination with the health care sector

The absence of a functional and complementary interaction between the healthcare sector (in particular hospitals) and care homes represented one of the most critical features during the development of the pandemic.

At the national level, the extraordinary plans of hiring implemented by central government to increase the staff level in the healthcare sector had a negative 'drain effect' on the care home sector. As a result, many doctors and nurses opted to leave their employment in nursing homes (la Repubblica, 2020), given the opportunity of being employed in the healthcare sector where contractual conditions and wage levels are more generous.

In Lombardy, the critical conditions of care homes were further exacerbated by decisions of the regional government over the discharge of hospitalised patients to care homes and the hospitalisation of sick nursing home residents. In this region, the pressure on hospitals became very strong during the pandemic's peak. As a result, the health authorities focused on increasing emergency units' capacity in hospitals, which also meant deciding where to find additional intensive care beds.

In this attempt to locate beds outside hospitals, on 8 March 2020, the regional government in Lombardy introduced the possibility of discharging hospital patients (including those affected by COVID-19 but in a less critical condition) to nursing homes, guaranteeing specific standards in terms of protocols and isolation.[19] Nursing homes were not obliged to accept these patients, but several of them agreed to do so. However, despite requesting specific standards and protocols, several media have reported weak control and monitoring that could have favoured the spread of the infection (Andreis et al, 2020; Di Feo, 2020).

A second critical aspect was the severe limitation on hospitalising care home patients. In Lombardy, according to a regional resolution on 30 March,[20] the hospitalisation of older patients (over 75) and in conditions of frailty or comorbidity was not allowed, leaving the responsibility to care homes. Furthermore, only patients over 75 with abnormal oxygen saturation values and 'fair health' could be sent to hospitals. While public authorities claimed that this decision was to avoid further risks of deterioration of highly vulnerable patients, the measure adopted denied proper medical care to many residents in care homes (Corriere Della Sera – Milano, 2020a).

Final considerations

Overall, the policy strategy adopted at the national and regional levels could have been more potent, not reactive, and problematic in coping with the emergency in care homes during the first wave of the pandemic. A national lockdown of care homes regarding the access of relatives and external visitors – a crucial measure to prevent possible infection transmission – was established only on 4 March 2020, about two weeks after the infection had begun spreading. Furthermore, for many weeks inadequate attention was paid to testing and monitoring activities among healthcare staff and patients in care homes: a priority for implementing such preventive activities was established only at the beginning of April 2020. Finally, the Minister of Health only published an ad hoc circular containing specific organisational guidelines for prevention and control strategies on 18 April 2020. These include the limitation of external access to facilities; the provision of special isolation spaces for new patients admitted to the NHS; testing activity; the restrictions on sending the elderly to the hospital for specialist visits and instrumental examinations; the use of masks and hand hygiene also in the case of external suppliers; and the early detection of suspected cases of infection both among the elderly and among operators.

In other words, while the pandemic invaded care homes, these institutions were unable not only to prevent or limit the entry of the virus into their structures, but also to provide personal protective equipment for their workers and adequate medical care to their COVID-19 patients, and very often unable to send them to hospitals. As a result, care home patients were on lockdown in institutions that could not take care of them.

This critical situation was not only due to the priority given to hospitals in the anti-pandemic policy, but also further reinforced by the structural weaknesses affecting care homes *before* the onset of the COVID-19 pandemic. Indeed, as described earlier, these institutions had specialised over the years in the intensive treatment of seriously dependent older patients without adequate staff and financial resources due to the lack of public investment in these structures.

Against this background, the issue of care homes started to be recognised in the public arena only due to claims and protests by relatives and workers, highlighting the deteriorating situation in this sector. Data were collected, and death statistics in care homes were published only in late April 2020. Only in April, therefore, could care homes get out of the invisibility that had characterised their situation for one month since the onset of the pandemic, and the number of deaths became a highly disputed public issue.

Further evolution and challenges for the future

In general, our evidence supports the conclusion that the pandemic crisis (especially during the first pandemic wave) in Italy, particularly in the Lombardy region, had a dramatic impact on residential institutions.

Our interpretation of that refers to policy legacy factors connected to the low public investments in residential structures *before* the outbreak. We have shown that prolonged institutional inertia in LTC policy peculiarly characterises Italy. In such a context, nursing homes faced internal and external problems during the pandemic. On the internal side, they had to face the entry of the virus into their structures with inadequate medical staff, resources and capacity to implement preventive actions. They were also unable to provide adequate health care to their COVID-19 patients and often could not send them to hospitals. On the external side, their situation was ignored for a long time by policymakers, who were mainly focused on handling the emergency in hospitals.

We argue that most of such criticalities are due to the pre-existent complex condition of these institutions. Nursing homes had been entrapped in a paradoxical situation for many years: the more they specialised in the intensive treatment of severely impaired older patients, the lower the quality of their services. This situation was mainly due to their precarious financial conditions, co-determined by the lack of adequate public funding and public regulation. The COVID-19 emergency has not only determined the death of thousands of nursing home patients. However, it has also shown the structural weakness of this sector, the main critical problems affecting it, and the need for better recognition of the strategic importance of nursing homes within the NHS.

Despite limited empirical evidence, the second pandemic wave (October to December 2020) confirmed the previous trends, involving more care homes located in different regions with the same dynamics. Improvements were found in the provision of PPE and the lockdown procedures. However, testing was still minimal, paving the way for the spread of the infection in many care homes (mainly brought by asymptomatic staff). Moreover, due to weak testing, a lack of data and information about the contagion and the number of related COVID-19 deaths persisted. This fact hampered the monitoring of the progress of the infection within care homes. Multiple organisational deficiencies were also reproduced, such as the lack of staff, the prolonged impossibility of patients having contact with their relatives, and the consequent worsening of their psychological conditions. Finally, many low-quality, private residential structures remained critical and operated under scarce public controls.

Since 2021, nursing homes had priority in the vaccination campaign in the country. In a few months, almost all patients in such structures completed the first vaccination round, drastically reducing COVID-19 mortality to zero. Care home patients were also prioritised in the further vaccination rounds, de facto banishing the pandemic from these structures. However, if the priority given to residential facilities in the vaccination campaign marked a vital turnaround, the public intervention has not gone beyond a purely emergency approach.

Alongside the significant results achieved by the vaccination campaign, there has been no honest public discussion on the need for a structural reorganisation of the sector. There has yet to be a discussion of the need for higher public expenditures to reduce fees, increase quality, or proceed with more stringent regulation of operational standards. On the contrary, an idea has taken ground in the public discourse that the massive number of deaths in the first wave occurred mainly because of the segregationist characteristics of facilities and their non-compliance with the standard rules, which expose inpatients to deplorable living conditions and assistance (shown by their high exposure to the contagion and mortality). Suppose this vision captures elements of reality (which also emerged from systematic investigations on residential structures). In that case, it also does not consider the criticalities due to the problematic institutional setting that structures must cope with.

In this context, the Italian Recovery and Resilience Plan (PNRR), funded by the EU, does not provide any public financial investment in nursing homes and concentrates investments only on in-home care assistance and alternative sheltered housing for the older. However, in more recent times, as PNRR foresees an overall reform in the national LTC system, so the requalification and upgrading of nursing homes, together with a reconsideration of the public financing and regulatory system, entered the public agenda.

Following this trend, a national coalition of social actors (trade unions, civil society organisations, disability groups, social service providers, and umbrella organisations of private residential institutions) – called 'Patto per un Nuovo Welfare sulla Non Autosufficienza' (Pact for a New Welfare on Long-term care) elaborated an LTC reform proposal. In this proposal, nursing homes are re-introduced in the reform process with a specific funding and regulatory responsibility given to the national level. The traditional cash-based model of the Italian LTC system is supposed to be progressively overcome by growth in professional home care services, reducing its gap with the mainstream LTC model developed in Western European countries.

The LTC reform proposal has mainly been incorporated in a draft law approved by the national government in October 2022 and sent to Parliament for examination and final approval. In the same month, however, a political change happened at the national level in the wake of the results of the national election and the subsequent establishment of a new right-wing government. Therefore, while this aspect represents a new condition, no apparent signs of change emerged in the political discussion. It has to be considered, however, that the difficult financial situation in the country may undermine the implementation of the LTC reform.

To conclude, our analysis has shown that the high mortality rate found in nursing homes during the first year of the pandemic was ultimately favoured by a substantial inability of national policy to consider the critical organisational conditions of residential structures and to guarantee, through rigorous and timely regulation, an adequate safety net. Secondly, our analysis indicates that this 'relative downgrading' of the residences in the emergency phase (Daly et al, 2021) has mirrored the great structural weakness of residences already in place before the onset of the pandemic – a situation determined by substantial inertia of LTC national policy. The progressive ageing of the population has, in fact, contributed to an increase in the demand for highly specialised long-term residential services, providing high-intensity healthcare treatments to very old, highly fragile patients. The inaction of public intervention, both in the forms of financial support and in regulation and control, has contributed to determining those conditions of low quality in the management of services that have favoured the dramatic impact of the pandemic in residential institutions described in this chapter.

Notes

1. https://mappe.protezionecivile.gov.it/it/mappe-e-dashboards-emergenze/dashboards-coronavirus/
2. https://ltccovid.org/
3. Istat online data warehouse: http://dati.istat.it/
4. https://www.oecd.org/en/publications/covid-19-and-well-being_1e1ecb53-en.html
5. https://www.istat.it/en/tag/care/

6 https://www.istat.it/en/tag/care/

7 Lombardy Regional Council Resolution (DCR) no. XIII/216 of 2 October 2006, 'Piano Pandemico Regionale di preparazione e risposta per una pandemia influenzale secondo le direttive del Ministero della Salute'.

8 Lombardy Regional Government Resolution (DGR) no. IX/1046 of 22 December 2010, 'Conclusione fase 6 pandemia influenzale da virus A/H1N1: valutazione e indicazioni operative'.

9 Order of the Health Ministry, 23 February 2020, 'Misure urgenti in materia di contenimento e gestione dell'emergenza epidemiologica da COVID-19. Regione Lombardia'.

10 Lombardy Region, 24 February 2020, 'Chiarimenti relativi all'applicazione dell'Ordinanza del Ministro della Salute di intesa con il Presidente di Regione Lombardia del 23 febbraio 2020'.

11 Decree of the President of the Council of Ministers, 4 March 2020, 'Ulteriori disposizioni attuative del decreto-legge 23 febbraio 2020, n. 6, recante misure urgenti in materia di contenimento e gestione dell'emergenza epidemiologica da COVID-19, applicabili sull'intero territorio nazionale'.

12 Decree of the President of the Council of Ministers, 8 March 2020, 'Ulteriori disposizioni attuative del decreto-legge 23 febbraio 2020, n. 6, recante misure urgenti in materia di contenimento e gestione dell'emergenza epidemiologica da COVID-19'; Decree of the President of the Council of Ministers, 9 March 2020, 'Ulteriori disposizioni attuative del decreto-legge 23 febbraio 2020, n. 6, recante misure urgenti in materia di contenimento e gestione dell'emergenza epidemiologica da COVID-19, applicabili sull'intero territorio nazionale'.

13 Circular of the Health Ministry, 27 February 2020, 'Documento relativo ai criteri per sottoporre soggetti clinicamente asintomatici alla ricerca d'infezione da SARS-CoV-2 attraverso tampone rino-faringeo e test diagnostico'.

14 Circular of the Health Ministry, 25 March 2020, 'Aggiornamento delle linee di indirizzo organizzative dei servizi ospedalieri e territoriali in corso di emergenza COVID-19'.

15 Circular of the Health Ministry, 3 April 2020, 'Pandemia di COVID-19 - Aggiornamento delle indicazioni sui test diagnostici e sui criteri da adottare nella determinazione delle priorità. Aggiornamento delle indicazioni relative alla diagnosi di laboratorio'.

16 Circular of the Health Ministry, 25 March 2020, see note 10.

17 Law decree no. 18, 17 March 2020, 'Misure di potenziamento del Servizio sanitario nazionale e di sostegno economico per famiglie, lavoratori e imprese connesse all'emergenza epidemiologica da COVID-19'.

18 Circular of the Health Ministry, 25 March 2020, see note 10.

19 Lombardy Regional Government Resolution (DGR) no. XI/2906 of 8 March 2020, 'Ulteriori determinazioni in ordine all'emergenza epidemiologica da Covid-19'.

20 Lombardy Regional Government Resolution (DGR) no. XI/3018 of 30 March 2020, 'Ulteriori determinazioni in ordine all'emergenza epidemiologica da Covid-19 - Indicazioni per gestioni operative per le RSA e le RSD'.

References

Amnesty International Italia (2020) *Abbandonati. Violazione del diritto alla vita, alla salute e alla non discriminazione delle persone anziane nelle strutture sociosanitarie e socioassistenziali durante la pandemia in Italia* [online], Available from: https://d21zrvtkxtd6ae.cloudfront.net/public/uploads/2020/12/report-rsa-anziani-.pdf

Andreis, E. and Santucci, G. (2020) Le case di riposo come frullatori: 'Qui tutti mischiati e il virus è esploso', *Corriere della Sera – Milano*, 8 April.

Arlotti, M. and Ranci, C. (2021) The impact of COVID-19 on nursing homes in Italy: the case of Lombardy, *Journal of Aging & Social Policy*, 33(4–5), 431–43.

Arlotti, M., Parma, A., Ranci, C., and Sabatinelli, S. (2020) Lavoro di cura. Una nuova frontiera della diseguaglianza sociale, *La Rivista delle Politiche Sociali*, 3, 97–127.

Altems (2020) *Analisi dei Modelli Organizzativi di Risposta al COVID-19. Focus su Lombardia, Veneto, Emilia-Romagna, Piemonte e Lazio*, Instant report 1: 31 March [online], Available from: https://altems.unicatt.it/altems-report.pdf

Ascoli, U. and Pavolini, E. (eds) (2015) *The Italian Welfare State in a European Perspective: A Comparative Analysis*, Bristol: Policy Press.

Bettio, F., Simonazzi, A., and Villa, P. (2006) Change in care regimes and female migration: the 'care drain' in the Mediterranean, *Journal of European Social Policy*, 16(3), 271–85.

Bettoni, S. and Santucci, G. (2020) Subito i tamponi, poi più nulla. I focolai 'sconosciuti' nelle Rsa, *Corriere della Sera – Milano*, 27 April.

Brera, P. G. (2020) Coronavirus, il grido delle Marche. 'Due calamità in tre anni. Ora rischiamo il collasso', *la Repubblica*, 17 March.

Casti, E. and Riggio, A. (2022) *Atlante COVID. Geografie del Contagio in Italia*, Roma: A.Ge.I [online], Available from: https://www.ageiweb.it/eventi-e-info-per-newsletter/pubblicazioni/atlante-covid-19/

Comas-Herrera, A., Zalakain, J., Litwin, C., Hsu, A.T. and Fernandez-Plotka, J.-L. (eds)(2020) Mortality associated with COVID-19 outbreaks in care homes: early international evidence, LTCCOVID.org, International Long-Term Care Policy Network, CPEC-LSE, 17 April [online], Available from: https://ltcCOVID.org/wp-content/uploads/2020/04/Mortality-associated-with-COVID-17-April-2.pdf

Corriere della Sera – Milano (2020a) Ospedali pieni, 118 in tilt. Commissione di verifica, *Corriere della Sera – Milano*, 11 April.

Corriere della Sera – Milano (2020b) 'Ats assente: lasciati in autogestione'. Don Gnocchi, sospesi dopo le denunce, *Corriere della Sera – Milano*, 22 April.

Daly, M., León, M., Pfau-Effinger, B., Ranci, C., and Rostgaard, T. (2021) COVID-19 and policies for care homes in the first wave of the pandemic in European welfare states: Too little, too late?, *Journal of European Social Policy*, 32(1), 48–59.

Da Roit, B. (2007) Changing intergenerational solidarities within families in a Mediterranean welfare state: elderly care in Italy, *Current Sociology*, 55(2), 251–69.

Da Roit, B., Le Bihan, B., and Österle, A. (2016) Cash-for-care benefits, in C. Gori, J.-L. Fernández, and R. Wittenberg (eds) *Long Term Care Reforms in OECD Countries: Successes and Failures*, Bristol: Policy Press, pp 143–66.

Di Feo, G. (2020) Coronavirus, pazienti smistati, accuse al Trivulzio: 'Non controllava se erano contagiati', *la Repubblica*, 25 April.

Fargion, V. (1997) *Geografia Della Cittadinanza Sociale in Italia*, Bologna: Il Mulino.

Fattore, G. (2019) Cost containment and reforms in the Italian National Health Service, in E. Mossialos and J. Le Grand (eds) *Health Care and Cost Containment in the European Union*, London: Routledge, pp 513–46.

Gori, C. and Gubert, E. (2021) L'indennità di Accompagnamento, in Maggioli (ed) *Network Non Autosufficienza,* L'Assistenza agli Anziani non Autosufficienti in Italia, VII rapporto, Adelphi: Punto di non Ritorno, pp 83–100.

ISS (2020a) *Survey Nazionale sul Contagio COVID-19 Nelle Strutture Residenziali e Sociosanitarie*, Terzo report, Aggiornamento 14 aprile ore 20.00 [online], Available from: https://www.epicentro.iss.it/coronavirus/pdf/sars-cov-2-survey-rsa-rapporto-3.pdf

ISS (2020b) *Survey Nazionale sul Contagio COVID-19 nelleSstrutture Residenziali e Sociosanitarie*, Report finale, Aggiornamento 05 maggio ore 20.00 [online], Available from: https://www.epicentro.iss.it/coronavirus/pdf/sars-cov-2-survey-rsa-rapporto-finale.pdf

ISTAT - ISS (2020) *Impatto dell'Epidemia COVID-19 sulla Mortalità Totale della Popolazione Residente. Periodo Gennaio-Maggio 2020*, 9 July [online], Available from: https://www.istat.it/it/archivio/245415

la Repubblica (2020) Sanitari reclutati dall'Asl. Le Rsa ora chiedono aiuto, *La Repubblica*, 18 March.

León, M., Arlotti, M., Palomera, D., and Ranci, C. (2021) Trapped in a blind spot: the COVID-19 crisis in nursing homes in Italy and Spain, *Social Policy and Society*, 22(3), 495–514.

Marocchi, G. and Pasquinelli, S. (2020) COVID nelle Rsa: la strage silenciosa, *Welforum*, 2 April [online], Available from: https://welforum.it/il-punto/emergenza-coronavirus-tempi-di-precarieta/tempi-di-precarieta/COVID-nelle-rsa-la-strage-silenziosa/

Ministerio della Salute (2020) Piano Strategico-operativo nazionale di preparazione e risposta a una pandemia influenzale (PanFlu) 2021–2023, Roma, Avilable from: https://www.salute.gov.it/imgs/C_17_pubblicazioni_3005_allegato.pdf

Noli, M. (2020) 'RSA e COVID-19, una drammatica realtà', *Lombardia Sociale* [online], 23 April, Available from: http://www.lombardiasociale.it/2020/04/23/rsa-e-COVID-19-una-drammatica-realta/

OECD (2020) *Who Cares? Attracting and Retaining Care Workers for the Elderly*, Paris: OECD Health Policy Studies, OECD Publishing [online], Available from: https://www.oecd.org/fr/publications/who-cares-attracting-and-retaining-elderly-care-workers-92c0ef68-en.htm

Pasquinelli, S. and Pozzoli, F. (2021) *Badanti Dopo la Pandemia. Vent'anni di Lavoro Privato di Cura in Italia*, Quaderno WP3 del progetto 'Time to care', Milano [online], Available from: http://www.qualificare.info/upload/RAPPORTO%20BADANTI%202021.pdf

Pavolini, E., Ranci, C., and Lamura, G. (2017) Long-term care in Italy, in B. Greve (ed), *Long Term Care for the Elderly in Europe: Development and Prospects*, London: Routledge, pp 75–92.

Pesaresi, F. (2020) Il COVID-19 nelle strutture residenziali per anziani, *I Luoghi della Cura*, 27 June [online], Available from: https://www.luoghicura.it/dati-e-tendenze/2020/05/il-COVID-19-nelle-strutture-residenziali-per-anziani/

Saraceno, C. (2016) Varieties of familialism: comparing four southern European and East Asian welfare regimes, *Journal of European Social Policy*, 26(4), 314–26.

Saraceno, C. and Keck, W. (2010) Can we identify intergenerational policy regimes in Europe?, *European Societies*, 12(5), 675–96.

SIAARTI (2020) *Raccomandazioni di Etica Clinica per l'Ammissione a Trattamenti Intensivi e per la Loro Sospensione, in Condizioni Eccezionali di Squilibrio tra Necessità e Risorse Disponibili*, 6 March [online], Available from: https://www.sicp.it/documenti/altri/2020/03/siaarti-raccomandazioni-di-etica-clinica-per-lammissione-a-trattamenti-intensivi-e-per-la-loro-sospensione/

Sparaciari, A. (2020) Il disastro coronavirus in Lombardia era già scritto in un audit del 2010, mai applicato, *Business Insider Italia*, 6 April [online], Available from: https://it.businessinsider.com/il-disastro-coronavirus-in-lombardia-era-gia-scritto-in-un-audit-del-2010-mai-applicata-anzi-una-delle-colonne-su-cui-si-basava-asl-e-stata-smantellata/

Tidoli, R. and Melzi, A. (2019) Rette RSA: cosa si 'nasconde' dietro ai numeri?, *Lombardia Sociale*, 20 June [online], Available from: http://www.lombardiasociale.it/2019/06/20/rette-rsa-cosa-si-nasconde-dietro-ai-numeri/

van Hooren, F. (2014) Migrant care work in Europe: variety and institutional determinants, in M. Léon (ed) *The Transformation of Care in* European societies, Basingstoke: Palgrave MacMillan, pp 62–82.

11

Government response to the COVID-19 pandemic in long-term care residences for older people: preparedness, responses, and challenges for the future in Luxembourg

Robert Urbé and Cristina Font Haro

Introduction

Luxembourg established in 1999 its system of long-term care (LTC) insurance when the law of 1998 came into effect (Grand-Duché de Luxembourg, 1998a), which recognised dependency as a new social security risk, similar to a disease, work accidents, and old age disability. Even though the care system implies home and residential care, the general preference is for home care.

Luxembourg is a small country with a population just a bit higher than 600,000 and 52 residences for the elderly; their system does not count multiple structures. Moreover, there are no regional authorities; apart from the national ones, there only exist ones at the municipal level. That is why evaluating COVID-19's impact, and political response is much easier than it would be in the case of a larger country.

The Luxembourg government started to evaluate the situation in China on 22 January 2020, and an inter-ministerial working group was installed 7 days later. The first two people showing symptoms were only tested 1 month later, on 24 February 2020, and 5 days later the first infected person tested positive.[1] The first two deaths were noticed on 17 March 2020.

The impact until 31 May 2020 was 4,019 COVID-positive out of 78,265 people tested; 110 died, of which 59 were residing in residential care homes. The death toll reached the maximum of 110 on 26 May 2020, of which 62 were men and 48 were women. On 31 May 2020, 29 hospitalisations were counted, out of which three were in intensive care. On 4 April 2020, the hospitalisations peaked at 190, while the intensive care patients arrived at the maximum twice on 3 April 2020 and 15 April 2020 (35 in total). On 31 May 2020, Luxembourg was among nine European countries showing a cumulative incidence of more or less 400 cases per 100,000 population.[2]

The number of 110 deaths was reached on 26 May 2020 (and stayed unchanged till 10 July 2020). It corresponds to 18.1 reported deaths per 100,000 population, which was more than the ratio for Germany (10.8) and Austria (7.9), but considerably less than for the other neighbouring countries France (44.5) and Belgium (85.2), and also less than the Netherlands (35.4).[3] Nevertheless, Luxembourg was the European country with the highest reported cases of infected people (698.0 per 100,000 population).

The high number of cases may depend on the fact that Luxembourg tested from the beginning much more than other countries. For example, data from 26 April 2020 inform that, whereas the mean number of people tested per 1,000 population was 27.7 for the OECD, it was 11.1 for France, 13.2 for the Netherlands, 30.0 for Belgium, 30.4 for Germany, and 30.5 for Austria, and it was 75.8 for Luxembourg (being second after Iceland with 147.6 and before Lithuania as third with 52.0).[4]

This advance in the number of tests increased, especially since the beginning of the large-scale testing programme, which started on 27 May with a testing capability of 20,000 tests per day, aimed at testing the whole population within 6 weeks.[5] The project was set up to last until the end of July. By the end of June, some 170,000 people had been tested, and 4,245 of them had been tested COVID-positive. Furthermore, on 29 May started the test activity at the Luxembourg airport[6]: every person could request a test upon arrival.

Like most European countries, Luxembourg decided on an almost total lockdown in response to the COVID-19 pandemic, leading to an economic downturn and heavy social consequences.[7] Nonetheless, during the first stage of the pandemic, there was a great deal of agreement between the government and the opposition; the vote in parliament to extend the state of emergency by 3 months was even unanimous. Moreover, the lack of knowledge about the virus made the population agree to the political measures and the lockdown.

However, critical voices increased with the duration of the lockdown. Predominantly economic actors expressed their impatience to be able to reopen as soon as possible. The easing of the emergency state caused the loss of agreement between the parties. The opposition criticised the government for the easing measures and proposed others; furthermore, it complained of a lack of transparency and could not access all the information.[8]

No opinion surveys have been conducted on the COVID-19 sanitary crisis and the measures taken by the government. However, a periodically conducted survey about the popularity of the politicians, organised by the largest daily newspaper and the largest radio and television station, published in June 2020, showed that in addition to the prime minister, especially the health minister, who had only been at that time in office since February, had improved their approval.[9] Therefore, it could lead to the assumption that, according to most of the population, they had done an excellent job.

After this brief introduction, where the social and political effect of the pandemic is explained, the second section develops a comprehensive descriptive analysis of LTC before the pandemic. It deals with the evolution of the LTC model and the debate surrounding its establishment. The third section looks at Luxembourg's response to the pandemic. The level of preparation in the country and the effects on the health system in general, particularly in residences, will be analysed. Finally, to improve preparation and future response, the conclusions of this study are drawn.

Description and analysis of the role of the residential care sector for their older-age population within the broader LTC arrangements (pre-COVID 19)

Evolution of LTC to the current model

When the law on compulsory LTC insurance, commonly known as 'dependency insurance' (*assurance dépendance*) was established in 1999, Luxembourg started to recognise dependency as a new social security risk, like disease, work accidents, and old age disability.[10] The law set up four guiding principles: (i) the priority of rehabilitation on care; (ii) the priority of home care on residential care; (iii) the priority of in-kind over in-cash benefits; and (iv) the guarantee of continuity of care. The goal of dependency insurance is to provide compensation for the expenses generated through third-party assistance to perform activities of daily living (ADL, *actes essentiels de la vie* – AEV). Therefore, it applies not only to the needs of older persons but also to the needs of disabled people.[11]

Entitlement and eligibility for the Luxembourg LTC system are neither income- nor asset-based. Age, too, is not a criterion. The only requirement for entry into the system is the evaluation of needs done by the Administration for Evaluation and Control of dependency insurance (*Administration d'évaluation et de contrôle de l'assurance dépendance* – AEC).[12] As a result of this evaluation, AEC determines the applicant's needs and translates them into a care plan, enumerating the different acts to be performed (and invoiced).

The need for care must be regular and represent a minimum of 3.5 hours per week. The status of dependency must be irreversible or last for at least 6 months.

Affiliation to dependency care insurance is mandatory, and access to continuous insurance benefits is guaranteed from the first day of membership. In addition, voluntary insurance is possible, for which a qualifying period of 1 year is applied. Dependency insurance applies the distribution of expenses with constitution of a reserve. This is essentially financed by three resources: (i) a dependency contribution levied on the income of insured persons; (ii) an annual contribution from the State, currently set at 40 per cent of the total expenses of the dependency insurance, including the working capital endowment (legal reserve); and (iii) an insurance licence fee from the energy sector.

The organisation of the LTC insurance has been entrusted to two bodies, namely the National Health Fund (*Caisse Nationale de Santé* – CNS) and the Evaluation and Orientation Unit (*Cellule d'Evaluation et d'Orientation* – CEO). The CEO was newly created and started its work of evaluating requests from dependent persons. During the initial phase, efficient procedures for assessing the needs of the applicants had to be developed. Other concerns at this early stage was a lack of beds in care institutions and how to meet the needs for technical adaptations in the homes of dependent persons. As a public service placed under the authority of the Ministry for social security and attached to the Inspectorate General of Social Security (*Inspection Générale de la Sécurité Sociale* – IGSS), CEO's mission was to ascertain the level of dependency and establish a care plan incorporating the help and care required by the dependent.

Care is provided by a set of community and residential care providers who practise by an authorisation issued by the supervisory ministry after an accreditation process. Providers may either be public or private, for-profit or non-profit. On demand of the beneficiary, part or all the care may be provided by an informal carer who has to be evaluated and recognised by the AEC as able to perform the tasks required. In this case, benefits-in-kind are replaced with cash benefits, which are paid to the beneficiary who may conclude a contract with the informal carer. In the case of a low number of hours and remuneration, these contracts may be concluded following a simplified formula.

The first modification of the law on LTC was carried out in 2005 and came into force 2 years later, which further specified and slightly amended the benefits package. The different acts to be rendered became hourly durations. The maximum duration of assistance is, in principle, set at 24.5 hours per week. However, in applying the law of 2005, the ceiling for essential life acts can be increased from 24.5 hours to 38.5 hours for severe situations (IGSS, 2019).

The LTC insurance law was amended in 2017 and 2018 (Grand-Duché de Luxembourg, 2017a, 2018). Concerning the financing of LTC insurance, in 2017, the contribution rate increased to 1.4 per cent on (more or less) all earnings without any upper threshold.

With the 2018 reform, greater flexibility was put in place with regards to activities of daily living through the introduction of flat-rate billing (instead of billing per provided acts) as well as changes in the organisation and time allocated for activities, support, domestic chores, and counselling (replaced by independent support activities, coaching, and home support activities) and the possibility of individual home care at night. In addition to these services, it also includes help and cares for activities of daily living in personal hygiene, nutrition, and mobility, products needed for help and care, technical aids, and accommodation conversions.

On the issue of transparency, a new list of more explicit dependency and support categories was defined in 2017. Specific categories of support were redefined to make the ambition of integration in the home setting more visible. The scope of services was widened, with more time for guidance and social integration in addition to personal care and housekeeping.

Care may be provided at the beneficiary's home or in institutions

Care may be provided at the home of the beneficiary or in institutions. There are four categories of care providers:

1. help and care networks (*résaux d'aide et de soins* – RAS: 22 networks as of the end of 2018);
2. semi-stationary centres (*centres semi-stationnaires* – CSSTA: 54 centres as of the end of 2018). These could either be day care or night care centres, although there are currently no night care centres in Luxembourg;
3. continuous care facilities accommodating dependent people day and night and providing them all the assistance and care required for their degree of dependency (*établissements d'aides et de soins à séjour continu* – ESC: 52 centres as of the end of 2018);
4. support and care establishments for intermittent stays (*établissements d'aides et de soins à séjour intermittent* – ESI: 43 establishments as of the end of 2018). Equally accommodating dependent people day and night and providing them with all the assistance and care required according to their degree of dependency, but allowing an alternation between the stay in the centre and the stay in a private home. This category responds predominantly but not exclusively to the needs of people with disabilities.

The first two incorporate care at home, the latter belong to the residential care sector. In 2018, 67.5 per cent of the 14,209 beneficiaries were provided for in the home care sector and ESI, whereas 32.5 per cent stayed in ESC. As a result, the number of LTC beds in 2017 was 8.28 per 100 population aged 65 and over (see OECD, 2019). Further to this, and as it has been said previously, providers may be public or private, for-profit or non-profit; they need accreditation by the supervisory ministry.

There are no data available about the market shares of these three forms of providers. However, after comparing data of the ICSS, the CNS, and COPAS, the market shares can be approximately defined as shown in Table 11.1.

Table 11.1: Estimated market shares of different forms of LTC providers, end 2018

Categories/Forms of providers	Public	For-profit	Non-profit
RAS	0.0%	25.0%	75.0%
CCSTA	12.5%	5.0%	85.5%
ESC	40.4%	9.6%	50.0%
ESI	4.5%	0.0%	95.5%

Source: Own calculations using data from IGSS (2020b), CNS and COPAS (data collected by phone).

The total workforce in the care sector that the providers mentioned was 9,641 FTE (full-time equivalents, *équivalent temps plein* – ETP) at the end of 2018, of which 70.1 per cent or 6,754 FTE were care workers; for the year 2017 these numbers are 9,485 and 6,702, and for 2016 they are 9,393 and 6,596 respectively. Among the different providers' employees, 27.9 per cent work for help and care networks, 4.5 per cent work for semi-stationary centres, 56.1 per cent for continuous care facilities, and 11.5 per cent for support and care establishments for intermittent stays.

Otherwise, there is limited data on the number of informal carers. It should be noted, however, that 7.6 per cent of the dependency insurance expenses were paid in cash in 2018, and should have served to remunerate the informal carers. Moreover, statistics show that out of 8,675 beneficiaries cared for at home, 1,270 opted for cash benefits, and 5,006 have opted for a combination of cash and in-kind benefits, which gives a potential number of 6,276 informal carers. Another, although limited, insight into the prevalence of informal carers can be given by the fact that, between 1999 and 2019, dependency insurance took over the social contributions to the pension insurance for 3,772 informal carers, as the law foresees this possibility. Nevertheless, not all informal carers have a contract and a salary, and not all are registered for pension insurance. Moreover, statistics for some of these workers show that most are women (72 per cent, except those aged 80+, see IGSS, 2020).

From the economic point of view, total public spending on LTC in 2018 was €664.1 million, from which 43.5 per cent was dedicated to home care, 50.3 per cent to care in institutions, and the other 6.2 per cent for several kinds of expenses (administration costs, cash benefits, benefits abroad, contribution transfers, other expenses). Beneficiaries are not obliged to any co-payment for LTC, except lodging costs (accommodation and services like meals, essential domestic services, laundry, among others) when residing in an institution. However, beneficiaries who cannot afford these costs may get means-tested support from the National Solidarity Fund (*Fonds National de solidarité* – FNS) called '*accueil gérontologique*'. This supplementary payment by the FNS is calculated to safeguard the beneficiary's pocket of €475.81 per month. In 2019, 615 persons benefited from this, to a total amount of €7.9 million (Ministère de la Famille, de l'Intégration et à la Grande Région, 2020).

Public debates and LTC challenges

There is no debate in Luxembourg between institutionalisation and home care. On the contrary, since the introduction of LTC insurance, one of the guiding principles has been the priority of home care over residential care. No one questions this principle.

There is also a social consensus about the priority of in-kind over in-cash benefits, the latter being disbursed to the beneficiaries but going at the end to informal carers.

On the contrary, trade unions presented elements to the public debate, such as the maintenance of the care level for the dependent persons and the level of employment. The reform law's forecast for future expenditures mentions: 'The presented results refer only to the protected resident population because the information about non-residents is insufficient'. The problem that only a limited amount of social spending for LTC goes to cross-border and other mobile workers has been and remains a concern. The LCGB trade union mentioned the pending problem of 175,000 cross-border workers (among which 40,000 from Belgium), who contributed to financing the LTC insurance system from the very start, but only benefited from it in a limited way.

Furthermore, the Luxembourg LTC system faces several challenges from before the pandemic, which need to be addressed in the future:

- a future constraint to access may come from the growing number of beneficiaries and hence the increased expenses for the LTC system (European Commission & Economic Policy Committee, 2018);
- this growing number of beneficiaries will also need more staff. At present, it is not easy to imagine where these workers might come from;
- a group of contributors largely excluded from LTC benefits is the cross-border workers: only a limited amount of social spending for LTC goes to cross-border and other mobile workers, despite their high percentage of the Luxembourg workforce (IGSS, 2020);
- another possible challenge with regards to the workforce is the potential decline in the number of persons willing to become informal carers; and
- language is another challenge concerning the workforce. Many cross-border workers, predominantly from Belgium and France, are employed in the Luxembourg LTC sector (about 60 per cent of all health professionals working in Luxembourg are foreign nationals – European Observatory

on Health Systems and Policies, 2019) and a large portion of these do not speak Luxembourgish, which causes a comprehension problem with older Luxembourg beneficiaries who often are not fluent in French.

On 11 February 2020, the Minister for Family and Integration tabled a draft law in parliament aimed at amending the 1998 law called 'ASFT' to improve the quality of institutions for the elderly. The ASFT law (Grand-Duché de Luxembourg, 1998b) regulated the relations between the state and the organisations working in social, family, and therapeutic fields. The draft law, which is currently in the legislative process (Chambre des Députés, 2020a), concerns the complete renewal of the section dedicated to services for the elderly. The objective is to clarify the definitions of the different kinds of services and guarantee their quality, flexibility, and transparency.

Analysis of the measures adopted to address the impact of the pandemic

Background of preparedness for the crisis

Luxembourg was not prepared at any level for a pandemic like the one experienced. Legally, Luxembourg was also not ready: the only legal provisions were a law from 1885 concerning 'the measures to be taken to prevent the invasion and spread of contagious diseases'. It was based on this ancient law that the first measures were taken: the ministerial decree ('*Arrêté ministériel*') on 'various measures relating to the fight against the spread of the COVID-19 virus' (Grand-Duché de Luxembourg, 2020a).

Another law was the one from 1980 on the Health Directorate ('direction de la santé': Grand-Duché de Luxembourg, 1980). This law defines the missions of the Health Directorate, including in particular public health, and more particularly to ensure compliance with the legal and regulatory provisions in the field of public health, to ensure the control of the health situation of the country, and to take the emergency measures necessary to protect health. To this end, the health department doctors have the capacity of judicial police officers in public health matters, and when it comes to preventing or fighting contagious diseases or contaminations, they have the right to issue binding prescriptions.

On a more practical level, the last time a pandemic plan had to be rolled out was the fight against influenza A (H1N1) in 2009–10. However, it was a simple plan of information, screening, detection, and monitoring, coupled with a vaccination campaign.[13] So, nothing specific could have guided those responsible for the present crisis.

As these instruments were not adequate to manage this type of situation, the government relied on paragraph 4 of article 32 of the Constitution, which since 2017 foresees the possibility of declaring a state of emergency

(Grand-Duché de Luxembourg, 2017b); this was initially intended to be able to react in the event of a terrorist attack.[14] This state of emergency gives the government the power to rule through regulations and to amend existing laws without consulting parliament.

One can doubt the constitutionality of the declaration of a state of emergency because of the text of Art. 32.4 of the Constitution provides as one of the conditions that 'after noting the urgency resulting from the impossibility of the Parliament to legislate within the appropriate deadlines',[15] which was not the case: the parliament extended the state of crisis for 3 months by passing a related law only 3 days later, and parliament met for a total of 21 sittings during the period of the state of crisis, and during this time, many laws were passed in record time.[16]

Other threats were both human resources and material ones. First, it was a lack of intensive care beds, masks, and other medical materials, actually as the Health Minister admitted in an interview, there was insufficient protective material at disposal initially, and even the ministry had no information about existing stocks, availability of intensive care beds and other capacities. On the other hand, Luxembourg depends on foreign staff because the health sector recruits about 45 per cent of its workforce from outside the country, primarily cross-border workers from France, Belgium, and Germany. However, the closure of borders and a possible requisitioning in their home country could have led to their unavailability for the Luxembourg health system.

At the organisational level, the Ministry of Health organised a range of special units, task forces, and working groups[17] to analyse, prepare, organise, monitor, and evaluate the evolution of the pandemic, the public response, and the effects on the population and in particular on the health sector. These units were formed from the employees of the Health Directorate, the Ministry of Health, and other ministries. In addition, the High Commissioner for National Protection also participated (even in a leading position),[18] as did the army, several secondments from globally operating companies, external consultants, and volunteers (pensioners, students). For example, one of the 'task forces' that advised the Ministry of Health was the 'Task Force for the Coordination of the Public Research Sector in the context of the COVID-19 pandemic'.

The government intended with all these measures to prevent the infection from spreading among large-sections of the population. Even though its first concern was the population, primarily the elderly, it wanted to prevent the overloading of the hospitals, particularly the intensive care units.

So, on 12 March 2020, the government took a range of decisions through the aforementioned ministerial decree, leading to a more or less total lockdown.

A range of regulations and laws followed in order to contain the pandemic and alleviate its consequences. Initially, there were plans to replace the ruling state of emergency with a new pandemic law replacing the one from 1885, but it turned out that this would have taken too long. For this reason, the government opted for a range of new specific 'COVID laws'. The plan for a new pandemic law will be followed up later, once the crisis is over.

The effects of the epidemic on the healthcare system

At a very early stage, the development of the crisis led to a total reorganisation of the health sector.[19,20] Hospitals started implementing two different systems (from reception to diagnostic stages through to treatment and floor care and intensive care) for 'normal' and corona patients. At the same time, all the surgical operations, and generally all the non-urgent treatments, were stopped, and the appointments already organised were cancelled (normal activities were resumed again from 4 May 2020).[21] In addition, some regular care beds were turned into supplementary intensive care beds to increase capacities. Supplementary respirators were ordered, and NATO provided Luxembourg with an additional capacity of around 100 beds flown in from Bari (Italy). Also, masks and other protection material arrived from China.

Outside the hospital sector, health care was organised alongside three lines of care or guard lines:

- guard line 1: medical care in Advanced Care Centres (CSA) and increased use of home visits in COVID patients;
- guard line 2: medical care by teleconsultation and home visits in non-COVID patients; and
- guard line 3: medical care for aid and care establishments (including care residencies for the elderly) and visits to aid and care establishments for COVID and non-COVID patients.

Three regional medical houses accommodating doctors on duty ('*Maisons médicales de garde*')[22] have to address the emergencies outside the opening hours of medical practices to relieve the emergency services of hospitals. In the first stage, these were now exclusively reserved for patients with symptoms of COVID-19. Then they were closed until 25 May 2020, while four newly implemented regional 'advanced care centres' ('*centres de soins avancés*' – CSA)[23] took over, starting between 22 and 25 March 2020. These new structures were designed operate by two strictly separate consultation channels: the first was designed to accommodate patients showing signs of infection with the COVID-19 virus; the second allowed patients with no sign of infection from the COVID-19 virus to come to the centre. In order to limit waiting times as much as possible, each consultation channel was provided for the care of several patients simultaneously. The intention was that these centres should be the entry point for anybody to the health system, with patients being dispatched from there for subsequent treatments. Therefore, these CSA also had two lines, one for 'normal' and one for corona patients. The staff for these CSA were recruited from those formerly present in the '*Maisons médicales*'. Other professionals were called on duty, too, while pensioners reactivated their professional status, and volunteers such as medical students were employed. As a result, the CSA functioned until 8 June 2020. After that, they were put on standby, with the possibility of reopening when the time comes.

General impact of the epidemic on the residential care sector and public responses

Studying the case of Luxembourg is interesting because, being one of the smallest countries, with a population of around 600,000 inhabitants, it only has 52 residences for the elderly. That is why there are no multiple structures or regional authorities except the national and the municipal ones. Besides, in the case of this study, the latter had no role to play in the questions under scrutiny. Therefore, the presentation of impact, responses, and coordination should be much clearer.

At the beginning of the crisis, the whole attention was focused on hospitals. However, when it came to protective equipment (masks, vests, overalls), there was initially too little available.[24] Since there was not enough material to supply the hospitals, there were even fewer supplies for other actors like resident doctors, pharmacies, and care residencies for the elderly (and disabled people too).[25] These actors, and even hospitals, tried to get additional protection material through private donations, volunteers tailoring masks, or through other channels.[26] However, even on 6 April 2020, a recommendation from the Health Directorate on the handling of protective materials, in particular masks, still gave advice to the medical and paramedical staff to handle the masks carefully and to minimise consumption (such as reducing the number of masks used, and limiting the use of masks by patients), which shows that the regular supply was not yet assured.

Access to care residencies for the elderly (and disabled) was also restricted to professional personnel (13 March 2020). Neither visitors nor suppliers were accepted. After the first infections had been discovered in some residencies, only on 30 March 2020, the Health Director ('*Directeur de la santé*') ordered that nursing staff should no longer be allowed into the residencies if they had signs of infection.[27]

Furthermore, only around 2 weeks later, a general testing campaign was launched: in response to health situations deemed critical in institutions for the elderly, tests were systematically offered to all residents and staff between mid-April and early June. These tests made it possible to stabilise the situation in this sensitive sector. As of 4 May 2020, tests were carried out in 49 of 52 residencies. Out of a total of 5,780 residents, 5,017 (91.8 per cent) were tested; 10 (0.2 per cent) showed a positive test.[28] However, testing in residential care did not continue in a systematic manner. Only when, in autumn, numbers of COVID-19 cases (and accordingly also deaths) began to increase significantly, a new wave of testing was deployed by the Ministry of Health.

Starting on 29 April 2020, visits were authorised again, but under restrictions and conditions, only in specially equipped rooms designated by the respective residence and only by prior reservation. Recommendations on handling the crisis in care residencies were edited by the Health Directorate and the Ministry for Families, Integration, and the Greater Region more or less on a 2-week basis.[29] One of the recommendations was to put residents in quarantine for 2 weeks if they returned from a necessary outing, such as for a medical examination. For this reason, some residents who were forced to go to the hospital for dialysis treatment regularly saw themselves almost permanently placed in quarantine.

The quarantine was heavily criticised by those affected and their families and even led to a parliamentary debate. Nevertheless, it was stopped after the ministry issued a new recommendation, drafted with the approval of the Health Directorate.[30] That is why, from 1 June 2020, outdoor visits were again allowed, and after 2 July 2020, visits in the residents' rooms.

The initial phase of around 6 weeks, when no visits were possible, and the following weeks with their restricted possibilities, led to distress situations for many residents, especially in the case of illness or death.[31] It was also a heavy burden for families not to be able to support their relatives in the event of illness or death. Many letters to the editor in the daily newspapers testify to this.

With the total reorganisation of the health system, a special guard line 3 was installed as part of the organisation of the health system during the COVID-19 pandemic to ensure medical care within the care residencies for the elderly themselves.[32] Thanks to this on-call line, each establishment had an on-call doctor. Guard line 3 operated 7 days a week, 24 hours a day, covering both visits to establishments and teleconsultations. The availability of doctors 24 hours a day contributed to the reduction in hospitalisations and visits to polyclinics, and to the development of continuous and personalised medical care within aid and care establishments.

Following the very positive results of the establishment of guard line 3 in aid and care establishments during the health crisis linked to COVID-19, the Government Council, to the satisfaction of all stakeholders, adopted in a meeting on 15 July 2020 the pilot project relating to the establishment of a service for the continuity of general medical care in the evenings, at night, at weekends, and on public holidays.[33]

This pilot project aims to perpetuate the care system put in place during the health crisis linked to COVID-19, better coordination and medical organisation to improve the quality of care and better continuity of care, and avoid unnecessary hospitalisations in the various structures of the country. This system will be applied from 1 September 2020 until 31 August 2022, therefore for 2 years, and provided by general practitioners. It will be organised by the Association of Doctors and Dentists (AMMD) with the collaboration and financial support of the state.

This guard line, as well as the reorganised healthcare system put in place, has contributed to the low mortality rate in Luxembourg compared to neighbouring countries, especially Belgium and France. Thus, accordingly to the mortality monitoring study at the European level, the excess mortality observed for Luxembourg during the acute phase of the crisis remains below the marked level of a substantial increase; it is also much lower than that observed in other European countries (Belgium, France, Ireland, Italy, Netherlands, Spain, Switzerland, UK).

Examples of development in specific care homes

For a better understanding of the situation experienced within the residences, a series of interviews have been carried out with three different subjects. The first two interviews were conducted with two senior members in the management of care residencies.

Both admitted that at the beginning, they had no precise idea about the virus and thought it would be limited to Asia, just as in previous cases. Moreover, when it became clear that it would affect the whole world, they felt unprepared and uncertain about the measures to adopt. The seriousness of the situation in Italy, on the one hand, and on the other the realisation that there was a lack of personal protective equipment and no longer any way to obtain it, were the starting points of increasing awareness.

Whereas one of them was contacted by the Ministry of Family, Integration, and the Greater Region as well as by the Health Directory, the other was not contacted during the first stage, which is why he called the Coronavirus Helpline of the Health Directorate. In the following, they contacted many authorities, such as the Health Directorate, the Ministries for Health, Education, Labour, Social Security and Family, and the National Health Fund and COPAS.

All residents were tested before and after periods of isolation during the large-scale testing process. The same happened to the staff. The Health Directorate, which manages the doctors in the residences, issued the requirement to test staff for COVID-19. At that time, in the case of the first interviewee, staff and residents were trained to handle the situation by the health directorate's hygienists. In contrast, the second interviewee received help from the diverse department's head and the Directorate of the residence.

Personal protective equipment was not provided in the first period; it was provided through the logistics unit of the crisis cell in the Health Ministry.

The visits to residents by family members were not allowed at the first stage and were limited afterwards, according to the official recommendations. Measures were taken to isolate those who were infected from those who were not: a separate department for isolations was built in extremis to ensure the best possible separation between positive and healthy residents. In both cases, the health reserve and volunteers reinforced the staff taking care of residents. Health care had to be adapted: in the event of infection, significantly intensified management was necessary along with increased monitoring of symptoms or warning signs; some treatments were not provided as a precaution, such as, for example, group physiotherapy activities.

When everything started, there were no actual recommendations yet. Guidelines existed before for managing infectious diseases (influenza, norovirus); these served as a basis for establishing more specific guidelines. More generally, the employees' knowledge of hospital hygiene enabled them to define a concept that was quite close to the subsequent recommendations of the Health Directory. Above all, they took measures to limit contagion and ensure the best possible functioning of their services. Their measures were subsequently revised to align them with the recommendations of the Health Directorate.

If an older adult was infected with COVID-19, they were automatically isolated. However, if there were several cases of infections, especially people who could not be isolated, such as people with dementia, the solution was 'cohorting': the infected people and the personnel who treated them were grouped together and scrupulously isolated from the other non-sick people. Regardless, physical contact with infected people was generally prohibited; contacts by phone, skype, facetime, and others were facilitated and encouraged. Even some exceptions have been made in the event of end-of-life, subject to stringent protection measures.

Older people have been infected by COVID-19 who have not been hospitalised so as not to overload hospitals, keep the elderly in their usual place of life, and guarantee them as much normalcy as possible; any hospitalisation not essential has been avoided. Instead, hospitalisation was medically ordered, and the decision was based on 'end-of-life guidelines' expressed by residents and their families.

A third interview was conducted with a senior manager, the head of the 'elderly' division at the Ministry of Family, Integration, and the Greater Region.

He admitted that at the starting point of the events, they lacked knowledge about the virus, how it spreads, and its contagiousness; their feelings were uncertain and concerned about news from neighbouring countries. Then, however, he realised for the first time the severity of the pandemic on 13 March 2020, the same day they decided about the closure of residential care facilities and the ban on visits for the relatives of the residents. They had been contacted, therefore, by the Ministry of Health, with which there has been a very close collaboration at all times of the situation, as well as COPAS (*Confédération des Organismes Prestataires d'Aides et de Soins*), the representative association of service providers in the field of LTC. This collaboration of the Ministry of Family with the Ministry of Health (and with COPAS) was based on joint working groups, where fast and pragmatic solutions and support positions for residency managers have been developed; for example, their recommendations have been repeatedly adapted during the sanitary situation. The Ministry of Family has also worked closely with the Sanitary Inspection (a Division of the Ministry of Health). While they provided the residencies with the necessary know-how through training on the subject of hygiene and infection control and by visiting the residencies individually together with the Ministry of Health and their specialists; they also provided them with information on how they might react in their situation and their premises if frequent infections were to occur. The houses were individually advised and cared for when they expressed a need.

The Ministry and COPAS established recommendations for the whole LTC sector; these measures were advised by the Ministry of Health each time. These recommendations included staff conduct, protective clothing, introducing and monitoring health measures, recognising symptoms, informing residents, and organising family visits.[34] The measures taken included, as already mentioned, the closure of residential care facilities, on the one hand, a ban on visits for the relatives of the residents, and on the other hand, a ban on going out for residents. In addition, visits to residents by family members were forbidden from 13 March 2020, limited from 28 April 2020, and there was an open phase 1 from 30 May 2020 and a phase 2 from the end of the state of crisis (24 June 2020). Besides, the residencies provided personal protective equipment to residents and visitors to ensure compliance with hygiene rules during the visits.

Despite that, residencies' directors were able at any time to give exceptions from the restrictions regarding visits, particularly at the end of life of a resident; some of them made little use of it, preferring to hide behind the Ministerial order. Only on 20 May 2020 did the order from the ministry provide more clarity.

Personal protective equipment for staff was provided by health authorities as soon as it was available, which was not the case from the start because of supply problems and a lack of stored material, a lack of preparation, and foresight.

Lessons learned?

Experiencing the pandemic in Luxembourg involved a great exercise in humility, since, as has been witnessed, one was not prepared for it. At the beginning of the pandemic, no legal framework would protect its citizens or indicate what measures to take. The action protocols also fell short since they had been designed for less contagious diseases. Moreover, materially, Luxembourg was only prepared to give aid to a small population of sick and older people.

The welfare state's fourth pillar, dependency, had already been developed in 1999, and its subsequent reforms in 2005, 2017, and 2018. However, it did not consider reorganising human and material resources to face a pandemic.

Although the legal framework dealt with pandemics, the 1885 law was too old and outdated, referring to a society with needs that no longer exist. During the first phases of COVID-19, they put a series of protocols in place; for example, health care was organised alongside three lines of care or guard lines, which met the objectives set. Nevertheless, again, it has been thanks to the prompt administrative response.

In Luxembourg, tough decisions such as total closure were made, given that the population and the various economic and political sectors acted in unison. Everyone accepted the seriousness of the situation and the need to be strict with the measures. Even so, the controversy resurfaced when the reopening and relaxation phases arrived. The harsh economic and social consequences took their toll on society. Furthermore, being a new situation, 'the easing phase', the government had not considered the consequences of this either.

Therefore, the main lessons learned are four for Luxembourg:

1. better preparedness of the health and care sector, stop to savings in the health sector;
2. elaboration of plans and response pathways in preparation for the next crisis;
3. assuring the material stocks necessary; and
4. stop the reliance on China for essential items.

While the legal framework is already being updated and the various action plans reorganise human resources, it is necessary to consider the material aspect of this problem. Or, in other words, the lack of it. Europe should provide masks, aprons, respirators, drugs, and vaccines instead of relying on China. During the crisis, the first reactions occurred: some companies converted to mask fabrication (textile), disinfectant production (paint manufacturers, distilleries), and some specialised and increased valve production for respirators or protective clothing. It could continue; however, subsidies will probably be necessary because of the wage gap between Europe and Asia.

There is also one issue on quality and reactivity in such a crisis. The management of the LTC system involves a range of actors: first, the CNS is responsible for contracting providers and the disbursement of payments; second, the AEC's mission is to ascertain the state of dependency and to establish a care plan incorporating the help and care required by the dependent, to monitor the quality of services provided and their adequacy in meeting the needs of dependents and informing and advising protected persons and bodies concerned with the prevention of addiction and the care of dependents; third, the IGSS provides control of social security institutions under the supervision of the Ministry for Social Security, which establishes the relevant laws for the sector. Fourth, the Ministry of Health and the Ministry for Family, Integration, and the Greater Region supervise the accredited providers. Fifth, the providers are responsible for correctly implementing the care system, combining human and material resources. Finally, COPAS is the representative organisation of care providers recognised as the collective bargaining party with the CNS (and the trade unions). As can be observed, the system shows remarkable complexity. Even though at this moment in time, there are no real complaints about its complexity and the multitude of actors, possible future budget constraints may require more rigorous management of the whole system in order to be competitive during or after the pandemic periods.

Furthermore, a general issue is how the sector can respond to the ever-growing demand (European Commission & Economic Policy Committee, 2018). It could put public finances under constraint, and there is also an issue of finding enough qualified staff within the borders who can speak the elderly's language. Again, during and after the pandemic, Luxembourg's dependency system must be consistently competitive.

Notes

1. These and the following information can be found on the government website: https://coronavirus.gouvernement.lu/fr.html and other sites registered there, as for example for the figures that stem from https://data.public.lu/fr/datasets/donneesCOVID19/, downloaded on 29 June 2020. Because of the narrow territory there now exist breakdowns of the numbers by region, age or social groups, and so on. Also, the first breakdowns on a regional basis were only published by end of July 2020.
2. This information stems from the World Health Organisation: https://www.euro.who.int/_data/assets/pdf_file/0006/445920/Week-22-COVID-19-surveillancer-report-eng.pdf
3. All these figures stem from https://www.ecdc.europa.eu/en/cases-2019-ncov-eueea, downloaded on 29 June 2020.
4. See: https://msan.gouvernment.lu/dam-assets/COVID-19/brochures/la-strategie-de-test.pdf, download on 29 June 2020.
5. See https://researchluxembourg.lu/COVID-19-taskforce/testing-strategy/, downloaded on 29 June 2020.
6. See https://coronavirus.gouvernement.lu/fr/communications-officielles.gouvernement%2Bfr%2Bactualites%2Btoutes_actualites%2Bcommuniques%2B2020%2B05-mai%2B29-bausch-luxairport.html
7. See Urbé (2020) for the description of the different measures.

8 See https://www.rtl.lu/news/national/a/1549500.html or https://www.wort.lu/de/politik/opposition-veraergert-wir-haben-es-satt-5f0eec1eda2cc1784e361a42
9 See https://www.rtl.lu/news/national/a/1546659.html or https://www.wort.lu/de/politik/politmonitor-das-feld-von-hinten-aufgerollt-5f06e919da2cc1784e361339
10 A global overview of the LTC insurance (Assurance dépendance) in Luxembourg can be consulted in IGSS (2019); Pacolet et al (2018) may also be consulted as well as Directorate-General for Economic Affairs (2019). There is also a practical guide to the LTC insurance before the 2017 reform (Ministère de la Sécurité Sociale, 2009).
11 If not indicated otherwise, all data and figures in this section stem from IGSS (2020).
12 During the time between the introduction of an application and the decision of the AEC, the dependency insurance covers a flat rate of 780 minutes of care per week.
13 See https://sante.public.lu/fr/actualites/2009/06/OMS-phase6/index.html
14 The text of article 32.4 reads literally as follows: 'In the event of an international crisis, real threats to the vital interests of all or part of the population or imminent danger resulting from serious attacks on public security' (translation by the author, original text: 'En cas de crise internationale, de menaces réelles pour les intérêts vitaux de tout ou partie de la population ou de péril imminent résultant d'atteintes graves à la sécurité publique').
15 Translation by the author, the original text reads: 'après avoir constaté l'urgence résultant de l'impossibilité de la Chambre des Députés de légiférer dans les délais appropriés'.
16 See https://chd.lu/wps/portal/public/Accueil/TravailALaChambre/Seances-Publiques/CalendrierSeances
17 See https://coronavirus.gouvernement.lu/fr/communications-officielles.gouvernement%2Bfr%2Bactualites%2Btoutes_actualites%2Bcommuniques%2B2020%2B04-avril%2B28-inventaire-groupes-travail.html
18 See https://gouvernement.lu/dam-assets/documents/actualites/2020/04-avril/28-inventaire-groupes-travail/MS-CC-COVID19-organigramme-Cellule-de-crise.pdf
19 Before the pandemic, the Luxembourg health system can be characterised in 2017 by the following indicators: 3 doctors per 1,000 population, 43 per cent being older than 55 years; 11.7 practising nurses per 1,000 population; 4.7 beds per 1,000 population, see OECD (2019).
20 See https://gouvernement.lu/dam-assets/documents/actualites/2020/04-avril/Organisation-systeme-de-sante-COVID.pdf
21 See https://coronavirus.gouvernement.lu/fr/communications-officielles.gouvernement%2Bfr%2Bactualites%2Btoutes_actualites%2Barticles%2B2020%2B04-avril%2B29-briefing-lenert-ammd.html
22 These are general practitioner offices covering out-of-hour care on evenings and weekends.
23 For more details, see https://statistiques.public.lu/catalogue-publications/Flash-COVID/2020/01-2020.pdf
24 See https://msan.gouvernement.lu/fr/actualites.gouvernement%2Bfr%2Bactualites%2Btoutes_actualites%2Binterviews%2B2020%2B06-juin%2B30-gaulier-lessentiel.html
25 See the results of a survey of institutions of palliative medicine: Association Luxembourgeoise de Médecine Palliative (2020).
26 See https://www.tageblatt.lu/headlines/xavier-bettel-und-paulette-lenert-zu-besuch-im-krankenhaus-auf-kirchberg/
27 See https://sante.public.lu/fr/espace-professionnel/recommandations/direction-sante/000-COVID-19/000-COVID-191-annexes/ordonnance-reseaux-soins-domicile-structures.pdf
28 See https://chd.lu/wps/PA_RoleDesAffaires/FTSByteServ-ingServletImpl?path=682BFE29A17F-0CE5BB8DA942A1BC4663AE7C-6CFF9722FFD9B499226E-B9A3A64378DDB2EE38B-06F94E857E8477B-CBBC45$B6A19C0CB81FA22F6-6963C9CB5BB6B81

[29] See https://sante.public.lu/fr/espace-professionnel/recommandations/direction-sante/000-COVID-19/index.html

[30] See https://sante.public.lu/fr/espace-professionnel/recommandations/direction-sante/000-COVID-19/000-COVID-191-annexes/recommandations-CIPA.pdf

[31] See https://www.wort.lu/de/politik/wie-im-gefaengnis-senioren-fuehlen-sich-eingesperrt-5ee8f661da2cc1784e35fcc1

[32] Normally care residents, who are considered to be 'at home' in their residence have the free choice to call in their personal doctor, the residence is not organising medical care.

[33] See https://msan.gouvernement.lu/fr/actualites.gouvernement%2Bfr%2Bactualites%2Btoutes_actualites%2B-communiques%2B2020%2B07-juil-let%2B15-continuite-soins-COVID.html

[34] See https://sante.public.lu/fr/es-pace-professionnel/recommandations/direction-sante/000-COVID-19/index.html and https://mfamigr.gouvernement.lu/fr/dossiers/faq/faqnew.html

References

Association Luxembourgeoise de Médecine Palliative (2020) *Pandémie et Soins Palliatifs: Impact du COVID19 sur la Prise en Charge des Patients Palliatifs au Luxembourg*, Luxembourg: Association Luxembourgeoise de Médecine Palliative.

Chambre des Députés (2020) *Projet de loi Portant sur la Qualité des Services pour Personnes Âgées et Portant Modification de: 1° la loi Modifiée du 16 mai 1975 Portant Statut de la Copropriété des Immeubles Bâtis; 2° la loi Modifiée du 8 Septembre 1998 Réglant les Relations entre l'Etat et les Organismes Œuvrant dans les Domaines Social, Familial et Thérapeutique*, Document parlementaire N°7524, Luxembourg: Chambre des Députés.

Directorate-General for Economic and Financial Affairs (2019) *Joint Report on Health Care and Long-Term Care Systems & Fiscal Sustainability*, European Economy No 105, June, pp 415–21 [online], Available from: https://ec.europa.eu/info/sites/info/files/economy-finance/ip105_en.pdf

European Commission & Economic Policy Committee (2018) *The 2018 Ageing Report: Economic and Budgetary Projections for the 28 EU Member States (2016–2070)*, European Economy Institutional Paper, No. 079.

Grand-Duché de Luxembourg (1980) Loi du 21 novembre 1980 portant organisation de la direction de la santé, *Journal Officiel du Grand-Duché de Luxembourg*, Mémorial A 79 du 27 novembre 1980, Luxembourg.

Grand-Duché de Luxembourg (1998a) Loi du 19 juin 1998 portant introduction d'une assurance dépendance, *Journal Officiel du Grand-Duché de Luxembourg*, Mémorial A 48 du 29 juin 1998, Luxembourg.

Grand-Duché de Luxembourg (1998b) Loi du 8 septembre 1998 réglant les relations entre l'Etat et les organismes œuvrant dans les domaines social, familial et thérapeutique, *Journal Officiel du Grand-Duché de Luxembourg*, Mémorial A 82 du 24 septembre 1998, Luxembourg.

Grand-Duché de Luxembourg (2017a) Loi du 29 août 2017 portant modification 1. du Code de la sécurité sociale; 2. de la loi modifiée du 15 décembre 1993 déterminant le cadre du personnel des administrations, des services et des juridictions de la sécurité sociale; 3. de la loi modifiée du 25 mars 2015 fixant le régime des traitements et les conditions et modalités d'avancement des fonctionnaires de l'État, *Journal Officiel du Grand-Duché de Luxembourg*, Mémorial A 778 du 1 septembre 2017, Luxembourg.

Grand-Duché de Luxembourg (2017b) Loi du 13 octobre 2017 portant révision de l'article 32, paragraphe 4 de la Constitution, *Journal Officiel du Grand-Duché de Luxembourg*, Mémorial A 908 du 16 octobre 2017, Luxembourg.

Grand-Duché de Luxembourg (2018) Loi du 10 août 2018 modifiant 1. le Code du travail; et 2. le Code de la sécurité sociale en matière de maintien du contrat de travail et de reprise progressive du travail en cas d'incapacité prolongée, *Journal Officiel du Grand-Duché de Luxembourg*, Mémorial A 703 du 21 août 2018, Luxembourg.

Grand-Duché de Luxembourg (2020a) Arrêté ministériel du 16 mars 2020 portant sur diverses mesures relatives à la lutte contre la propagation du virus COVID-19, *Journal Officiel du Grand-Duché de Luxembourg*, Mémorial A 149 du 16 mars 2020, Luxembourg.

IGSS (Inspection Générale de la Sécurité Sociale) (2019) *Rapport Général sur la Sécurité Sociale 2018*, Luxembourg: IGSS.

IGSS (2020) *Rapport Général sur la Sécurité Sociale 2019*, Luxembourg: IGSS.

Ministère de la Famille, de l'Intégration et à la Grande Région (2020), *Rapport d'Activité 2019*, Luxembourg: Ministère de la Famille, de l'Intégration et à la Grande Région.

Ministère de la Sécurité Sociale (2009) *L'Assurance Dépendance: Guide Pratique, Cellule d'Évaluation et d'Orientation de l'Assurance Dépendance*, Luxembourg [online], Available from: http://sante.public.lu/fr/publications/a/assurance-dependance-guide-fr-de-pt-en/assurance-dependance-guide-fr.pdf

OECD (2019) *Health at a Glance 2019: OECD Indicators*, Paris: OECD.

OECD/European Observatory on Health Systems and Policies (2019) *Luxembourg: Country Health Profile 2019, State of Health in the EU*, Brussels: OECD Publishing.

Pacolet, J. and De Wispelaere, F. (2018) *ESPN Thematic Report on Challenges in long-term care, Luxembourg*, European Commission [online], Available from: https://ec.europa.eu/social/BlobServlet?docId=19858&langId=en

Urbé, R. (2020) *Luxembourg: Consequences of a General Economic Downturn due to the COVID-19 Pandemic*, ESPN Flash Report 2020/24, European Social Policy Network (ESPN), Brussels: European Commission.

12

The COVID-19 crisis as a 'hospital issue': the impact of COVID-19 measures on Dutch nursing homes

María Bruquetas and Anita Böcker

Introduction

The first confirmed COVID-19 case in the Netherlands was reported on 27 February 2020. Two weeks later, the number of new cases had risen to around 200. It was decided not to conduct contact tracing anymore for all identified cases because the regional public health services could not handle the caseload. Over March, the number of new cases continued to rise, and so did the number of hospital admissions and deaths, a problem for the Netherlands, a country with a relatively small number of hospitals and, especially, intensive care beds. On 13 March, only 2 weeks after the first confirmed case, 'code red' was promulgated for hospitals in the (catholic) province of Noord-Brabant – where Carnival turned out to have been a super spreading event. All non-emergency surgeries were postponed, and the leaves of care workers were revoked. Many hospitals in other parts of the county took the same measures, preparing for a large influx of COVID-19 patients. In addition, many GPs contacted their older patients – either on their initiative or asked to do so by hospitals – to talk with them about whether they wanted to be treated in an ICU in case they contracted COVID-19.

Consequently, the public and political debate in the Netherlands and government policies throughout this first wave revolved around hospital capacity and, in particular, the capacity of ICUs. As a result, lockdowns were promulgated to avoid collapsing the healthcare system and the hospital sector.

By 15 June, the cumulative number of confirmed cases was nearly 50,000 (281 per 100,000 population); the cumulative number of hospital admissions was nearly 12,000 (68 per 100,000); and the cumulative number of deaths of confirmed COVID-19 patients was 6,000 (35 per 100,000). However, Statistics Netherlands calculated that there were almost 9,000 more deaths than usual during the first 9 weeks of the pandemic, representing 32 per cent excess mortality.[1]

These aggregate figures conceal socio-demographic differences. The southern part of the Netherlands was hit hardest during this first pandemic wave. There were municipalities with three times more deaths than average. Excess mortality was relatively high among the elderly and highest among people aged 80 or older. Across all age groups, it was higher among men than among women. It was not higher among lower-income people than among higher-income groups. It was somewhat higher among people with an ethnic minority background than those with a Dutch background.[2]

However, in absolute and relative terms, excess mortality was exceptionally high among people receiving long-term care (LTC) in care and nursing homes. During the first 9 weeks of the pandemic, more than 15,000 people living in care and nursing homes died – 5,000 people (52 per cent) more than expected if there had been no pandemic. In the general population, nearly 21,000 people died, some 3,800 people (22 per cent) more than expected.[3]

In a recently published report, the Dutch Safety Board concluded that the focus of the crisis approach contributed to the excess mortality in care and nursing homes. The crisis approach focused on the hospital and ICU occupancy. Bottlenecks within the residential care sector remained underexposed during the first months of the pandemic also because this sector was not represented in the Outbreak Management Team (OMT), which advised the government on the crisis approach. Another factor contributing to the excess mortality in care and nursing homes is that there has been a trend in this care sector toward attaching more importance to a home-like environment, autonomy, and quality of life. Hygiene and infection prevention were receiving less – according to the Safety Board, too little – attention.[4]

These factors – which are more or less specific for the Netherlands – and the dilemmas confronting managers and care workers in care and nursing homes will be further analysed in the following sections. First, we describe the organisation of LTC in the Netherlands, specifically the residential care sector. Next, we analyse the approach of the government and other involved actors to the pandemic, with a particular focus on the residential care sector. Finally, we describe this sector's developments in the pandemic's following phases, focusing on lessons learned.

Paving the way for the crisis: residential care sector for the older-age population and LTC arrangements

Policy reforms, reduced state's responsibility, and deinstitutionalisation

In 1968 when mandatory social insurance was impulsed to cover all Dutch residents for non-insurable health risks, the Dutch LTC system was founded. The Exceptional Medical Expenses Act (AWBZ) meant that people in need of LTC or ongoing care – related to old age, chronic illness, or disability – no longer depended on the discretion of municipalities, as LTC became an insured right. Furthermore, the system provided in-kind benefits rather than cash transfers, funded mainly through income-related contributions and, to a lesser extent, through taxes. Initially, it was entitled to residential care (nursing, personal, and medical care in institutions), but in 1970 non-residential care was added (Mot, 2010; Companje, 2015).

The expansion of the scope of the AWBZ in the following decades triggered increasing concerns about the system's sustainability. That inaugurated a long process of policy reforms. Deinstitutionalisation was actively promoted from the late 1980s, and throughout the 1990s and 2000s, legislative changes sought to stimulate the creation of care markets.[5] After two decades of discussion, the government passed a reform in 2015 to reduce state responsibilities and stimulate the re-familiarisation and informalisation of care (Grootegoed & Van Dijk, 2012; Maarse & Jeurissen, 2016; Van den Broek, 2016). Broadly, the reform comprised expenditure cuts, a shift from residential to non-residential care, and decentralisation of non-residential care (Van Ginneken et al, 2015). Care at home became an explicit policy goal, arguing that it coincides with people's preferences and is more efficient than care in institutions (Da Roit, 2012; Companje, 2015). The new policy promotes 'self-reliance'[6] and is underpinned by a framing of a 'participation society' that expects citizens to care for each other (Grootegoed & Tonkens, 2012).

The reform restricted access to residential care and excluded lighter forms of home care support from LTC funding. Arguing that the AWBZ expansion had made people overly dependent on public assistance, the government launched the Social Assistance Act (WMO, 2007), which made entitlements to social care conditional to the non-availability of informal care (Grootegoed et al, 2015) In addition, the new Long-term Act (WLZ, 2014) limited entitlement to LTC for persons with continuous and severe care needs, and strict needs-assessment procedures were introduced. As a result, most *residential homes* for the elderly were closed down, keeping *nursing homes* for people with severe care needs.[7]

Restricted universalism

From its outset, the Dutch LTC system has been characterised as a universalist LTC regime that provides universal access to state-supported services for those in need (Da Roit, 2012, 2013; Van den Broek, 2016). Against a regular healthcare system where risks are privately insured, the LTC system is based on a logic of universal entitlement to cover significant expenses that would not be feasible for private insurance. However, the reforms have turned the system into an example of 'restricted universalism' (Ranci & Pavolini, 2015). Although LTC is still seen as a social right and a citizenship entitlement, more emphasis has been placed on individual responsibility, and access to institutional care is needs-tested (Da Roit, 2012; Grootegoed & Van Dijk, 2012). Access to the system is still universal and not means-tested, although user charges have been raised.

Nowadays, and despite the reforms, public responsibility is still strong. The system features a decisive regulating role of the state, a high level of public spending, and in-kind services as a significant instrument (Maarse & Jeunissen, 2016). The Dutch public expenditure on LTC as a percentage of GDP (3.7 per cent in 2017) is more than twice the OECD average (1.7 per cent in 2017); by contrast, the share of private expenditure (co-payments and out-of-pocket expenses) in total spending on LTC services is relatively low.

The system provides extensive need coverage with a broad range of health and social care services, including residential and home-based care.[8] While residential care is now reserved for people with severe and continuing care needs, those with lighter care needs are entitled to home care. From 2015 on, the regulation of the services previously under the AWBZ was split between the Long-term Care Act (WLZ, 2014), the Social Support Act (WMO, 2015), and the Health Expenses Act (ZVW, 2008). The WLZ focuses mainly on residential care and consists of a mandatory insurance scheme, redistributive and open-ended in nature,[9] that ensures care for those who need it regardless of their income level. The ZVW covers, particularly, nursing care and personal care provided at home. The WMO covers the remaining home-based care, comprising what is known as 'social care' (assistance with daily living activities) and domestic help (cleaning).

Residential care was, from the outset, an essential part of the system. Seventy five per cent of public spending is allocated to LTC residential care, as reflected in the relatively large number of LTC beds in such facilities (OECD, 2019). Cash-for-care schemes were a late addition to the system, responding to LTC clients' demands and the wish to encourage the development of markets in the LTC sector. Since 2003, it has been available to all LTC clients, but most LTC (WLZ) beneficiaries still opt for in-kind benefits.[10] In 2016, only 4.7 per cent of LTC (WLZ) recipients aged 65 and over had a personal care budget (MLZ, 2018).

Fragmented governance pattern dominated by the State

Although the state plays a central role in the Dutch LTC system, private actors and subnational administrations are also prominent. Public regulation and financing are combined with private service delivery – non-profit or for-profit. In the Netherlands there are no government-owned care providers; all providers are private, although the majority are not-for-profit (Mot, 2010). For-profit providers can operate in the home-based care sector, while only non-profit providers are permitted in the LTC regulated sector.

Policy reforms have entailed essential changes in the governance pattern, particularly in marketisation and decentralisation. Since 2015, the LTC system has been partially deregulated.[11] While residential care remains more strictly controlled, non-residential care has been devolved to private insurers or municipalities. Health insurers have gotten more responsibility in LTC provision: the implementation of the WLZ is delegated to care offices run by a single care insurer as the representative of all insurers in a region. The remaining home-based care has been decentralised to local authorities,[12] including what is known as 'social care', managed and financed by municipalities under the Social Support Act (WMO, 2015).

This fragmented governance pattern has brought about tensions and inconsistencies among the different actors involved in the implementation. Mainly, coordination problems arise because the LTC system now comprises three different financial regimes, each with its implementing agencies, budgets, and incentives (Non et al, 2015; Maarse & Jeunissen, 2016).

Underlying the policy reform is the idea that private insurers and municipalities can organise LTC more efficiently than the care offices which organised LTC under the previous AWBZ.[13] In addition, municipalities are now responsible for providing a wide range of services and receiving a non-earmarked budget, so they have the incentive to limit spending (Mot et al, 2010). As a result, cutbacks have had significant consequences on the price and availability of services, leading municipalities to negotiate a lower tariffs or contract lower volume of care, which on its part, has triggered a deficit among many care providers (Maarse & Jeunissen, 2016).[14]

Measures for the impact of the pandemic on the residential care sector for the older-age population

Efficiency logic and scarce preparedness for a pandemic

The Netherlands had a national pandemic action plan before the COVID-19 outbreak.[15] The plan was drawn up in 2014 by the national council for infectious disease control (LOI).[16] The pandemic action plan is aimed at public health services and describes which measures should be taken in each crisis phase and who is responsible for determining the phase.

There must be regional and, if necessary, national coordination during a crisis.[17] Measures to be taken in response to a crisis or pandemic are discussed within the 11 regional councils on acute care (ROAZ) and 25 regional medical assistance organisations (GHOR).[18] The ROAZ organisations have drawn up an escalation model in which the required cooperation and coordination of care is described for various situations or phases: from green (potential mapping bottlenecks, for example, at the start of the flu season) to yellow to orange to red to black (supra-regional coordination required). For example, measures in response to the COVID-19 outbreak were first coordinated at the regional level in the province of Noord-Brabant. The national institute took over coordination for public health (RIVM) as the outbreak of COVID cases became widespread. Moreover, an outbreak management team (OMT) was set up to advise the government on how to tackle the outbreak.[19]

All hospitals in the Netherlands are obliged to prepare for disasters and crises such as influenza pandemics by drawing up a 'hospital disaster relief plan' (ZiROP), which describes the measures the hospital will take in the event of a large influx of victims or patients.[20] In addition, every ICU is obliged to have a care policy plan, which states with which regional hospitals it has agreements and what they entail. Furthermore, the national association of ICU physicians (NVIC) developed its own specific pandemic action plan for ICUs, using colour codes from green (standard care) to orange (upscaling) to red (crisis care). As of 30 March, 'code red' has been applied (mentioned earlier).[21]

Despite all these plans and organisations, several experts noted that the Netherlands needed to prepare for a pandemic. They pointed out that since the Ebola outbreak in West Africa in 2014, the Dutch government had been advised several times to pool knowledge and expertise about pandemics, seek international cooperation, and create buffers for ICU capacity, respirators, and medicines. However, more was needed to be done with these recommendations.[22] A crisis expert pointed out that disaster exercises and the 2018 influenza epidemic had shown that the available capacities would quickly fall short in the event of a pandemic. However, solving these capacity problems would be highly costly.[23] Another expert characterised the Dutch preparations for a pandemic as 'mainly symbolic', pointing out that national risk analyses had been made and all kinds of plans had been written, 'but materially, we were not prepared'. According to this expert, the costs involved were the main factor: 'It is a cost-benefit consideration. That is why those national risk analyses that predicted a pandemic were decoupled from policy a few years ago. It prevented the departments from having to do anything with the results of those analyses'.[24]

A journalistic investigation based on interviews with dozens of stakeholders and public and internal documents concluded that the illusion that the Netherlands was well prepared for an outbreak led to an underestimation of the coronavirus. For example, in the worst-case scenario of the GGDs, there would be a 'large' introduction of up to 20 patients simultaneously – a scenario proved untenable within 2 weeks after the first known infection. According to this journalistic investigation, the shortages were the logical consequence of decades of pursuit of economy and efficiency in Dutch health care: 'This is called "sensible care" in policy language. Empty IC rooms, large stocks, and extensive diagnostics must all be avoided. It has resulted in a system that in normal times offers just enough care for everyone'. However, the COVID-19 crisis made it clear that such a system also comes at a price.[25]

Specific provisions for nursing homes

The national pandemic action plan is generic but contains several appendices relevant to care homes and nursing homes. These appendices provide detailed guidelines for how nursing homes and other institutions should deal with outbreaks of gastroenteritis,[26] norovirus,[27] scabies,[28] and respiratory infections.[29] It is difficult to say to what extent and which of these pre-existing guidelines helped respond to COVID-19 outbreaks in nursing homes and whether and to what extent they were consulted and followed by nursing homes during the first weeks of the COVID epidemic when there were not yet specific COVID-19 guidelines for nursing homes. However, the circumstances were unfavourable: there was limited testing capacity and limited knowledge about symptoms that could indicate a COVID-19 infection and the modes of transmission of the virus.

During the pandemic, the RIVM developed a series of national COVID-19 guidelines, some aimed at the LTC sector. On 20 March, the first guidelines on the use of personal protection equipment by care personnel outside hospitals were published.[30] Moreover, on 24 March, the first guidelines for deploying and testing non-hospital care workers with symptoms or with family members with symptoms were issued.[31] According to these first versions, using personal protection equipment by non-hospital care workers caring for patients who were not infected was unnecessary and (given the scarcity of this equipment) was also not desirable. Non-hospital care workers who had only mild symptoms could not be tested (because of the limited test capacity) and had to continue working to prevent staff shortages due to high absenteeism. In the following months, these guidelines were revised repeatedly. However, it took longer to solve the shortages of personal protection equipment (discussed earlier). Nursing homes with an urgent shortage of protective equipment and (possibly) infected residents were advised to contact the ROAZ in their region.

Again, it is difficult to say to what extent these RIVM COVID-19 guidelines were followed. What is clear, however, is that they were challenging to follow for many nursing homes for many reasons, which were, to a large extent, beyond the control of the homes. The latter is the case for the limited testing capacity and availability of personal protection equipment and the intense focus of policymakers and policy advisers on supplying hospitals as a priority. The repeated adjustments to the guidelines also made it difficult to keep an overview, and it was only in a version published on 1 May that the RIVM acknowledged that 'these guidelines … require further elaboration per sector, taking into account context and target group. If the specific situation requires it, healthcare workers can deviate from these principles based on their professional insights and experience'.[32]

Management capacity

The Netherlands has a relatively small number of ICU beds. When the epidemic began, there were about 1,150 ICU beds (6.6 per 100,000 population), including 250 insulating beds. Usually, about 70 per cent of these beds are occupied. In the second week of April, more than 1,300 COVID-19 patients were treated in ICUs. During the epidemic, about 650 temporary extra ICU beds were created. The health minister and politicians wanted even more extra beds, but that was impossible. The main bottleneck was the number of ICU nurses. At the epidemic's peak, there was also an impending shortage of ICU equipment (private hospitals and the army provided respirators to hospitals with COVID-19 patients) and a shortage of anaesthetics (the Healthcare inspectorate temporarily approved a veterinary anaesthetic for use in humans to help solve this shortage).

ICUs were thus put under extreme strain. However, over time, the priority given to COVID-19 patients was criticised by medical specialists such as cardiologists and oncologists, who noted that it was detrimental to the interests of patients with other life-threatening diseases. Suspending regular care might cause casualties as well. This risk was exacerbated because many people hesitated to contact emergency services because they assumed that the emergency department was too busy with COVID-19 patients. They feared contracting COVID-19 in the hospital too.

Non-hospital care sectors (home care and nursing homes) were also under enormous strain. In addition, there was a scarcity of personal protection equipment, such as face masks. Therefore, a central allocation model was developed to assess the availability of protective garments and manage distribution. Initially, this model prioritised supplying hospitals, assuming they would receive most COVID-19 patients. What may also have played a role is that the LTC sector was hardly represented in the outbreak management team (OMT), the team of experts chaired by the director of the Center for Infectious Disease Control of the National Institute for Public Health (RIVM, www.rivm.nl), which advises the government on how to tackle the COVID-19.

Due to the scarcity of supplies, many care workers outside hospitals thus had to work without protective equipment. Moreover, suppose they had only mild symptoms. In that case, they could not be tested (because of the limited test capacity), and they had to continue working (to prevent staff shortages due to high absenteeism). These were guidelines of the RIVM applicable at the time.

Nevertheless, the situation in the residential sector did not aggravate the overburdening of hospitals and ICUs. It was instead the other way around. As interview four put it: 'Because (many) people die in the nursing home, the IC capacity was not under too much pressure. Unfortunately, because so many people are dying, we do not have to consider our capacity of beds as such a concern' (Interview 4).

Governance and the crisis as a 'hospital issue'

In the Netherlands, the COVID-19 crisis management has been criticised for its lack of leadership, inconsistency, and untransparent decision-making. The reactive attitude that the government has adopted reflects the subsidiary role that the Ministry VWS has within the semi-privatised and regionalised healthcare system. As a result, subsidiarity prevails (regional and private stakeholders must face the problem), while the Ministry VWS has a mere coordinating, supervising function.[33] This dominant governance pattern in healthcare has resulted in 'soft' crisis management and the absence of strong leadership. In this context, client politics under the influence of pressure groups and different actors in the healthcare scene have played a prominent role.

This overall management of the crisis partly explains the strong impact of the epidemic in the residential care sector. In managing the corona crisis, a cure has been put before care and prevention, focusing all attention on the hospitals and (especially) their ICU stations. As the third interviewee says, 'the position of the nursing homes was not acknowledged for a long time, despite the drama that was taking place there … Most of the dead did not fall in the hospitals but in the nursing homes, and they got no masks, no attention'. The LTC system, and the residential care sector in particular, was not represented in the group of experts that advised the government during the first phase of the crisis. Conversely, the influential part that the strong Dutch hospital lobby has played has been highlighted in all the interviews.

The fact that the Dutch healthcare sector (hospitals) is better organised as a lobby than the LTC sector (nursing homes) has been determinant in channeling a specific framing of the issue and related policy responses. The perspective of medical and emergency care has dominated the construction of the problem, contributing to a view of the COVID crisis as an 'emergency' and a 'healthcare issue', specifically affecting hospitals and ICU stations.[34] The hospital lobby has promoted such a policy frame through their role as policy advisors (top-down) and via their influence on the media. As this narrative of the issue effectively permeated Dutch society, the hospital lobby got to 'own the issue' (Petrocik, 1996). The COVID-19 issue became a 'hospital issue'. In the reality of figures and death tolls, and it was as much a 'nursing homes' issue.

Intersectional coordination

The coordination or lack thereof between the healthcare and the LTC systems has not been an issue in the Netherlands. According to a representative of the association of residential care organisations (Interview 4), nursing homes and hospitals have collaborated particularly for purposes of testing and for the transfer of clients. In addition, to reinforce personnel shortages, there have been regional exchanges, for example, nurses from nursing homes to hospitals or geriatric doctors supporting each other across regions. Nevertheless, such initiatives have been occasional and not been at a large scale because, at a general level, 'there has not been a need' and 'in terms of staff, we in the Netherlands have managed well. We do not see what we have seen in Italy or Spain' (Interview 4).

The (lack of) collaboration between the public and private residential care organisations has not been an issue, despite the latter being better resourced and equipped. Somehow, not much interaction was deemed necessary with the healthcare system, considering that nursing homes are well equipped to provide medical care for COVID-19 patients, as they count on their personnel[35] – besides nurses and care assistants, also GPs, geriatric doctors, and other specialists.[36] Customarily, elderly residents who get ill are treated within the nursing home, only exceptionally being transferred to a hospital. The same was applied to COVID-19 patients, most of whom were treated in their own nursing homes, rooms, or special sections specifically arranged. Only a minority of the residents severely affected by the virus were transferred to hospitals, following a path-dependent practice. According to the interviewees, due to the fast tempo of how the disease unfolds, there was virtually no time to transfer ill people, as most of them suddenly deteriorated and died. Many elderly patients showed no symptoms or only light ones and suddenly died.

The higher epidemic incidence in some regions also prompted more proactive initiatives and vital stakeholder coordination and collaboration. For example, care homes in the southern part of the country were affected more severely, most likely because COVID hit that region harder. In Brabant, a specific structure was created, agglutinating LTC actors (RONAZ) parallel to the emergency care network (ROAZ), which was later extended to other regions.

Assessment of the measures

The COVID-19 epidemic has dramatically impacted the Dutch residential care sector. By early April, it became public that the virus had severely hit nursing homes. At that point, the RIVM estimated that in about 40 per cent of all nursing homes, there were (or had been) outbreaks, with high mortality figures in some of these homes. By 15 May there had been 7,900 verified COVID-19 cases among residents of nursing homes, plus 4,550 unverified cases. About 7 per cent of the residents of nursing homes had been infected, and 2 per cent had died.[37]

The government's approach in the first wave of the COVID crisis paved the way for the spread of the virus in care homes.[38] Notably, two early policy choices can be associated with high infection and mortality rates in the sector: the test policy and the distribution of protective material. Access to COVID tests was subjected to very restrictive conditions from the offset; only persons who had been in Wuhan (China), presented fever (above 38 degrees Celsius), and two other symptoms of the illness were entitled to be tested.[39] This very restrictive test policy was held until June because of shortage of test capacity.[40] In addition, care homes were at the end of the cue for receiving protective equipment since its distribution was administrated by the regional networks of emergency care (ROAZ), dominated by hospitals.[41] The ROAZ focused on scaling up hospitals and the ICU. As a result, although nursing homes had more infected people than the hospitals and the ICU, the masks were divided between hospitals and nursing homes in a ratio of 90 per cent to 10 per cent. Interviewee 1 described that, instead of providing them with protective equipment, the ROAZ went so far as to ask them to 'make our protective equipment available to the hospitals'.

The scarcity of protective material for personnel in nursing homes was an apparent spreading factor, aggravated by RIVM guidelines establishing that those professionals with mild symptoms had to continue working. Paradoxically, this rule, established to prevent staff shortages, contributed to the high incidence of infection and absenteeism among personnel. While official figures of COVID-19 incidence among healthcare professionals are not disaggregated by sector,[42] our interviewees report high levels of sick leave among staff (10–12 per cent), well above regular rates.[43] Consequently, nursing homes struggled with labour shortages, which in many cases were covered by hiring temporary personnel (Interview 3) or by intensifying the working hours of regular employees by, for example, asking them to work more days or not to take days off (Interview 1). Likewise, nursing homes with many infected care workers got assistance from nurses from the Dutch army; in some homes, the army must take (over) the reins of the institution. No emergency legislation related to the health system has been issued other than relaxing to some extent the registration requirements for healthcare personnel involved in COVID-19 care.[44]

On 20 March, the minister of health decided that all care homes and nursing homes had to close their doors to all visitors. The decision was taken on the advice of the OMT and Verenso, the association of specialists in geriatric medicine, and after consultation with the RIVM and Actiz, the umbrella organisation of LTC providers.[45] As far as we have been able to ascertain, nursing homes across the country have implemented this measure with immediate effect.

Evolution of the situation in the following phases of the pandemic and challenges for the future of the care home sector

Lessons learned?

During the first COVID-19 wave, it slowly became clear that a 'silent disaster' was unfolding in nursing homes. As a result, the Lower House of Parliament passed a motion on 4 June 2020 asking the government to quickly draw lessons on the measures taken and policies to be implemented in nursing homes shortly and during a possible second wave.[46]

After consulting parties from the LTC sector, the Minister of Health described the lessons learned concerning nursing homes in a letter to Parliament dated 17 July 2021. In this letter, he acknowledged, among other things, the dilemma between safety on the one hand and quality of life and humanness on the other.[47] This dilemma was described as follows by the Council for Government Policy (WRR) in an advisory report on sustainable care published in 2021: 'The one-sided focus on safety, but at the same time the lack of preparation for the risks in this regard became poignantly clear during the first wave of the COVID-19 pandemic. Not only was nursing home care not included in the contingency plans of the Ministry of Health and the RIVM, but personal protection measures and testing equipment were also scarce, resulting in many infections and, consequently, deaths in nursing homes. Furthermore, the lockdown measures, including the ban on visits, were strictly adhered to, causing many older adults to become lonely and their quality of life to suffer in other ways'.[48]

Parties from the LTC sector also formulated lessons from the first COVID-19 wave in a position paper dated 30 June 2020.[49] Both the minister and the sector emphasised the importance of:

- an excellent national and regional positioning of nursing home care ('care' not to be seen separately from 'cure');
- ensuring sufficient personal protective equipment and testing capacity;
- scope for customised visiting rules (in consultation with care professionals); and
- basic safety in all nursing homes, with an emphasis on quality of life and hygiene, and infection prevention.

The results of our interviews with two managers of nursing homes and two policy advisors of the employers' organisation of nursing homes, conducted between June and August 2020, were mainly in line with these policy documents. At the time of the interviews, some demands for more discretionary space for nursing homes and their organisations had already been granted. Another lesson emphasised by the respondents was the need to increase coordination across sectors and levels, particularly more local and regional coordination (Interview 3), better collaboration between interest groups (in particular ACTIZ and VERENSO), and more coordinated work between hospitals and nursing homes' geriatric doctors and more support for the last ones (Interview 2).

The need for customised visiting rules in nursing homes during a COVID-19 outbreak was also emphasised by academic researchers. In the future, a national visiting ban should be avoided, and there should be scope for a regional approach, with nursing homes and residents involved in the decision-making, according to two teams of researchers from various universities.[50] In October 2020, managers from the LTC sector and academics published a manifesto in which they argued that quality of life must prevail over safety; closing the nursing home doors would strip away much of what makes the life of residents worthwhile.[51] In December 2020, the government issued stringent lockdown measures in response to a dramatic increase in infections and hospitalisations. However, it did not announce a visiting ban for nursing homes. Nursing homes reacted differently to outbreaks of the – very contagious – British COVID variant. Some closed their doors to visitors completely, and others tightened their visiting rules but did not close their doors altogether.[52]

In September 2020, new guidelines for testing and face masks were published for nursing homes. Nursing homes should have all residents and staff tested weekly if a fellow resident is found to be infected with the coronavirus. This guideline follows the results of a study into the spread of the virus in four Dutch nursing homes, which showed that many residents were carrying the virus without showing any COVID-19 symptoms. The OMT also recommended stricter measures to prevent the virus from entering a nursing home. Nursing home staff should be trained better in recognising COVID-19 signals. As soon as the number of infections in the vicinity of a nursing home increases, staff and visitors should start wearing preventive protection equipment. The nursing home should consider having its residents and staff tested at random.[53]

The Netherlands was confronted with a second COVID-19 wave from September 2020 to January 2021. Again, there was excess mortality in nursing homes, but less than during the first wave. During this second wave, 4,900 more people died in nursing homes than expected if there had been no pandemic.[54] A third period of excess mortality occurred among nursing home residents and the general population in the last months of 2021. Measured over the whole year 2021, the relative excess mortality among residents of nursing homes was lower than in 2020, while that among the rest of the population was higher.[55] That was probably thanks to the high vaccination uptake among nursing home residents. From mid-January onwards, nursing home residents could be vaccinated, and as soon as 1 month later, the effects on the number of infections and deaths were visible.[56]

Until April 2021, national guidelines stated that if 80 per cent of a nursing home's residents had been fully vaccinated, a resident could receive a maximum of two visitors per day; if less than 80 per cent of residents had been fully vaccinated, a resident could receive a maximum of one visitor per day. Since April 2021, there are no national guidelines for visiting policies for nursing homes anymore, and individual homes can set their policies.[57]

The future of the residential care sector

A dilemma that will probably continue to exist is between the quality of life on the one hand and safety (including infection prevention) on the other. Unfortunately, safety standards applied to the entire healthcare sector may be too rigid for nursing homes.[58]

The biggest challenge for the sector will undoubtedly be attracting and retaining staff. More than 40 per cent of new care employees leave the sector within 2 years. Reasons include the low starting salary of care workers, the work pressure and working hours, the lack of career prospects, and the need for a culture of investing and learning.[59] In addition, since the second wave of the COVID-19 pandemic, the sector has been struggling with high levels of absence due to illness.[60]

Concerning the positioning of LTC, it is worth noting that the government which took office in January 2021 was the first to have a minister for LTC. In the coalition agreement, however, the nursing home sector was not mentioned at all. In May 2022, the minister wrote in a letter to parliament that the growth of the number of jobs in the care sector must be slowed down to prevent that. By 2040, one in four employees will work in this sector. According to the minister, other forms of work are needed, focusing on shared regional employment and providing care through technology that reduces work pressure and the retention of care workers.[61]

Notes

1 CBS (2022a).

2 De Visser et al (2021).

3 CBS (2022a).

4 Onderzoeksraad voor Veiligheid (2022: chapter 7).

5 To allow for greater competition between care providers, care was split into different 'care functions' (nursing, personal care, domestic care, assistance) which could be purchased separately.

6 In Dutch: '*eigen regie*'.

7 The percentage of people aged 65 and older living in institutions dropped from 7.2 per cent in 2004 to 6.5 per cent in 2010 (Alders et al, 2016). Nursing homes nowadays concentrate the most vulnerable old-age population.

8 Extensive need coverage is coupled with high social contribution (12 per cent of work-related income in 2011).

9 In practice, however, each government makes estimations of the LTC expenses for the coming 4 years, and the Ministry of Health, Welfare and Sport (VWS) is responsible for making expenditures stay within this budget. To adjust expenses they may introduce increases in co-payments, reductions in coverage and tariff cuts for the providers (Mot et al, 2010).

10 Cash benefits are nevertheless relevant for the present study, as they are also used to finance small-scale housing initiatives (*'kleinschalige wooninitiatieven'*) for elderly people.

11 The functioning and competition of the LTC markets is monitored by the Dutch Healthcare Authority (NZa); only in the part that is still regulated (residential care) the NZa makes rules and supervises providers' compliance.

12 This includes services for older persons, persons with disabilities, drug addicts, and persons with psychiatric problems.

13 The expenditure cuts in the WMO and ZVW were politically sold as 'efficiency cuts', and amounted to €0.7 and €0.4 billion, respectively (Maarse & Jeunissen, 2016).

14 Particularly, many providers for housekeeping have stopped their activities.

15 https://lci.rivm.nl/draaiboeken/generiek-draaiboek

16 The LIO was established in 1995 and is composed of representatives of the regional public health services (GGDs), the four major cities, the healthcare inspectorate, the national coordination centre for travel advice (LCR) and other organisations.

17 https://nvic.nl/sites/nvic.nl/files/Draaiboek%20Pandemie%20deel%201%20versie2.0%20-%20160620%2012.pdf

18 https://richtlijnendatabase.nl/covid-19.html

19 www.covid19healthsystem.org/countries/netherlands/livinghit.aspx

20 www.ggdghorkennisnet.nl/?file=34383&m=1497268853&action=file.download

21 https://nvic.nl/sites/nvic.nl/files/Draaiboek%20Pandemie%20deel%201%20versie2.0%20-%20160620%2012.pdf

22 Kabinet negeerde adviezen over pandemie-aanpak, *Trouw*, 15 April 2020.

23 Onze voorbereidingen op een pandemie waren symbolisch, NRC, 27 March 2020.

24 Onze voorbereidingen op een pandemie waren symbolisch, NRC, 27 March 2020.

25 Hoe Nederland de controle verloor, NRC, 20 June 2020.

26 https://lci.rivm.nl/draaiboeken/gastro-enteritis-en-voedselvergiftigingen

27 https://lci.rivm.nl/richtlijnen/norovirus

28 https://lci.rivm.nl/richtlijnen/scabies

29 https://lci.rivm.nl/draaiboeken/generiek-draaiboek

30 https://lci.rivm.nl/covid-19/PBMbuitenziekenhuis

31 https://lci.rivm.nl/lci.rivm.nl/covid-19/bijlage/zorgmedewerkersinzetentestbeleid

32 https://lci.rivm.nl/covid-19/PBMbuitenziekenhuis

33 For instance, talking about the possible shortage of protective material, the Minister of Healthcare said that it was not necessary to purchase large stocks of masks. In his own words, he must limit itself to follow the developments and call the attention of care providers and private insurances in case that there are incidental shortages (Hoe Nederland de controle verloor, NRC, 19 June 2020). This is also consistent with the general approach of the government's coalition (VVD, D66, and so on).

34 Following McBeth et al (2010), we can analyse the narrative behind many of these public discourses in terms of a story with actors, victims, and villains. This construction of the issue depicts IC's personnel as the 'health heroes' struggling against the coronavirus (the villain), to save COVID-19 patients (the victims). Nursing homes are absent from this narrative.

35 In the Netherlands, care homes with accreditation for WLZ care are responsible for the organsation of the medical care of their residents, which includes both general medical care or specific LTC (WLZ).

36 Interviews showed that nursing homes even count with specialists in other areas, such as infectious diseases (Interview 1) or lungs (Interview 3).

37 Bijna 8000 coronagevallen in verpleeghuizen, ruim 2500 doden, Telegraaf, 20 mei 2020.

38 Moreover, different actors warned about the wrong assumptions underlying the Dutch approach (in the first 2 months). Among others, the association of microbiologist doctors warned that because of the restrictive test policy, the RIVM data gave an inaccurate view of the spreading of the virus in the country.

39 RIVM guidelines. In fact, the Outbreak Management Team emphatically advised people with symptoms, but who fell outside the definition, not to get a test. Otherwise 'we could end up testing everybody with a cold' (Hoe Nederland de controle verloor, NRC, 19 June 2020).

40 Later on, it was known that the test capacity was actually pretty high, and had been unused (NRC, 2020).

41 These coordinating bodies prioritised the needs of hospitals and IC departments; often, nursing homes were not even members of the network.

42 According to RIVM, since the outbreak began 16,973 healthcare workers have been diagnosed with COVID-19, 529 healthcare workers have been hospitalised and 11 have died (data from 6 June).

43 Interviewee 3, from an organisation that suffered a dramatic COVID outbreak, reports that during the whole period (March–June) 119 employees were tested positive.

44 https://www.covid19healthsystem.org/countries/netherlands/livinghit.aspx?Section=5.1%20Governance&Type=Section

45 https://www.rijksoverheid.nl/documenten/mediateksten/2020/03/19/persconferentie-minister-president-rutte-en-minister-de-jonge-over-aftreden-minister-bruins-en-het-bezoek-aan-verpleeghuizen

46 Tweede Kamer, vergaderjaar 2019–20, 25295, nr. 396.

47 Kamerbrief 'Lessen verpleeghuizen met het oog op een eventuele tweede golf', kenmerk 1709971-207318-LZ, 16 July 2020.

48 WRR (2021: 151).

49 Position paper ActiZ, V&VN, Verenso en Zorgthuisnl – geleerde lessen langdurige zorg Covid-19, 30 June 2020.

50 Verbeek et al (2020); Van Tol et al (2021); Verbeek-Oudijk and Koper (2021: 78).

51 'Manifest: doe verpleeghuizen niet meer op slot', *Trouw*, 10 October 2020.

52 'Verpleeghuizen weer dicht voor bezoek', *Friesch Dagblad,* 4 January 2021; 'Duikt Britse mutant op? Dan blijven bezoekers welkom', *De Stentor*, 16 January 2021.

53 'Kabinet: verpleeghuizen moeten bij één besmetting iedereen testen', *de Volkskrant*, 2 September 2020.

54 Schürmann et al (2022).

55 CBS (2022b).

56 'RIVM ziet eerste effecten van vaccin bij ouderen', *Trouw*, 25 February 2021.

57 International Long-term Care Policy Network 2021.

58 WRR (2021).

59 SCP (2021: 77); WRR (2021).

60 'Conny Helder: "De rek is uit de verpleeghuiszorg"', *Skipr*, 9 December 2020, Available from: https://www.skipr.nl/partnernieuws/waardegedreven-organiseren-veel-meer-dan-uitkomsten/?daily=1

61 Hoofdlijnenbrief Toekomstbestendige Arbeidsmarkt Zorg, kenmerk 3360942-1028444-MEVA, 13 May 2022.

References

Alders, P., Comijs, H., and Deeg, D. (2016) Changes in admission to long-term care institutions in the Netherlands: Comparing two cohorts over the period 1996–1999 and 2006–2009, *European Journal of Ageing* [online], Available from: https://repub.eur.nl/pub/95503/Alders-2016-Changes-in-admission-to-LTC.pdf

CBS (2022a) *Gezondheid in Coronatijd* [online], Available from: www.cbs.nl/nl-nl/visualisaties/welvaart-in-coronatijd/gezondheid-in-coronatijd

CBS (2022b) *10 Procent meer Mensen Overleden dan Verwacht in 2021* [online], Available from: www.cbs.nl/nl-nl/nieuws/2022/04/10-procent-meer-mensen-overleden-dan-verwacht-in-2021

Companje, K. P. (2015) 'Financing high medical risks in the Netherlands: Healthcare, social insurance and political compromises' in Companje, K. P. (ed) *Financing high medical risks. Discussions, developments, problems and solutions on the coverage of the risk of long-term care in Norway, Germany and the Netherlands since 1945 in European perspective*, Amsterdam: Amsterdam University Press, pp 101–76.

Da Roit, B. (2012) The Netherlands: The struggle between universalism and cost containment, *Health and Social Care in the Community*, 20(3), 228–37.

Da Roit, B. (2013), Long-term care reforms in the Netherlands, in Ranci, C. and Pavolini, E. (eds) *Reforms in long-term care policies in Europe: Investigating institutional change and social impacts*, New York: Springer, pp 97–115.

De Visser, M., Kunst, A., Stoeldraijer, L., and Harmsen, C. (2021) *Sociaal-Demografische Verschillen in COVID-19-Sterfte Tijdens de Eerste Golf van de Corona-Epidemie* [online], Available from: www.cbs.nl/nl-nl/longread/statistische-trends/2021/sociaal-demografische-verschillen-in-COVID-19-sterfte-tijdens-de-eerste-golf-van-de-corona-epidemie

Grootegoed, E. and Van Dijk, D. (2012)'The return of the family? welfare state retrenchment and client autonomy in long-term care, *Journal of Social Policy*, 41, 677–94.

Grootegoed, E., Van Barneveld, E. and Duyvedak, J. W. (2015) What is customary about customary care? How Dutch welfare policy defines what citizens have to consider 'normal' care at home, *Critical Social Policy*, 35(1), 110–31.

Grootegoed, E. and Tonkens, E. (2016), Voluntary care: A deficient alternative, *Nederlands tijdschrift voor Geneeskunde*, 160, D243–D243.

Hoe Nederland de controle verloor, NRC, 19 June 2020, Available from: https://www.nrc.nl/nieuws/2020/06/19/hoe-nederland-reageerde-op-het-nieuwe-virus-uit-china-van-niks-aan-de-hand-tot-blinde-paniek-a4003075

International Long-term Care Policy Network (2021) Current situation in relation to 'visiting' in care homes and outings for residents, *LTCCOVID International Overviews of Long-Term Care Policies and Practices in Relation to COVID-19*, 2, August [online], Available from: https://ltcCOVID.org/2021/08/05/current-situation-in-relation-to-visiting-in-care-homes-and-outings-for-residents-ltcCOVID-international-overviews-of-long-term-care-policies-and-practices-in-relation-to-COVID-19/

Maarse, J. A. M. and Jeurissen, P. P. (2016) The politics and policies of the 2015 long-term care reform in the Netherlands, *Health Policy*, 120(3), 241–45.

McBeth, L. et al (2010) Buffalo tales: interest groups policy stories in Greater Yellowstone, *Policy Sciences*, 43(4), 391–409.

Mot, E. (2010) CPB document no. 204: The Dutch system of long-term care, The Hague: CPB.

Mot, E. et al (2010) The Long-Term Care System for the Elderly in the Netherlands. ENEPRI Research Report No. 90, Brussels: Centre for European Policy Studies.

Non, M. et al (2015) Keuzeruimte in de Langdurige zorg, The Hague: CPB and SCP.

OECD (2019) Health at a Glance 2019: OECD Indicators, Paris: OECD Publishing.

Onderzoeksraad voor Veiligheid (2022) *Aanpak Coronacrisis. Deel 1: tot September 2020*, Den Haag: Onderzoeksraad voor Veiligheid.

Petrocik, J. R. (1996) Issue ownership in Presidential Elections with a 1980 case study, *American Journal of Political Science*, 40(3), 825–50.

Ranci, C. and Pavolini, E. (2015) Not all that glitters is gold: Long-term care re- forms in the last two decades in Europe, *Journal of European Social Policy*, 25(3), 270–85.

Schürmann, R., van der Toorn, J., and Stoeldraijer, L. (2022) *Ontwikkelingen in Sterfte in 2020 en 2021* [online], Available from: www.cbs.nl/nl-nl/longread/diversen/2022/ontwikkelingen-in-sterfte-in-2020-en-2021.

Van den Broek, T. (2016) Supporting ageing parents: Comparative analyses of upward generational support, Rotterdam: Erasmus University Rotterdam, Available from: https://repub.eur.nl/pub/93509/

Van Ginneken, E. and Kroneman, M. (2015) Long-term care reform in the Netherlands: too large to handle, *Eurohealth*, 21(3), 47–50.

Van Tol, L. S., Smaling, H. J. A., Groothuijse, J. M., Doornebosch, A. J., Janus, S. I. M., Zuidema, S. U., Calijouw, M. A. A., Achterberg, W. P., and de Waal, M. W. M. (2021) COVID-19 management in nursing homes by outbreak teams (MINUTES) – study description and data characteristics: a qualitative study, *BMJ Open*, 11(11): DOI: 10.1136/bmjopen-2021-053235.

Verbeek, H., Gerritsen, D. L., Backhaus, R., de Boer, B. S., Koopmans, R. T. C. M., and Hamers, J. P. H. (2020) Allowing visitors back in the nursing home during the COVID-19 crisis: a Dutch national study into first experiences and impact on well-being, *Journal of the American Medical Directors Association*, 21(7), 900–4.

Verbeek-Oudijk, D. and Koper, I. (2021) *Het Leven in een Verpleeghuis*, Den Haag: SCP.

WRR (2021) *Kiezen Voor Houdbare Zorg. Mensen, Middelen en Maatschappelijk Draagvlak*, Den Haag: WRR.

Interviews

Interview 1. Trudy Prins, nursing home De Rijnhoven (Utrecht).

Interview 2. Jacqueline Joppe, ZGE (former ACTIZ), lobby/interest association of care employers.

Interview 3. Martin den Hartog, nursing home AxionContinu (Utrecht).

Interview 4. Frank Hagelstein and Charlotte Vromans, ZGE (former ACTIZ), lobby/interest association of care employers.

13

Portugal: structural weaknesses of nursing homes network exposed by the pandemic

Luis Capucha, Alexandre Daniel Calado, and Nuno Nunes

Introduction

This chapter is about the COVID-19 pandemic in long term care residences (LTCR) in Portugal from 2 March 2020, to 15 July 2020. It was a dramatic period in which Portuguese society faced a threat unprecedented in the memory of people and institutions, about which little or nothing was known.

One of the most disconcerting facts that occurred was how the pandemic spread to the elderly and, in particular, those who were institutionalised in LTCR. However, this being the focus, we will only deviate from the topic and the fixed period when there is a need to frame them, namely regarding the pandemic's evolution and the LTCR network's evolution.

Although the period under analysis in this chapter is the four and a half months between 2 March 2020, when the first case of infection was detected, and 15 July 2020, when the first cycle of the pandemic ended, it is worth looking at its evolution from a broader perspective. This perspective reveals a much higher incidence of the disease after autumn 2020 than until then, as shown in Figure 13.1. The daily new cases recorded by the Directorate-General for Health were 53 per day at the beginning of March 2020, increasing to around 350 per day by July of the same year and coming close to 750 cases per day in early October 2020.

At that time, a wave of large proportions emerged, reaching a peak of almost 7,000 cases per day in mid-November and 15,000 per day in late January 2021. There are two crucial phenomena to register: first, the relationship between policies, population behaviour, and how people perceive the evolution of SARS-COV2 infections. The effect of the 2 months of confinement after the first wave of April–May 2020 and the opposite effect of the lifting of restrictions after the confinement that followed the summer and, later, Christmas and New Year, combined with the appearance of new, more contagious, strains of the virus, in a context still without the effects of vaccination, produced moments of euphoria for the success in the fight

Figure 13.1: Evolution of the COVID-19 pandemic in Portugal (from 2 March 2020 to 4 September 2022)

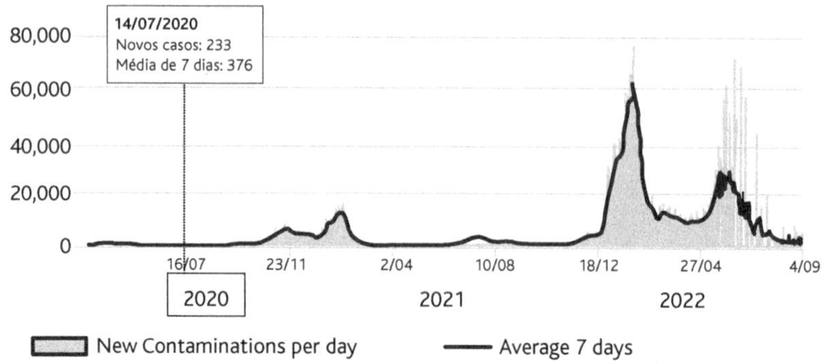

against the pandemic, alternated with moments of panic at the verification of the inability to control its growth.

After February 2021, the incidence dropped again to daily values between 200 and 600, and then, in December, a new wave began, reaching daily values of around 45,000 in January 2022. During 2022, the daily infections ranged between 12,000 and 25,000, almost until the summer, when they declined to 2,000 and 4,000.

Interestingly, when there were fewer infections, fear prevailed at the beginning, while society started to live normally with the disease when the infection reached its highest value. The fact that little was known about the disease and how to fight it, the unpreparedness of services, and the morbidity up to July 2020 explain the fear, while the arrival of vaccines and then the appearance of new strains, more contagious but less lethal, explain the 'normalisation'.

In total, 5,430,000 people were infected in Portugal between March 2020 and September 2022 (52.7 per cent of the population). Of these, 24,865 died, which represents 0.46 per cent. The daily means of infections was 5,777. Looking at the period between 2 March 2020 and 15 July 2020, 47,426 people were infected, averaging 351.3 per day, but of these, 1,676 people died, or 3.5 per cent. The fear did not come, at this time, only from the images of what was happening in China, Italy, and Spain. It also came from the lethality of the disease.

More than half of these deaths occurred in LTCR. Therefore, it justifies the need to understand what happened in these structures that should take care of the well-being of the elderly but appeared to be the most dangerous places they could be.

This chapter is divided into three parts, the first will address the structure and evolution of the social facilities network for the elderly, the second will address the measures adopted to combat the pandemic, especially in the

LTCR, and in the third we will present how health and social services were articulated in the LTCR and what lessons can be learned for the future.

Care sector for the elderly in Portugal: a poor coverage of legal and non-legal facilities with contrasting quality

Portugal is the fourth most-aged country in the European Union, after Italy, Germany, and Greece. Rapid ageing, both at the top and the bottom of the age pyramid, is one of the most characteristic features of the processes of change in Portuguese society, as is the case throughout the world (Capucha, 2014; Silva & Pereira, 2015; Calado et al, 2019).

The ageing rate in Portugal (number of residents over 65 years old per hundred residents under 15 years old) went from 30 in 1971 to 161 in 2019, registering a growing trend in all decades. Likewise, the percentage of people over 65 has grown steadily from 9.5 per cent in 1971 to 22.0 per cent in 2019 (Figure 13.2).

The percentage of the population aged 75 and over grew even more rapidly, from 3.1 per cent in 1971, or 6.7 per cent in 2000, to 10.7 per cent in 2019. Additionally, the 'big elderly' segment, of people aged 85 or more, multiplied their weight by six, from 0.5 per cent in 1971 to 3.1 per cent in 2019.

Women are the majority among the elderly. At all age groups, there are 52 per cent of women versus 48 per cent of men. However, women in the older segments represent 60 per cent of the total population. The 'big elderly' contribute the most since 574,674 women are between 65 and 74 years of age, and 593,066 are in the group of 75 years or more.

After the Democratic Revolution of 1974, better living conditions permitted accelerated ageing (Capucha, 2005; Botelho et al, 2015). The country's infrastructure in terms of electricity, sewerage, and access to

Figure 13.2: People aged over 65, 75, and 85 years old as a percentage of the total population

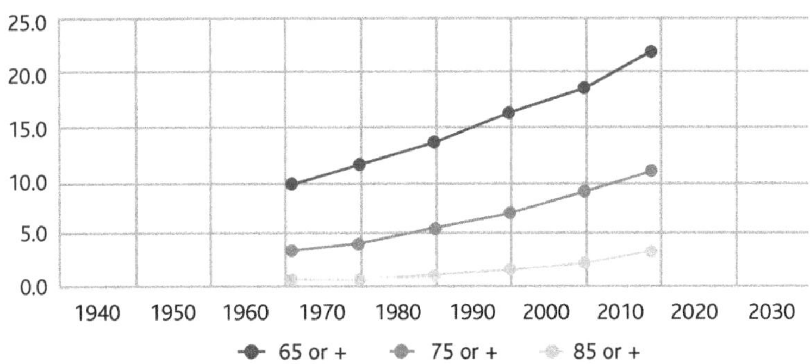

Source: Pordata, 15 July 2020

drinking water at home, alongside the extraordinary development of the national health system and the creation of the universal social protection system, are the main factors that explain this ageing trend.

However, progress also brought new problems, such as the elderly dependency rate and its impact on the pension system (Ocampo & Stiglitz, 2018). As lives get extended, situations of dependency to carry out daily tasks become common. In addition, there are other delicate issues, namely the provision of care to older people when they live alone or with another older person. The isolation of the elderly is, moreover, a reality that is proliferating (Mauritti, 2011). The number of households of isolated people in 2019 was 934,100, representing 22.5 per cent of the total households. Of that total, 513,200 (54.9 per cent) were people aged 65 or over.

Thus, dependent older people without family support (or with deficient support, including the frequent practice of domestic violence) are left with the existing responses promoted by the market (Esping-Andersen, 1990) or by civil society organisations (private institutions of social solidarity – IPSS), partially financed by the State.

Evolution of long-term care: a sector managed by civil society organisations supported by the State, with a trajectory of growth, but still too short

In 1984, the first Social Security Basic Law was published and revised in 2007. The Pillar of Social Action was defined in the Basic Law and integrated into the Solidarity Subsystem in 2007. It includes social facilities promoted by the State, the solidarity sector (comprised mainly of IPSS connected in different ways with the Catholic Church), and the market. The system is highly centralized. Regional centres of social security inform processes of licensing and control of facilities and social responses. However, they have been increasingly losing autonomy, and now they act simply as applicants of the national central directives. The state supports the IPSS in the construction of facilities and by financing services for the lower-income segments of the population. They form a vast network of civil society organisations functioning locally, depending on the National Institute of Social Security. Their scope is local, and they follow national policies and guidelines.

In 2000, the Department of Studies, Prospective and Planning of the Ministry of Labour and Solidarity (DEPP-MTS) published the first characterisation of the social facilities network in Portugal, the Social Charter (DEPP-MTS, 2000). The publication included all the existing 7,068 equipment, with its 14,208 facilities serving 250,894 citizens. The number of social facilities for the elderly was 4,483, and it welcomed 142,532 older adults. The characterisation comprised only the licensed social facilities network of the Portuguese mainland (the autonomous regions of the

Azores and Madeira are not under the tutelage of the national government in this field).

The typology of social facilities for the elderly in Portugal from the mid-1970s to 2000 was as follows:

1. Day centres (DC) and convivial centres – appeared as experimental areas in the mid-1970s, intending to keep people at home. In 2000, there were 1,339 DCs, of which 253 started their activity between 1975 and 1985, 727 between 1986 and 1995, and 281 between 1996 and 1998 (Table 13.1). There were 399 convivial centres in 2000, 20 created before 1974, 106 between 1975 and 1985, 198 between 1986 and 1995, and 75 between 1996 and 1998 (Table 13.1). The DCs had a capacity of 45,946 users in facilities from the solidarity sector and 327 users in facilities from the market sector. The State did not promote DC facilities. By 2000, DC's capacity represented 3.2 per cent of the population aged 65 and over and 8.3 per cent of those aged 75 and over. However, the occupancy rate was 78.5 per cent, corresponding to 36,328 users. The convivial centres had a capacity for 29,670 users in the solidarity sector and 162 users in the profit sector, representing 2.1 per cent of the population aged 65 and over and 5.3 per cent of the population aged 75 and over. The utilisation rate was 85.3 per cent, corresponding to 25,315 users. The most significant demand is among people between 70 and 74 years old (24 per cent), followed by people between 65 and 69 years old (21 per cent), and people between 75 and 80 years old (20 per cent). Over that age, the values decrease to 14.5 per cent. Women are 59 per cent in both types of social facilities.
2. LTCR for the Elderly (ERPI) – the historical origin of LTCR is the nursing homes. Before 1974, they welcomed, without any dignity, the elderly without a family. Nowadays, the situation is quite different since the number of older people is much more significant, and the demand in the search for well-being is also greater. Individual social homes have a minimal expression (there were only 33 in the solidarity network and six profitable in 2000). Homes are collective residences that aim to provide housing in a humanised environment, provide permanent personal and health services, ensure basic needs, and create conditions that allow for preserving family relationships without dependence on the elderly from their relatives. In 2000, the officially licensed facilities were constituted by 805 LTCR of the solidarity network and 376 LTCR of the profitable network. The installed capacity was 49,934 users, distributed by 41,951 in the solidarity network and 7,108 in the profitable network. These numbers corresponded to 3.5 per cent of the population aged 65 and over and 9.0 per cent of those aged 75 and over. The occupancy rate in the solidarity network was 95.9 per cent, while in the profitable network,

it was 85.2 per cent. About 72 per cent of users were aged 75 or over (5.7 per cent in this segment), while 48 per cent were 80 or older (9.2 per cent of the total population in that group). Women represented 64.5 per cent of users. In terms of the activities organised in these facilities, approximately 75 per cent of LTCR organised trips for their users, 50 per cent ateliers and occupancy activities, and 65 per cent other cultural and recreational activities. Regarding health assistance, 88 per cent had medical and/or nursing support. The medical staff consisted of employees, personnel hired as independent services providers (48 per cent of medical support and 43 per cent in nursing), or through protocols with public health services (22.7 per cent of medical staff and 17.9 per cent of nursing were in this condition). In 2000, of the 10,900 people who provided services in LTCR, only 2,400 were technical personnel, of which 27 per cent were nursing personnel, 21 per cent medical personnel, 4 per cent social workers, 1 per cent psychologists, 6 per cent monitors, 5 per cent therapists, and 36 per cent directors or coordinators. The non-technical staff, comprising the remaining 8,500 employees, were 19 per cent family helpers, 60 per cent auxiliary, 1 per cent drivers, 4 per cent administrative staff, 1 per cent barbers, 8 per cent cooks, and 7 per cent 'others'.

3. Home support service (HSS) – this measure aims to provide specialised home care to families and individuals who, due to illness or disability, cannot meet their basic needs and, simultaneously, avoid isolation by maintaining elders at home. In 2000 there were 1,269 responses (Table 13.1). They cared for 38,022 people, corresponding to 2.6 per cent of people over 65 and 6.8 per cent over 75. The average utilisation rate was 90 per cent. Those over 80 years old represent 34.5 per cent of users, those between 75 and 80 years old represent 27 per cent, and those between 70 and 74 years old represent 19 per cent. Women represented 57 per cent of users.
4. Family care for the elderly – this measure aims to provide the elderly with Ann social environment alternative to the family of origin. In 2000, it was in the embryonic stage, with only 110 foster families (Table 13.1). Ninety-four per cent of beneficiaries were over 70 years old, and two-thirds were women.
5. Holiday centres – this measure is residual. In 2000 there were 12 holiday centres with 393 beds in mainland Portugal (Table 13.1).

Long-term care nowadays – consolidates the scarce network that provides continuing care services

After the revision of the Social Security Act (2007), the State withdrew from the system. The option was to reinforce the financing of the IPSS, and in return, they would practice 'social prices' for the poorest segments

Table 13.1: Evolution of the number of social facilities for the elderly in Portugal*, from before 1974 to 2000

	Before 1974	1975–1985	1986–1995	1996–1998	2000
Day centres	–	253	980	1,261	1,339
Convivial centres	20	126	324	399	399
LTCR for the elderly	154**	334**	651**	787**	1,181
Home support service	15	154	902	1,269	1,269
Family care for the elderly	–	–	–	–	106
Holiday centres	–	–	–	–	12

* Data regards mainland Portugal

** Data regards only the solidarity network

Source: Social Chart, MTSS

of users (Ferreira, 2015). As these responses are markedly insufficient for the growing needs of the population, clandestine LTCR residencies proliferated in the informal market, often operating in very precarious conditions and without supervision.

In 2018, according to the Social Charter, the Social Services and Equipment Network included, for all categories, 11,500 pieces of equipment, which represents a growth of 62.7 per cent when compared to 2000. The promoted facilities were around 17,900, representing an increase of more than 3,500 compared to 2000. Owners grew from 4,000 to 6,500, 71 per cent of which were non-profit entities, and 29 per cent were market entities. Considering the number of equipment, the percentage in the third sector increased to 83.4 per cent. Of the 18,400 existing facilities, 41.2 per cent (about 7,600) were aimed at the elderly. The growth in the number of responses was higher than the average, with 67 per cent of the new equipment created between 2010 and 2018 being LTCR (36 per cent), home support services (17 per cent), and DCs (14 per cent).

In 2006, the PARES Program was implemented, whose goal was to finance the expansion of social facilities in Portugal promoted by third-sector entities with public support for construction and operation. The planning, coordination, and financing of social action policies are central, while local authorities participate by granting land to build the facilities. As a result of the PARES Program, the installed capacity in the Network of Services and Social Equipment grew drastically between 2000 and 2018, from 400 thousand to 1.1 million available facilities and a little more than 400,000 users (with over occupation) to 900,000 users. However, the exponential growth of the population aged 65 years or older prevented a considerable coverage rate increase. In 2018, the occupation rate in homes for the elderly was 93 per cent.

Regarding services and equipment for the elderly, there has been an increase in the type of social facilities, which have come to be named: 'residential structures for the elderly (ERPI)' (LTCR and Residences), day centres (DC) and social centres (CS), home support for the elderly (ADI), family reception (AF) and the new measure of night centres (CN). The number of responses grew sharply in the 20 years between 1998 and 2018 (around 89.3 per cent, corresponding to an additional 3,400 new responses), with the most accentuated increase being in ADI – the primary response in the community environment – with a 108 per cent growth, and in ERPI with 105 per cent growth. In 2018, there were 7,300 responses in the ERPI, ADI (the two most frequent valences), and DC.

In 2018, DC provided 23.6 per cent (65,000) of facilities for the elderly. However, only 64 per cent of the capacity of those facilities was used. LTCR covered 36.5 per cent of facilities for the elderly, HSS covered 40 per cent of the capacity of facilities for the elderly, and DC provided 23.6 per cent of facilities for the elderly. LTCR's capacity was close to full use (93 per cent), with about 63 per cent of users covered by cooperation agreements, through which the State finances the institutions that host them. HSS and DC registered around 62 per cent of people under the age of 80, while LTCR users were, in half the cases, people aged 80 years or older.

As summarised in Table 13.2, the total capacity of the facilities in 2018 was close to 274,000 users, representing an increase of 104 per cent compared to 1998 (139,200 available seats). However, these places provide a coverage rate for the population aged 65 and over, only 12.6 per cent.

It is important to note that the network for expanding the social facilities was renewed in 2020, under the PARES Program 3.0, with an investment of 110 million euros.

The PARES Program also aimed to increase the inspection and closure of private structures, some clandestine and other legal, which did not meet the requirements for operation, set out in the Law. The more common issues are the dimensions of the facility and its rooms, the guarantee of users' privacy, the qualification and number of technicians and employees, the conditions of accessibility, and the security of the infrastructure.

Table 13.2: Social services for the elderly, Portugal, 1998 and 2018

	Facilities	Users	Places	Coverage Rate (%)*
1998	4,310	132,240	139,200	6.2
2018	7,600	254,820	274,000	12.6

* Population aged 65 or more/Places

Source: Social Chart, MTSS

Continuing care, a social and health facility addressed to people who need intense and daily health care for the rest of their lives but not needing inpatient hospital services, is not considered in this typology. Nevertheless, according to the Director of a Misericórdia interviewed, they are extensions of LTCR. This official also argued that this issue needs urgent clarification by the Government. The fact that LTCR is at present functioning partially as health services in the field of palliative care impacts negatively on their capacities to respond to the pandemic appropriately.

Several problems with the LTCR network were already identified before the pandemic. However, the measures taken during the pandemic were aimed at something other than solving these problems. The processes were facilitated by allowing the facilities to start operating through a simple communication to the Ministry of Labour and Social Security instead of a double license (one of the municipalities for use and another of the MTSS for operation) that was previously required. Unfortunately, the simplification of procedures aimed at streamlining processes and combating illegal facilities was not accompanied by an update of the requirements for operation, to be established later. That is why the leaders of the institutions operating in the sector wonder if the effect of reducing illegal activity will be verified.

It is estimated that more than 3,500 illegal LTCRs are currently in operation in Portugal. The situation of generalised and little-repressed clandestine facilities became evident to the municipalities, through the civil protection commissions, with their emergency responses to COVID-19 (which, fortunately, were never necessary). As a result, many municipalities conducted inspections of these structures, often almost invisible, and the list of known cases of illegal LTCR has increased. There are even counties where it has doubled. At that time, attention was drawn to the need to know how many of these 'social facilities' exist, how many people live there, and under what conditions, for an effective fight against the pandemic, in the context in which it was most reproducing.

According to the testimonies collected, when people have to place their families in private LTCRs, they first look for those whom social security supervises. However, frequently they cannot pay the prices requested for private LTCR with quality. Then they look at the other options, usually of poor quality and, in fact, largely clandestine. The difference in quality crosses all domains, from the material conditions of residence to the services provided, to the qualification and quantity of personnel to the type of approach, with the substitutive human relationships of the family being decisive.

Role of families in long-term care

Traditionally, the woman provides the care needs for dependent older adults inside the family. However, daughters and daughters-in-law are less and less available, as female participation in the labour market is high. The female activity rate has been above 54 per cent since 2002, reaching 54.7 per cent in 2019. The female employment rate was 50.8 per cent in the same year (55.3 per cent). Even so, in cases of illness, it is estimated that the family provides 80 per cent of the continued care for the elderly (Nogueira, 2012), the vast majority by other older adults, whether spouses or sons aged 65 or over (Herlofson & Brandt, 2020).

Families are still the primary resource on three levels: (1) partial financing (as a supplement to pensions) of the LTCR frequency; (2) the provision of care, mainly by daughters and daughters-in-law; and (3) the provision of services by spouses who are also elderly. The problem with the first solution is that, in a crisis, many of these families bring the elderly to their homes to use their income as a 'resilience' strategy (Estevão et al, 2017). The second solution's problems are the frequency of domestic violence, the low quality of services, and the double workload of women who provide care alongside their professional activity. The big problem of the third is the precariousness and low quality of the services provided, although the affectivity tends to be great.

Long-term care debates before the pandemic

In Portugal, the debate on the social services system for the elderly revolves around three main issues. Firstly, the problem of supply and coverage rates. Scarcity is significant and widespread around the country. The question, therefore, is of the possibilities for supply growth.

Second, the issue of average quality and its control is pressing. The main problem is that clandestine private homes of poor quality (both in terms of conditions and services) proliferate due to the scarcity of supply in the face of demand. The inspection is largely tolerant since the State does not have alternatives for families. Therefore, their impact is residual despite campaigns to close homes in terrible conditions. This situation allows many private homes to be maintained without conditions, even when they are legalised and licensed. In addition, there are also many problems regarding the quality of services provided on the social network, namely in health care and entertainment activities, given the limited funding by the State.

Finally, there is a debate around governance, which takes two directions. One focuses on the effects of the monopolisation of the system by social network structures favoured by the State to the detriment of other more flexible community-based responses supported by neighbourhood networks. The other criticises the State's delegation of its responsibilities to third sector organisations, with gains for the budget (mainly because they practice lower salaries than in the public sector) but with less control over the supply quality.

For this reason, the debates tend to concentrate on the level of financing by the State, with minor consideration of quality, in terms of network and number of facilities or the services they provide.

Policies to combat the pandemic in the long-term care sector in Portugal

Health services had never reached a situation of such disruption as during the COVID-19 pandemic. Neither had their professionals ever had to decide between two patients, which one would be in intensive care or connected to a ventilator. Only at the end of 2020 were some doctors warning of a danger of saturation of the health system in the Lisbon and Tagus Valley (LVT) region. Afterward, by December 2020 to January 2021, hospitals were close to exceeding their capacities. However, they have yet to reach the limit. The percentage of patients who required hospitalisation was 9 per cent.

From an early stage, in the first half of March (with only 785 infected), 'the entire hospital network was ready to receive patients. This means creating circuits inside the same hospital, in which patients are divided into two large groups (with and without symptoms)', informed the Director General of Health. The care models introduced for COVID-19 were established, compelling people who felt symptoms to seek help through the telephone service, from where they were referred to the health services, if necessary. That avoided congestion at hospitals and other emergency services. As a result, health services have proved that they are able to respond to several hospitalised patients that do not exceed around 450 cases, at the peak point of the two first vacancies of the pandemic.

Early policies to combat the pandemic consisted of public investment in the public health system (SNS), purchasing equipment such as ventilators and personal protection, and stimulating the intervention of local governments to create 'campaign hospitals' that were spread all over the country. It was a priority because SNS had been under solid financial pressure and staff shortages. However, the Council of Public Finances, an entity that monitors State accounts created during the crisis of 2011–14, emphasised that the pandemic had exposed the fragility of the SNS and its financial stability. The accumulated deficit of €2,796 million between 2013 and 2019 was at stake, and so was the suppliers' debt, which equalled €1,589 million in 2019.

Still, it was necessary to hire 1,800 professionals. As a result, the number of beds in intensive care increased by 35 per cent between 1 March and 2 May (from 528 to 713). In addition, 500 ventilators were purchased from China, the first 100 of which arrived between 19 and 23 May 2020. On the other hand, on 16 March 2020, the SNS suspended scheduled activities so that on the 19th of the same month, almost 1.4 million consultations and 51,000 surgeries had been postponed.

The macroeconomic situation supported this strategy. In 2019, for the first time in the history of Portuguese democracy, the State budget balance was positive. Moreover, external debt was in the process of marked reduction. Both factors created conditions for the government to invest in strengthening the health system, preventing redundancies, and destroying the productive fabric. However, the reports presented to the Portuguese Parliament in the third week of July 2020 pointed to a 9 per cent drop in GDP. It is estimated that the State had revenue losses of around €2,423 million and expenditure increases of €1,319 million. In 2019, public debt was estimated at €117.7 per cent of GDP, increasing to 135.9 per cent. The European response to the crisis has become indispensable (Eurofound, 2020).

Internally, there is a problem of a government that matters. There is virtually no link between health and social security authorities. The regulations and norms related to health conditions in LTCR and other social facilities for older people were initially defined in the law with contributions from Health authorities (based on the Protocol of Action for Social Support), but the collaboration ended there. The decisions to support the promoters, licensing, and inspection were entirely the responsibility of social security.

However, at the local level, the institutions articulated with the Health Centres. It translates into providing outpatient nursing support to users of Home Support Services and monitoring users of LTCR for elderly people to consult. This collaboration was focused on routine and preventive health care, vaccinations, and advice. It was mainly performed by nurses, although many LTCR facilities also have had contact with doctors. So, health services assist the Nursing Homes when problems arise, as with any other institution or individual citizen, but there is no permanent collaboration plan. Furthermore, facilities are required to have, at most, very tight internal health services, and more is needed to improve collaboration.

During the pandemic, cooperation was naturally strengthened by the circumstances: the LTC residences were where the very vulnerable population was and constituted critical points of contamination, which forced double care of attendance and reinforced prevention, but only while the pandemic lasted. With its demise, some LTC services were reinforced with crisis response structures (for example, quickly deployable rear beds). However, both systems proved resilient, returning to their normal state and staying apart.

Description and analysis of the measures adopted to address the impact of the pandemic on the residential care sector for the elderly

Preparedness for the crisis in the long-term care system

The pandemic, an enormous health crisis, took Portugal entirely by surprise. There is no notice of any prevention approach to a pandemic or type of crisis management plan or protocol. There were plans to fight against other risks, mainly natural and associated with buildings and equipment, but not against a pandemic. There was no national plan to deal with this kind of situation. All the actions were taken under the pressure of a dramatic situation. That was something that the LTCR system, like other sectors, had to face unexpectedly, and all the answers were to be found after the disease arrived.

Exceptionally, 1 year before the pandemic, the General Inspection of Health promoted a visit of a pedagogical nature to several LTCRs. During these visits, it was noticed the existence of facilities with insufficient levels of health care; the lack of rigour in the documentation, such as records of nursing acts; the absence of systems for regular assessment of the degree of dependence of users or lack of monitoring of users in their night shifts; the lack of definition of the medication circuit; and the shortage of nursing staff, given the residents' problems. The report that resulted from it re-emerged as early as mid-July 2020, given the visibility that the problem had gained. The situation of 'Portugal at the tail of Europe', in the number of formal caregivers per 100 elderly people, was then added to the diagnosis. Only Poland and Greece were in a worse position (OECD, 2020; Tello et al, 2020).

Policy measures to combat the pandemic and its impact on the long-term care system

Even before the first case was registered in Portugal, the Social Security and the National Health Department, by 27 January 2020, presented orientations to all social facilities, which were revised and updated on 29 February and 4 March. In addition, measures regarding health services, and the creation of 'dedicated areas' in all emergency services in hospitals and health centres (community health units existing in all municipalities) were part of the strategy to combat the pandemic right from the start. Unfortunately, however, equipment that would be considered decisive was not available.

When the epidemic started to be perceived as a real threat, the government's main objective was to keep the infection levels relatively low, between 0.9 and 1 infected by each patient. The strategy was to 'flatten the curve'. It would be decisive, on the one hand, to avoid the collapse of the Health Services and, on the other hand, to create good conditions for the resumption of economic activity, something that was then thought to be a quick process, taking into consideration the evolution of the pandemic in China.

The first phase of the political response to COVID-19 was called the 'mitigation phase' and lasted from 2 March to 17 March 2020. Visits to hospitals and prisons were suspended, day centres for the elderly were closed, and institutions (universities, schools, companies, and public services) started to define 'contingency plans' according to the instructions from the Health General Directorate. In addition, people with symptoms were required to test and, in the case of a positive test, were kept in quarantine, under police control.

On 11 March 2020, the WHO declared the state of the pandemic. On the same day, the General Health Department published an orientation report regarding the procedures of the LTCR, to the Integrated United of Continuous Care (UCCI), to the National Network of Continuous Care (RNCCI), and other social responses for elders, and institutions of care for at-risk children and youngsters. In addition, the District Centres of Social Security implemented a plan for the IPSS to develop and implement contingency plans. As a result, visits to structures of residential care were suspended by 14 March 2020.

On 18 March 2020, a state of 'national emergency' was declared by the Portuguese government. It was the first time this constitutional rule was declared. The national emergency state reinforced the measures taken before and added confinement of people at home. However, there were a few exceptions: (i) health professionals and other workers who work in essential activities, such as transporting patients, selling food, sanitation, cleaning, and public safety; (ii) all workers who were unable to stay on lay-off, or telework (for example, cleaning services, civil construction, manufacturing industry; and (iii) leaving home to go shopping for food, walk pets, physical exercise, and care for dependent family members. Universities, schools, and daycare centres were closed, and medical consultations and non-urgent treatments were postponed. Bars, clubs, show venues, beaches, and other leisure spaces, libraries, archives, museums, monuments, art galleries, concert halls, auditoriums, hairdressers, manicures, and the like, as well as commercial spaces, except for those selling food, pharmacies, and other essential goods, were closed. The frequency of public transport was significantly reduced, while the means of transport on service should do so with only two-thirds of the seats, which was materially impossible to fulfil. In some counties, a 'sanitary belt' was imposed. One thousand two hundred prisoners were released. Funerals were limited to a maximum of five persons attending.

Regarding the residential care sector, day centres were closed, and visits to LTCR were prohibited. It was enacted to maintain very restrictive rules for spatial distance. Infringements could be punished with fines. The borders were closed, reopening only on 1 July 2020, with pomp and circumstance.

In terms of future impacts, along with the confinement and closure of schools and social facilities for children, the most emblematic measures were the advice of telework, both in the private sector and in the State, and the creation of special rules for simplified lay-off in companies.

Distance education was even more controversial since most teachers needed to prepare for this educational modality's pedagogical and technological requirements. Moreover, many students needed electronic equipment to follow the classes and perform the proposed exercises. At any rate, the system worked, and some of the solutions, like 'tele-school' – school on TV, were welcomed by the families and pupils, while many teachers rapidly acquired new e-learning competencies.

By May 2020, the leading indicators of the pandemic had dropped to levels that were considered consistent with the strategy's objectives, which led the government to enact the end of the national emergency and the beginning of a deconfinement phase. So far, the strategy's success has contributed to the Public Health Service and the media. There was a severe compromise to support the objectives of combating the pandemic and appealing to citizens to comply with all indications from the government and health authorities, from the political parties that have refrained from making politics around the pandemic, and from the government that has promoted transparency of information and the involvement of all political agents in the consensus of the measures to be taken, suggested by experts.

The new phase was planned to be divided into two periods – one until 18 May 2020, and the next after an assessment of what happened. What happened was an increase in the number of cases of infection in LVT. Thus, in June 2020, the country started to be in a 'state of alert', except for this region, which was in a 'state of calamity'. For example, clusters of more than 20 people were not allowed in the streets, reduced to 10 in the AML and 5 in 14 of its parishes. The Rt remained around 0.9 (1.07 in the AML).

Visits to LTCR were resumed, but with new rules – one visitor per user, by appointment, and at most for 20 minutes.

The Portuguese mainland entered the second phase of deflation, which foresaw the lifting of several restrictions. For example, visits to prisoners and young people hospitalised in educational centres were resumed, and the telework regime was no longer mandatory, except for groups at risk. Unfortunately, many people misperceived the signals sent as the end of special care and organised parties that generated contamination outbreaks. The rate of contamination among young people doubled after the deconfinement. Other outbreaks appeared in industrial companies among the less qualified workers, many of them immigrants, in neighbourhoods of social housing, and, in continuation of what had happened before, in nursing homes.

After the deconfinement, the numbers skyrocketed. They did not reach the numbers at the beginning of March 2020, but still a frequency above the desired. The image of the successful country fighting the pandemic was followed by another one, marked by panic due to the decisions of other countries, in particular the United Kingdom, to impose quarantine on those traveling from Portugal, strongly affecting tourism.

The government's initial message, pressured by international comparisons and with different European countries closing borders for those traveling from Portugal, was that the increase in cases was due to an increase in testing. Testing went from 490,000 on 6 May 202 to more than 1,500,000 on 26

July 2020. Still, the fact was that the number of positives was increasing and not decreasing.

The LTCR sector benefited from a special testing effort, as would later happen with vaccination, which was a priority.

On July 2020, the Minister of Labour announced the adoption of more agile measures for the licensing of LTCR while referring to the joint number of tests carried out on employees of social facilities (120,000) as proof of the consideration that Portugal was one of the most proactive countries applying tests. However, at the end of June, Parliament passed a measure to pay 100 per cent of the wages to workers discharged by COVID-19.

Challenges for the future of LTC: lessons to learn from the COVID-19 pandemic in Portugal

The pandemic brought a situation in which there is no memory in the homes of the elderly and the promoting institutions. The total closure of DC left users unresponsive, and the routines were changed in LTCR and Home Support Service. In addition to the negative effect of ending family visits.

On the other hand, the financial impact on promoters is high due to the costs of protective materials in the context of speculation in the market. 'This was all very fast. Nobody was prepared. However, in our case, we already had previous procedures, and a code of conduct, so it was not difficult to implement an emergency plan', said the person responsible for an LTCR that performed well in the context of COVID-19. In the case of an LTCR that performed poorly, certain disbelief and disorientation were revealed. Not everyone was prepared the same way, and the virus showed it. Nevertheless, in the good-performing case, the difference was mainly due to adopting more strict rules of visits and contact with the outside world.

When the pandemic was declared, there were no clear views about what had to be done. For example, the initial message from the General Direction of Health was that masks were not recommended since they created a false sense of security (anyhow, there were no masks available in the market). It took much work to acquire them when they were recommended. Finally, companies started to produce them voluntarily and distribute them to LTCR centres through the Union of the IPSS of Portugal. The municipalities also decided, in all places, to acquire masks and other equipment, and distribute them to health services, LTCR, and other services. That was an essential help since the LTCR promoters faced difficulties in supporting equipment and test costs.

A criticism that emerged strongly in this field was directed at the policy measure taken in 2012, during the intervention of the Troika formed by the European Commission, the IMF, and the European Bank, to authorise the accommodation of three older adults per room in the LTCR. Subsequent governments, while proclaiming an end to austerity, maintained most of the measures then taken, which proved fatal during the pandemic. Moreover, there needed to be more specific financial support from the government. Only municipalities have allocated small sums to purchase equipment and cover urgent expenses. Private entities have also donated, mainly for protective equipment. From the State, the LTCR only received guidelines and rules to follow.

An article published in June (Gil, 2020) on the performance and working conditions of 'home helpers' shows that overwork, poor working conditions associated with the lack of training, and the excessive turnover of human resources, have adverse consequences on the quality of care that these professionals provide, but also on their physical and mental health, and employment.

The system was not prepared to respond effectively to a pandemic like this. According to one of our interviewees, the problem is structural. Most people institutionalised in LTCR are very old, have illness problems, and have extreme disabilities. They needed health support that LTCR could not provide. Continuing Care Units are the structures that, due to their nature, should respond to the real needs of most 'interned' in LTC. However, in this area, the responses are very scarce. On the other hand, home support is insufficient to accommodate all the elderly who can remain in their homes. Thus, people residing in LTCR become particularly exposed to the pandemic. Particularly those from LTC, who contributed to 50 per cent of deaths.

The mortality numbers, as well as the incidence of cases in LTCR that are accessible, are proxies since the collection of data on the field has been problematic, not being assured common standards in terms of coverage of all types of residences (particularly the clandestine network), timeline considered in the input of data, and the classification of cases. The situation regarding data collection is illustrative of the extension of the stress that the pandemic poses to LTCR, the lack of coordination between institutions and actors on the field, and the lack of existing policies and instruments to monitor and evaluate the LTCR system.

The heads of LTCR promoted by IPSS go further and question the model governing social action policies in social facilities. The State limits itself to inspecting and subsidising the promoting institutions (without actually cooperating with them) to which it transfers contributions according to the number of users with lower incomes. Nevertheless, these reimbursements are far from covering operating costs. The problem is that the State, more than money, transfers responsibilities. According to the sector's representatives, this contributes to keeping low wages. That is to say, the State handed over social facilities to the third sector because it practices far lower wages than those paid to public workers with the same qualifications and equivalent work. Even so, for example, wages absorb 70 per cent of the revenues of the Misericórdias, an essential sector of third sector organisations, which for that reason are obliged to offer places in the market, with which, together with other revenues (including patrimonial) they finance the social component of the responses.

Thus, a fundamental overhaul of social action policies is an urgent need. With a lack of resources less exposed than health services, the LTCR network has deficiencies and weaknesses that strongly expose its users to frequently unworthy living conditions, and increased health risks.

The few discussions about the impact of COVID-19 in social facilities conclude that a large-scale program for the rehabilitation of social housing to fight the factors of poverty among residents, policy measures to promote access for the most disadvantaged and least qualified to technologies, and the revision of social facilities policies and model of governance are unavoidable social and health requirements.

All developed countries face ageing scenarios, particularly in Europe, although with varying degrees of incidence. In the Portuguese case, the weak social support to the elderly by the State stands out. The State mainly delegates responsibilities to families or institutions partially supported by social security services. It creates a context in which the market fulfils the demand for a residential care home. This sector needs to improve the number of care workers and specialised health and social services, mainly without supervision and quality control. These structural features have manifested in how the elderly care sector has dealt with and is currently dealing with the COVID-19 crisis.

References

Botelho, M. d C., Nunes, N., Mauritti, R., and Craveiro, D. (2015) Tendências de mudança das funções do Estado em Portugal, in: A. F. Costa and R. M. Carmo (eds) *Desigualdades em Questão. Análises e Problemáticas*, Lisbon: Mundos Sociais, pp 59–75.

Calado, A., Capucha, L., and Estevão, P. (2019) Welfare state development in Portugal: From 'stage zero' to the postcrisis 'leftist' compromise against austerity, *Comparative Sociology*, 18(5), 658–86.

Capucha, L. (2005) *Desafios da Pobreza*, Oeiras: Celta Editora.

Capucha, L. (2014) Envelhecimento e políticas sociais em tempos de crise, *Sociologia, Problemas e Práticas*, 74, 113–31.

DEPP-MTS (2000) *Carta Social*, Lisboa.

Esping-Andersen, G. (1990) *The Three Worlds of Welfare Capitalism*, Princeton, NJ: Princeton University Press.

Estevão, P., Capucha, L., and Calado, A. (2017) Resilience: moving from a 'heroic' notion to a sociological concept, *Sociologia, Problemas e Práticas*, 85, 9–26.

Eurofound (2020) *COVID-19: Policy Responses Across Europe*, Luxembourg: Publications Office of the European Union.

Ferreira, S. (2015) New paths for third-sector institutions in a welfare state in crisis: the case of Portugal, *Nonprofit Policy Forum*, 6(2), 213–41.

Gil, A. P. (2020) Estruturas residenciais para pessoas idosas: relação entre qualidade dos cuidados e qualidade do emprego, *Cidades, Comunidades e Territórios*, 40: 67–87.

Herlofson, K. and Brandt, M. (2020) Helping older parents in Europe: the importance of grandparenthood, gender and care regime, *European Societies*, 22(3), 390–410.

Mauritti, R. (2011) *Viver Só: Mudança Social e Estilos de Vida*, Lisboa: Mundos Sociais.

Nogueira, M. A. (2012) A doença e dependência na família, in C. Moura (ed) *Processos e Estratégias do Envelhecimento – Intervenção para um Envelhecimento Ativo*, Euedito, Lisboa.

Ocampo, J. A. and Stiglitz, J. (2018) *The Welfare State Revisited*, New York: Columbia University Press.

OECD (2020) *Who Cares? Attracting and Retaining Care Workers for the Elderly*, Paris: OECD Publishing.

Silva, P. A. and Pereira, M. T. (2015) *Cuidar do Futuro – Os Mitos do Estado Social Português*, Lisboa: Clube do Autor Editora.

Tello, J. E., Pardo-Hernandez, H. R., Rodrigues, S., Ilinca, K., Leichsenring, I., Aguirre, Y., Huber, M., and Barbazza, E. (2020) A services delivery perspective to the provision of long-term care in Portugal, *Portuguese Journal of Public Policy*, 5(1), 8–27.

14

Long-term care for older people during the COVID-19 pandemic in decentralised Spain

Jorge Hernández-Moreno, Roberta Perna, Manuel Pereira-Puga, and Gibrán Cruz-Martínez

Introduction

Long-term care (LTC) for older people has been a traditionally under-developed social policy area in Spain, with national measures addressing situations of dependency and care needs in a somewhat fragmented way until the early 2000s. The creation of the System of Autonomy and Dependency Care (SAAD, by its Spanish acronym) in 2006 attempted to provide a coherent answer to increasing demands for dependency care. However, its practical implementation has been hindered by several structural problems: vertical and horizontal fragmentation across actors in the health and social service domains, weak coordination, precarious employment conditions, and shortages of professional caregivers. As highlighted in the following pages, the outbreak of the COVID-19 pandemic, which hit Spain early and severely, exacerbated these structural problems, (re-)opening a public and political debate on the weaknesses of the LTC system for older people in the country.

The chapter is structured as follows. The first section presents an overview of the country's evolution and key features of the LTC system. In contrast, the second section provides the key facts and figures concerning the evolution of the COVID-19 pandemic and its impact on the Spanish health and care sectors. The next section delves into the institutional and organisational measures adopted to prevent and minimise the impact of the health crisis on care homes for older people across the country. Finally, taking stock of the lessons learnt, the concluding section engages with a two-decades-long debate about the future of the care home sector in Spain. This debate stresses the need to strengthen this increasingly relevant policy domain's human, financial, and institutional resources and its coordination with the health system.

LTC policy and the care home sector for older people in Spain

Evolution of the system and current arrangements

Sharing the key features of the Mediterranean, family-based welfare and care regimes (Chapter 2 in this book), LTC in Spain has been a traditionally underdeveloped social policy area (Aguilar-Hendrickson, 2020). From the 1980s onwards, different reforms were articulated at the national level, although they were somewhat fragmented. The Law for the Social Integration of the Disabled (1982) and the National Gerontological Plan (1982) stand out. From an extra-sectoral point of view, other measures such as the General Law on Health (1986), the Concerted Plan for the Development of the Basic Provision of Social Services by Local Authorities (1988), or the Non-Contributory Pensions Act (1990), have also tried to address situations of dependency and care needs.

Consequently, until 2006 LTC was structured in two basic levels. On the one hand, a very restricted national social security system granting limited cash transfers to workers under 65 years of age with dependency due to work-related accidents or to people with a disability of more than 65 per cent. On the other hand, a residual regional and municipal social services system to protect the most disadvantaged groups aimed at funding dependency care through institutionalised care homes. This second level was characterised by significant territorial heterogeneity in the scope of services (Arlotti & Aguilar-Hendrickson, 2017). Due to these structural weaknesses, the public LTC system served only a tiny proportion of the population. Against such residual state intervention, the responsibility and tasks related to the care of dependent people fell mostly on informal female carers – family members and migrant workers, the latter often in an irregular situation (Da Roit et al, 2013; Spijker & Zueras, 2020).

Despite these limitations, it was in the 2000s that the issue of LTC entered the political agenda. Pressures from different venues – socio-demographic (ageing and growing dependency rate, progressive incorporation of Spanish women in the labour market), domestic (concerning the structure of organisation and provision), and international (LTC reforms taking place in other European countries) – triggered a substantial reform of the Spanish LTC system (Spijker et al, 2022). Facilitated by favourable macroeconomic trends, and the relatively healthy state of Spain's public finances at that time, the reform resulted from a long process of political debate. As well as the development of *sui generis* coalition of interests between the different levels of government, social partners (employers and trade unions), social actors (such as NGOs), and professionals (see Moreno Fuentes, 2015).[1] Such debate resulted in the adoption of the 39/2006 Act on Promotion of Personal Autonomy and Attention to People in a situation of Dependence (the so-called 'Dependency Law'), which established the current SAAD.

The approval of the Dependency Law significantly transformed the previously existing LTC policy framework in the country. As a result, access to the SAAD became configured as a subjective, universal right to social protection for any person who can prove stable residence in Spain for at least 5 years (regardless of age) and who presents one of the degrees of dependency envisaged in the law. Unlike the previous configuration, the LTC system is mainly oriented towards service provision, including prevention services for dependency situations and promoting personal autonomy, remote care service, and home care service. Exceptionally, the system also foresees cash transfer programmes for purchasing care services on the market, hiring an assistant, or financially compensating a family member or a non-professional caregiver.

Historical institutional inertia of regional and local social services schemes, budgetary constraints experienced during the Great Recession, the change of the political cycle in 2011, and the ideological preferences of some regional policy-makers all contributed to the salience of cash transfers despite the norm's preference for direct service delivery (see Deusdad et al, 2016). Nevertheless, this initial trait of the new LTC system has been progressively changing towards a growing service provision role in recent years. Thus, in 2009 cash transfers accounted for 58.22 per cent of the system's benefits, but in 2022 they represented 42.29 per cent (compared to 57.70 per cent of direct service provision; IMSERSO, 2022a).

LTC multi-level governance and funding mechanisms in Spain

With the 2006 Dependency Law, the governance of the SAAD has been structured as a complex multi-level system of shared competencies. The central government is responsible for regulating the primary conditions of the system to ensure equal access throughout the national territory and the management of the information system (SISAAD). Autonomous communities (ACs) remain responsible for the operational structure and day-to-day running of the system, granting benefits, assessing the degree of dependency, and accreditation of centres and services, among other issues. Since 2013, the role of the municipalities has varied significantly depending on the delegated competencies attributed to them by regional laws. In general, local authorities supplement the benefits basket (mostly home care) with resources and with funds transferred by regional governments.

To strengthen coordination across levels of administration, the Dependency Law created the SAAD Territorial Council, composed of the central government's Minister for Social Affairs, the corresponding regional ministers, and local authorities (via the Spanish Federation of Local Governments, FEMP). This Council is responsible for establishing the distribution of funding criteria, the intensity of services, the conditions and amounts of financial benefits, as well as for defining the scale for the recognition of the situation of dependency. Furthermore, each AC must transpose the agreements reached by the Territorial Council into its regional legislation. Since its creation in 2007, this intergovernmental body has shown high levels of activity and institutionalisation. Its meetings have become regular throughout different legislative periods, showing central governments' willingness to use this cooperation instrument (Ministry of Territorial Policy, 2022). However, the ideological opposition between central and regional governments, and the different levels of political commitment and 'institutional loyalty' of regional authorities to the deployment of the Dependency Law, have often created coordination problems and difficulties in ensuring equity in access to the benefits of the SAAD across the country (Marbán Gallego, 2019).

For what concerns the central government and the ACs fund the financing of the LTC system, the SAAD, with funds obtained through general taxation, complemented by a co-payments system based on the type and cost of the service and users' income and wealth levels. There are three levels of public funding. First, the central government is supposed to assume and guarantee a minimum level of funding for the whole State, transferring the corresponding funds to the ACs according to need, the social characteristics of the territories, the number of people requiring care assistance, and other specific geographic conditions. The central and regional governments agree upon supplementary funds.[2] Each level of the administration is supposed to contribute similarly. Finally, there is an additional level set and financed by each AC voluntarily and from their budgets. In relative terms, in 2020, the central government bore 15.1 per cent of the overall cost of the system, users (through co-payment) 20.6 per cent, and ACs the remaining 64.3 per cent (AEDGSS, 2021). These percentages are far from the initial forecasts established in the Dependency Law since the central government was expected to bear about one-third of the system's total costs.

Main features of the LTC system for older people in Spain

Although there is no official register of residential centres for older adults in Spain, statistics compiled by *Envejecimiento en Red-CSIC* indicate that in September 2020, there were a total of 5,567 centres, accounting for 384,251 beds.[3] This means that there were 4.2 beds for every 100 older people, although with significant differences across ACs (Abellán-García et al, 2021a). Therefore, it is estimated that in September 2020, these facilities represented the habitual place of residence for 312,668 older adults (Abellán García et al, 2021b).

Regarding the public-private mix, it should be noted that the private sector plays a significant role in the Spanish LTC system, with most beds (73.2 per cent) being located in privately owned care homes (Abellán-García et al, 2021a). However, a significant percentage of places in private care homes are financed by public resources through agreements signed between public administrations and private providers (the so-called '*conciertos*'). According to recent estimates, subsidised places account for 32.7 per cent of all private places (Muñoz Díaz et al, 2021).

Spanish care homes vary considerably, from tiny centres to extensive facilities. The latter are of great importance: according to CSIC data, 51.3 per cent of places are in care homes with 100 or more beds (Abellán-García et al, 2021a). This fact is especially relevant to understanding the differential impact of the COVID-19 pandemic on Spanish care homes. The size (number of beds) and occupation level of these facilities have been proven to correlate positively with the lethality of COVID-19 during the first wave of the pandemic (Barrera-Algarín et al, 2021).

Another organisational feature of the Spanish care home sector relates to the characteristics of the workforce. Unlike the health sector, there is no official caregiver's register in Spain. At the same time, estimates indicate the presence of approximately 320,000 workers in the sector, the vast majority of whom are women (83 per cent) (Jiménez-Martín & Viola, 2020). Like other EU countries (OECD, 2020), employment in the Spanish care sector is characterised by low wages, temporary contracts, high turnover, and part-time employment. Also, due to these unappealing working conditions, there are shortages of professional care workers. At the same time, a significant proportion of caregivers are low-qualified (Hernández-Moreno & Pereira-Puga, 2021). These weaknesses in staffing levels and in the degree of professionalisation of the sector are particularly problematic due to the multiple vulnerabilities that affect older people in care homes. Almost 80 per cent of residents are 80 years or older (IMSERSO, 2020), increasing the probability of being dependent on caregivers. Likewise, they often suffer from co-morbidities. For example, in Murcia, a recent study shed light on the profile of older adults in care homes: 45.4 per cent suffer from severe dementia, 43.7 per cent are dependent, and 72.9 per cent use diapers (Novoa Jurado et al, 2022).

Evolution of the COVID-19 pandemic

From the state of emergency to the 'new normality'

On 30 January 2020, the WHO declared the outbreak of the new coronavirus a Public Health Emergency of International Concern. The day after, the first official case of COVID-19 was confirmed in Spain. Following the multiplication of cases, the central government assumed the existence of community transmission on 9 March. Finally, on 11 March, the WHO formally declared the existence of a pandemic. Three days later, the Spanish government declared a 'state of emergency' by Royal Decree 463/2020. The decree empowered the Minister of Health as temporarily delegated authority to manage the crisis in health care, being able to adopt all measures deemed appropriate to reinforce the decentralised national health system (*Sistema Nacional de Salud*, SNS).

Throughout the first state of alarm (March–June 2020), the central government and the ACs made significant coordination efforts in healthcare (González Gómez, 2021). During that period, the Interterritorial Council of the SNS, the leading intergovernmental political body in this domain, composed of the central government and ACs' health authorities, met 40 times. Technical committees (such as the Public Health Commission) were also very active, with 70 meetings. However, despite these coordination efforts, central government initiatives were often criticised for not including ACs in their decisions (the Ministry of Health approved more than 75 orders in little more than 3 months) and for the alleged ineffectiveness of its measures to manage the crisis. Moreover, some ACs, such as Madrid and Catalonia, showed an aggressive attitude towards the central authorities (Mattei & del Pino, 2021), politicising the pandemic for partisan competition reasons.

On 9 June, with more favourable epidemiological data on the table, the Royal Law-Decree 21/2020 established the conditions for the 'new normality', identifying the criteria that ACs and their territories had to comply with to soften the restrictions set by the state of alarm progressively. On 21 June, after the National Parliament validated six extensions, the alarm state was lifted. A new phase in intergovernmental relations began at this point (Navarro & Velasco, 2022). The ACs fully recovered their competencies in health matters, while the coordination powers of the Ministry of Health were strengthened.[4]

Differently from coordination efforts in healthcare, no similar dynamics took place in the LTC sector. Neither the Royal Decree 463/2020 and its successive renewals, nor State instructions appointed the Second Vice-President and Minister of Social Rights and Agenda 2030 as delegated authority to manage the COVID-19 crisis in the LTC sector and care homes. Instead, the Ministry of Health at the national level established the criteria for managing and coordinating care centres with other administrations. The ACs and local governments retained their usual powers of dependency management throughout the pandemic. In fact, the social service intergovernmental body (the SAAD Territorial Council) had much lower activity levels than its health counterpart (Hernández-Moreno, 2021).

At the regional level, although the 'single command' in crisis management was usually centred in the Health departments, an intense dynamic of coordinated work developed in many ACs between the departments of Health and Social Services. For instance, socio-sanitary coordination plans and joint action protocols were drawn up in Galicia and Castile-La Mancha.

In the Canary Islands and Asturias, the Regional Ministries of Social Rights and Health developed a shared system to monitor the epidemiological situation in all care homes. However, inter-sectoral coordination problems were clearly identified regarding which Ministry – national or regional – was responsible for the care home sector (including more technical issues such as collecting and publishing data on infections and deaths) (del Pino et al, 2021).

Key figures: impact on the health system and care home sector

In terms of deaths, Spain was one of the first and most severely affected countries during the pandemic in the EU. The Ministry of Health confirmed 46,252 deaths caused by the virus from the start of the pandemic until November 2020 (Ministry of Health, 2020), while the National Institute of Statistics (INE) reported excess deaths of almost 80,000 people in the same period.

From the healthcare domain, the pandemic represented an unprecedented shock for all healthcare systems worldwide. It strained their material and human resources, operational capacities, and governance, including healthcare systems classified as high-performing and resilient to epidemic and pandemic outbreaks, such as the Spanish SNS (Legido-Quigley et al, 2020).[5]

Although Spain's diagnostic capacity was in line with the rest of the EU countries at the beginning of the pandemic, the lack of prepared laboratories, specialised personnel, and medical products for testing delayed the response to the crisis in the face of the high incidence of the virus (European Commission, 2021).

In terms of material resources, the shortage of personal protective equipment (PPE) – especially FPP2/FPP3 masks, goggles, and full PPE – as well as medical products and therapeutics used in intensive care units (ICU), primarily affected the operational capacity of the SNS, especially in the early stages of the crisis (Médicos sin Fronteras, 2020). While difficulties in purchasing PPE were reported globally, Spain lacked national stocks and a nationally based industryl able to produce them (Cáceres Armendáriz & Sierra Alonso, 2021), leaving the central and regional governments with unprecedented difficulties in finding such products in the markets.[6] Problems were also reported concerning the availability of medical equipment, particularly mechanical ventilators, which are crucial in treating patients with COVID-19. As a survey conducted at the end of May 2020 indicates, healthcare professionals rated the quantity and quality of available equipment very negatively (3.46 out of 10 points) (SATSE, 2020).

In a context characterised by these shortages, the incidence rate of the disease among healthcare workers was twice as high as in the general population (the highest rate in Europe) and accounted for 25 per cent of the total number of positive cases reported during the first wave of the pandemic.[7] This situation was aggravated by the fact that the SNS had to face the pandemic with a structural shortage of human resources, with only 3.4 medical and nursing professionals per 1000 inhabitants, a rate well below the EU average (5.74) and far from countries such as Germany (13.0), or Sweden (10.9) (Eurostat, 2022).

In operational terms, primary healthcare services, the main point of access to the SNS and an important triage and follow-up point for COVID-19 patients, were severely overstretched in terms of care capacity due to staff shortages and the closure of many healthcare centres (Amnesty International, 2021). In addition, although telemedicine was strongly promoted to deal with limitations on face-to-face care, this shift in the modes of primary care provision raised issues of equity and inclusion (for mobile, migrant, rural, and vulnerable populations), as it occurred in other countries (Sagan et al, 2021).

The pandemic also affected the operational capacity of ICUs (Ma & Vervoort, 2020). Spain was below the OECD average in ICU beds per 100,000 inhabitants in 2019 (10.4 vs. 14.1). Peak occupancy was reached on 5 April (6,576 ICU beds), with some ACs such as Madrid and Catalonia reaching their maximum capacity during the Spring of 2020. To deal with this overwhelming situation, ICU bed capacity was increased by using resources from other hospital units (such as post-surgical awakening units), adapting inpatient or surgical beds, and making all ICU beds in private hospitals available to the SNS, as indicated by the declaration of the 'state of emergency'. These decisions allowed the rapid doubling of the capacity of ICU beds in public hospitals, from 4,446 beds to 7,930 in only 2 months (OECD, 2021). However, this transformation implied inevitable costs for all non-COVID19 related hospital treatments.

Accordingly, another pandemic side effect is access to the SNS for patients with diseases other than COVID-19. During the first half of 2020, most of the scheduled surgeries were postponed or cancelled. In June 2020, patients waited an average of 170 days for surgery, almost 2 months longer than in December 2019. Delays for the first visit to a specialist increased by 34 days (Ministry of Health, 2021a). In addition, 25 per cent of the Spanish population reported forgoing a necessary medical test or treatment during the first 12 months of the pandemic (Eurofound, 2021). This situation led health professionals and authorities to worry about the worsening of certain diseases and delays in diagnosing new pathologies (Ministry of Health, 2021b).

For what concerns the impact of the pandemic on the care home sector, it has been widely recognised that these facilities accounted for a significant proportion of COVID-19 related deaths during the first wave. However, reliable estimates are difficult to obtain due to underdiagnosis and data reporting, among other factors. Nevertheless, IMSERSO (2022b) reported that between 14 March and 22 June 2020, 9,381 older people living in care homes died with confirmed COVID-19, while an additional 10,492 people died with compatible COVID-19 symptoms.[8] From a comparative perspective, Spain was one of the high-income countries which reported the highest proportion of care home resident population with COVID19-associated death (more than 5 per cent) (Comas-Herrera et al, 2021).

Beyond data about mortality, a significant number of older people residing in care homes suffered adverse effects on their health and quality of life due to the prevention and contention measures adopted in those facilities. For example, actions involving isolation and limitation of social contacts have been associated with the appearance of diseases related to sedentary lifestyles, the aggravation of pre-existing pathologies, and motivational and affective disorders (SEGG, 2020).

Minimising the impact of the pandemic in the Spanish care homes: preparedness, measures, and efficacy

The Spanish 1978 Constitution establishes that the general coordination of healthcare and public health is an exclusive competence of the central government and, specifically, of the national Ministry of Health. However, the Centre for the Coordination of Health Alerts and Emergencies (CCAES), created in 2004, prepares and develops Preparedness and Response Plans to address current or emerging public health threats. In addition, a National Early Warning and Rapid Response System (SIAPR, by its Spanish acronym) was set up in 2013, composed of regional liaison centres, responsible for coordinating response measures against potential health threats from a multi-sectoral point of view.

The Ministry of Health and the CCEAS developed several Preparedness and Response Plans within this framework (for influenza [2005], vector-borne diseases [2016], MERS-CoV coronavirus [2017], Ebola [2020], and West Nile fever [2020]), and ACs are in charge of developing and updating regional Preparedness and Response Plans. However, neither the National Strategies nor the existing pre-pandemic Preparedness Plans, included guidelines directly related to the care home sector. Consequently, with the outbreak of the COVID-19 crisis, the central government urged care homes to develop contingency plans to combat the pandemic. Accordingly, Royal Decree-Law 21/2020 of 9 June listed several urgent preventions, containment, and coordination measures to deal with the health crisis caused by COVID-19. Likewise, several ACs draw up various documents to guide care homes dealing with the COVID-19 pandemic (such as Aragon or Madrid), including the definition of contingency plans.

Throughout the first months of the pandemic, these protocols and contingency plans were continuously updated as new information and global guidelines became available (WHO, 2020a, 2020b). However, the weak vertical and horizontal coordination between the multiplicity of actors

Table 14.1: Closing of care homes: indications from employers' organisations and autonomic instructions

AC	Employers' organisation	First communication from the employers' organisation	Instruction from the competent authority
Catalonia	ACRA	25 February	12 March
Castile-La Mancha	ARTECAM	26 February	14 March
Aragon	ARADE	25 February	16 March
Valencian Community	AERTE	25 February	18 March
Castile and León	ACALERTE	1 March	13 March
Madrid	AMADE	6 March	15 March
Andalusia	CECUA	11 March	14 March

Source: CEAPs (2020)

involved meant that care homes were overburdened with regulations that could sometimes be difficult to implement.

In the context of unclear guidelines, several measures were adopted by both ACs and directors of care homes for older people (del Pino et al, 2021), often following a trial-and-error approach. Many of these measures resulted from the proactive role of directors of care homes or employers' organisations, which often assumed a leadership role in managing the crisis – particularly in its beginning – in the absence of clear indications from public authorities.

The closing to external visits represented one of the first and most common measures adopted by directors of care homes, often before the publication of instructions from the competent regional authorities, as Table 14.1 indicates. Similarly, the sectorisation and isolation of residents according to symptoms constituted another fundamental measure to stop the spread of the virus. However, its feasibility largely depended on the level of occupancy and the architectural characteristics of each centre (size, existence of shared rooms, organisation of shared spaces, and so on) (Martín López & Durán López, 2021), while its effectiveness was affected by the availability of both staff and diagnostic tests.

As mentioned before, the COVID-19 pandemic exacerbated pre-existing structural shortages in staffing levels in the Spanish care home sector, which dramatically increased due to sick leaves (in certain centres, involving up to 75 per cent of staff). It, in turn, led to overloading the workload, tasks, and responsibilities of available staff (Pérez-Raya et al, 2021). At the level of care homes, directors frequently adopted mechanisms of workers' rotation, sectorisation, and the concentration of working hours on fewer shifts to reduce potential contagion and turnover, as well as to facilitate the detection of positive cases among the staff (by allowing more time for potential symptoms to appear).

At the institutional level, several ACs created dedicated employment lists for people willing to work in the sector during the pandemic or made available workers from other public sectors that were not operational (such as nurses from the education system) to care homes in need of personnel. While representing an important measure to deal with such shortages, ad hoc employed persons often lacked the necessary training to adequately perform their job, even more so in the context of a pandemic. From this perspective, materials published by the WHO (2020b), the Ministry of Health, and several ACs, as well as the ones drafted by the same care home staff, were fundamental to rapidly train workers – although with difficulties derived from the development and continuous updating of documents as new information arrived.

What concerns the availability of diagnostic tests and PPE, the concentration of the demand in the international market, and the decision to prioritise their allocation to healthcare structures largely conditioned the availability of these diagnostic and protective instruments in care homes, particularly during the initial months of the pandemic. Some more extensive facilities had anticipated purchases of PPE already in January 2020, learning from the lessons of previous epidemics when the system suffered from severe supply problems. Nevertheless, most had to buy these materials at very high prices, reuse them beyond technical specifications, or even rely on non-approved PPE.

Specifically concerning diagnostic tests, the time elapsed between the request for PCR tests and the possibility of performing them was pretty significant, ranging from several days to more than a week (especially during March and the first half of April), and with relevant differences between ACs. In some cases, this time was even longer when receiving the test results, revealing the system's difficulty in simultaneously performing and processing a massive volume of tests. Furthermore, in addition to the availability of tests, changes in the indications received by the health authorities, often in a matter of days, and frequently incorporating new evidence as it was produced, contributed to confusion among the staff, leading to inefficient and ineffective use of diagnostic tests.

Due to the difficulties related to the isolation of COVID-19 infected residents within the same centre, some ACs set up specific structures to move these patients from the care homes where outbreaks had occurred (del Pino et al, 2021). This solution allowed care homes to reduce the risk of the spread of the virus among residents and staff and the slow but progressive re-establishment of 'normal' daily routines and activities. Moreover, it represented a necessary measure to deal with difficulties in accessing overwhelmed healthcare facilities, and overcoming fragmentation and interaction problems between the care home sector and the different parts of the SNS.

Access to primary and secondary healthcare was drastically limited during the first months of the pandemic, as mentioned earlier. In some ACs, it was challenging to access primary healthcare centres. These were either overcrowded by the general population or directly closed (for example, in the Community of Madrid, 7.8 per cent of primary care centres, and 53.3 per cent of local public practices, were closed in April). To deal with this limitation, some ACs opted for the 'medicalisation' of care homes, that is, sending human resources and medical material to care homes. In contrast, in others, the interaction of care homes with the SNS mainly took place with hospitals through the geriatrics service, as in Madrid or Valencia (Sáez-López & Arredondo-Provecho, 2021).[9] Moreover, given the pre-existing shortage of healthcare staff in most of the homes and the lack of medical training for care staff, nurses from the primary care centres often acted as crisis managers in the care homes themselves, supporting directors and staff in the development of contingency plans, coordinating positive and asymptomatic patients, or facilitating access to diagnostic tests, among other functions.

More generally, the pandemic exacerbated the structural, limited integration – or even fragmentation – between LTC and healthcare services in Spain, weakening the capacity of the system to rapidly and effectively manage the health crisis in care homes. Subordination of social services to healthcare services, fragmentation in the distribution of competencies and responsibilities, as well as the diverse organisational cultures and differences in status and social (self-)perception between healthcare and social professionals, have been identified as critical points of frictions and, at times, causes of blockage in the management of the pandemic. In this sense, the disregard for health authorities' peculiarities of care home facilities when applying hospital organisation and management criteria had a clearly negative impact on the physical and emotional health of elderly residents and their families.

After the first wave: learning processes and challenges for the future

The first wave of the pandemic was critical, particularly for older people and workers in care homes. The subsequent waves produced a lower incidence of COVID-19 cases in these facilities, which experienced a different distribution of cases compared to the general population.

On the one hand, the incidence and mortality rates in care homes improved thanks to mass vaccination, as infections in vaccinated older people were more likely to be controlled without requiring hospitalisation (Fernández Riquelme, 2021). As reported in an evaluation of the measures adopted in Catalonia (Parilla Valero, 2022), vaccinations reduced the incidence of

COVID-19 for older people in care homes during the third and fourth waves to levels below the average of the general population. With the arrival of the SARS-CoV-2 delta variant, the incidence and mortality increased, although nothing like during the critical moments of the first wave. According to the Catalan Health Department, vaccinations were the main reason for halting the incidence and mortality of the more contagious delta variant (Generalitat de Catalunya, 2021).

On the other hand, some lessons from the first wave were learned and implemented, namely: (i) the increase in the number of diagnostic tests; (ii) the development of appropriate contingency plans by care homes to mitigate future contagions; and (iii) the establishment of coordination mechanisms between the care home sector and primary health care by launching Nursing Homes Care Units. These liaison units might be used in the post-pandemic era to avoid the fragmentation of care between hospitals and care homes, to strengthen face-to-face visits to care homes, telemedicine sessions, and the coordination between the national healthcare service and the care homes (Menéndez-Colino et al, 2021).

Overall, the COVID-19 pandemic brought a two-decades-long debate about the future of the care home sector in Spain. As a result, the Congress of Deputies (2020) echoed various proposals by care home directors, formal caregivers, and trade unions in the Resolution of the Reconstruction Commission. Among these, we can highlight the following:

- The care home conditions and regulations need to be adjusted to the current profile of older adults. As described in the first section, care home residents arrive older (due to their preference to remain at home as long as possible) and become more dependent as time passes. It necessarily requires more coordination between the healthcare and social service professionals. The limited coordination between sectors is considered one of the main elements that conditioned the quality of the response to the COVID-19 pandemic in care homes (Novoa Jurado et al, 2022).
- The unanimous rejection by care home directors on the 'medicalisation' of care homes, claiming that these structures are the principal residence of older people that need the care to live a life as close to normal and as autonomous as possible, and not necessarily healthcare. Rather than medicalisation, coordination between the two sectors is deemed central. Accordingly, the level of coordination achieved throughout the pandemic is considered a clear step in normalising the links between care homes and the healthcare system (primary healthcare, hospitals, emergency facilities, public health, primary social services, and care homes). A recommended output is the development of medium to long-stay hospitals that accommodate older persons needing long-term medical attention.

- The need to professionalise care workers and to increase the offer of university training programmes for different profiles needed in the care home sector. Most importantly, the urgency to dignify and improve the working conditions and environment of care workers.
- The importance of considering the needs, perspectives, and preferences of older people in the design of care homes, fostering an internal re-organisation of care homes into cohabitation units where older people live together in smaller groups and with similar profiles. Gallego et al (2021) consider that these cohabitation units, combined with a reinforcement of home and community care, should be at the forefront of the transformation of the LTC system.

To achieve these goals, reforming the care home sector for older people – and of the LTC sector more broadly – requires a compromise by the different levels of government to increase the financial resources currently allocated to care for older people. Although regional governments have made significant efforts to increase the number of formal caregivers and strengthen primary healthcare during the pandemic, these are considered insufficient by organisations and workers in the care and health sector (Amnesty International, 2021). Moreover, according to trade unions, formal caregivers' wages and job quality must be improved, thus requiring more financial commitment to the sector. Hence, the big question arises: how do we fund the fiscal space needed to implement these reforms and transform Spain's LTC sector? Three visible options arise, which should be evaluated regarding political and economic viability: increase taxation, redirect current expenditure to this sector, or a combination of both strategies.

Notes

1 However, criticism was posed by some regional nationalist parties, and some ACs even reformed their regional Statutes of Autonomy to reaffirm their exclusive competencies in social services (such as Andalusia).

2 Through the National Reform Programme of 2012, the conservative central government suspended the supplementary funds and considerably reduced the minimum level of funding for the LTC system.

3 The number of beds is unknown for 11 of the 5,567 centres. Therefore, the total number of beds does not take into account these 11 LTC facilities.

4 A reform in June 2020 Law 16/2003 on Cohesion and Quality of the SNS introduced the Declaration of Coordinated Actions, which allows the central government to establish binding measures for all ACs.

5 The SNS was considered the most efficient healthcare system in Europe and the third in the world (Bloomberg Index).

6 In July 2020, the central government, in the 'Early Response Plan for the control of the COVID-19 pandemic' framework, established a national strategic stockpile as a support measure for ACs to guarantee the supply of commodities for at least 8 weeks. Nevertheless, care homes were not included among the structures receiving priority in allocating this national stock.

7 https://cnecovid.isciii.es/

8 These data refer to older adults living in care homes, regardless of the specific place of death (the care home where they lived or elsewhere).

9 For example, the Community of Madrid created Geriatrics Liaison Units in public hospitals in the following phases of the pandemic. Along with the Spanish Society of Geriatrics, these units informed care homes about prevention, early detection, and sectorisation. At the time of finalising this chapter (summer 2022), the new protocols for interaction between care homes and the 22 hospitals in the ACs (which have restricted access to these healthcare services for elderly patients suffering from COVID-19) have been legally challenged by several regional courts.

References

Abellán García, A., Aceituno Nieto, P., Ramiro Fariñas, D., and Castillo Belmonte, A. B. (2021a) *Estadísticas Sobre Residencias. Distribución de Centros y Plazas Residenciales por Provincia. Datos de Septiembre de 2020*, Madrid: CSIC.

Abellán García, A., Aceituno Nieto, P., Castillo Belmonte, A. B., Fernández Morales, I., and Ramiro Fariñas, D. (2021b) ¿Hacia un registro de personas institucionalizadas?, *EnR? Envejecimiento en Red* [online], Available from: https://envejecimientoenred.es/hacia-un-registro-de-personas-institucionalizadas/

Aguilar-Hendrickson, M. (2020) Long-term care in Spain: a reform failure or the regulation of a development path?, *International Journal of Sociology and Social Policy*, 40(11/12): 1301–17.

Amnesty International (2021) *La Otra Pandemia: Entre el Abandono y el Desmantelamiento: el Derecho a la Salud y a la Atención Primaria en España*, Madrid: Amnesty International.

Arlotti, M. and Aguilar-Hendrickson, M. (2017) The vicious layering of multilevel governance in Southern Europe: the case of elderly care in Italy and Spain, *Social Policy & Administration*, 52(3): 646–61.

Asociación Estatal de Directores y Gerentes en Servicios Sociales (2021) *XXI Dictamen Del Observatorio de La Dependencia*, March, AEDGSS [online], Available from: https://directoressociales.com/dependencia/

Barrera-Algarín, E., Estepa-Maestre, F., Sarasola-Sánchez-Serrano, J. L. and Malagón-Siria, J. C. (2021) COVID-19 and elderly people in nursing homes: impact according to the modality of residence, *Revista Espanola de Geriatria y Gerontologia*, 56: 208–17.

Cáceres Armendáriz, P. and Sierra Alonso, S. (2021) La crisis de los equipos de protección individual en la pandemia por la COVID-19 y el Instituto Nacional de Seguridad y Salud en el Trabajo, *Revista Española de Salud Pública*, 95(1): e1–e9.

CEAPs (2020) *Informe Analítico de Gestión en Centros Residenciales en España durante COVID-19, Comisión para la Reconstrucción Social y Económica, Grupo de Trabajo de Sanidad y Salud Pública*, 5 June [online], Available from: http://ceaps.org/wp-content/uploads/2020/06/INFORME-ANALI%CC%81TICO-GESTIO%CC%81N-COVID-V1.pdf

Comas-Herrera, A., Zalakaín, J., Lemmon, E., Henderson, D., Litwin, C., Hsu, A. T., Schmidt, A. E., Arling, G., Kruse, F., and Fernández, J- L. (2020) Mortality associated with COVID-19 in care homes: international evidence, *International Long-term Care Policy Network, CPEC-LSE*, 14 [online], Available from: https://ltcCOVID.org/2020/04/12/mortality-associated-with-COVID-19-outbreaks-in-care-homes-early-international-evidence/

Congress of Deputies (2020) *Dictamen*, Comisión para la Reconstrucción Social y Económica, 3 July, Madrid [online], Available from: http:// www.congreso.es/docu/comisiones/reconstruccion/153_1_Dictamen.pdf

Da Roit, B., Gonzalez Ferrer, A., and Moreno-Fuentes, F. J. (2013) The Southern European migrant-based care model: long-term care and employment trajectories in Italy and Spain, *European Societies*, 15(4): 577–96.

del Pino, E., Moreno Fuentes, F. J., Cruz-Martínez, G., Hernández-Moreno, J., Moreno, L., Pereira-Puga, M., and Perna, R. (2021) Governmental response to the COVID-19 pandemic in long-term care residences for older people: preparedness, responses and challenges for the future: Spain, *MC COVID-19 working paper*, 13/2021, DOI: 10.20350/digitalCSIC/13688

Deusdad, B. A., Comas-d'Argemir, D., and Dziegielewski, S. F. (2016) Restructuring long-term care in Spain: the impact of the economic crisis on social policies and social work practice, *Journal of Social Service Research*, 42(2): 246–62.

Eurofound (2021) *Living, Working and COVID-19*, COVID-19 series (Round 3: March 2021), Luxembourg: Publications Office of the European Union [online], Available from: https://www.eurofound.europa.eu/publications/report/2020/living-working-and-COVID-19

European Commission (2021) *State of Health in the EU: España: Perfil Sanitario Nacional 2021* [online], Available from: https://ec.europa.eu/health/state-health-eu/country-health-profiles_es

Eurostat (2022) *Nursing and Caring Professional* [online], Available from: https://appsso.eurostat.ec.europa.eu/nui/show.do?dataset=hlth_rs_prsns&lang=en

Gallego, V. M., Codorniu, J. M., and Cabrero, G. R. (2021) El impacto de la COVID-19 en la población mayor dependiente en España con especial referencia al sector residencial, *Ciência & Saúde Coletiva*, 26: 159–68.

Generalitat de Catalunya (2021) Anul•la l'anterior: salut fa una crida a reduir la interacció social per frenar els contagis de la COVID-19 per l'alta virulència de la variant Delta, Press release, 21 July [online], Available from: https://govern.cat/salapremsa/notes-premsa/412171/salut-crida-reduir-interaccio-social-frenar-contagis-COVID-19-lalta-virulencia-variant-delta

González Gómez, A. (2021) La coordinación del Sistema Nacional de Salud en España: regulación y resultados en tiempos de pandemia, in C. Colino (ed) *Retos de la Gobernanza Multinivel y la Coordinación en el Estado Autonómico: de la Pandemia al Futuro*, Madrid: INAP.

Hernández-Moreno, J. (2021) La gestión institucional de la crisis de COVID-19: coordinación intergubernamental e intersectorial en las políticas de Sanidad y Servicios Sociales, in C. Colino (ed) *Retos de la Gobernanza Multinivel y la Coordinación en el Estado Autonómico: de la Pandemia al Futuro*, Madrid: INAP.

Hernández-Moreno, J. and Pereira-Puga, M. (2021) *On the Corona Frontline – The Experiences of Care Workers in Spain*, Friedrich Ebert Stiftung [online], Available from: https://library.fes.de/pdf-files/bueros/stockholm/17762.pdf

IMSERSO (2020) *Servicios Sociales Dirigidos a las Personas Mayores en España. Informe a 31/12/2019*, Madrid: IMSERSO.

IMSERSO (2022a) *Datos de Gestión. Sistema para la Autonomía y Atención a la Dependencia (SAAD)*, Madrid: IMSERSO [online], Available from: https://www.imserso.es/imserso_01/documentacion/estadisticas/info_d/estadisticas/est_inf/index.htm

IMSERSO (2022b) *Actualización nº62. Enfermedad por Coronavirus (COVID-19) en Centros Residenciales*, 1 May, Madrid: IMSERSO [online], Available from: https://www.imserso.es/interpresent4/groups/imserso/documents/binario/inf_resid_20220501.pdf

Jiménez-Martín, S. and Viola, A. (2020) La asistencia residencial en España y COVID-19, *Estudios Sobre la Economía Española*, 2020/20, Madrid: FEDEA [online], Available from: http://documentos.fedea.net/pubs/eee/eee2020-20.pdf

Legido-Quigley, H., Mateos-García, J. T., Campos, V. R., Gea-Sánchez, M., Muntaner, C., and McKee, M. (2020) The resilience of the Spanish health system against the COVID-19 pandemic, *The Lancet Public Health*, 5(5): e251–e252.

Ma, X. and Vervoort, D. (2020) Critical care capacity during the COVID-19 pandemic: global availability of intensive care beds, *Journal of Critical Care*, 58: 96.

Marbán, G. V. (2019) *El Sistema Español de Atención a la Dependencia. Entre la Regresión y las Reformas*, Madrid: Fundación FOESSA [online], Available from: https://caritas-web.s3.amazonaws.com/main-files/uploads/sites/16/2019/06/paper-4.9.pdf

Martín López, L. and Durán López, R. (2021) A typological analysis of nursing home environments during the COVID-19 pandemic: risks and potential, in M.A. Montoya, A. Krstikj, J. Rehner, and D. Lemus-Delgado (eds) *COVID-19 and Cities*, Cham: Springer.

Mattei, P., and del Pino, E. (2021) Coordination and health policy responses to the first wave of COVID-19 in Italy and Spain, *Journal of Comparative Policy Analysis: Research and Practice*, 23(2): 274–81.

Médicos sin Fronteras (2020) Informe de Médicos Sin Fronteras sobre proteccion al personal sanitario resumen, Barcelona: Médicos sin Fronteras [online], Available from: https://www.msf.es/sites/default/files/documents/msf-informe-COVID19-proteccion-web01.pdf

Menéndez-Colino, R., Argentina, F., de Miguel, A. M., Marqués, M. B., Jiménez, B. C., Poblete, C. F., Alarcón, T., Peromingo, F. J. M., and González-Montalvo, J. I. (2021) La geriatría de enlace con residencias en la época de la COVID-19. Un nuevo modelo de coordinación que ha llegado para quedarse, *Revista Española de Geriatría y Gerontología*, 56(3): 157–65.

Ministry of Health (2020) *Actualización de Casos COVID-19* [online], Available from: https://www.sanidad.gob.es/profesionales/saludPublica/ccayes/alertasActual/nCov/situacionActual.htm

Ministry of Health (2021a) *Sistema de Información de Listas de Espera del Sistema Nacional de Salud* [online], Available from: https://www.mscbs.gob.es/estadEstudios/estadisticas/inforRecopilaciones/listaEspera.htm

Ministry of Health (2021b) *La Pandemia del COVID-19 y la Prevención y el Control del Cáncer* [online], Available from: https://www.sanidad.gob.es/gl/organizacion/sns/planCalidadSNS/pdf/PANDEMIA_DE_LA_COVID-19_Y_LA_PREVENCION_Y_EL_CONTROL_DEL_CANCER.pdf

Ministry of Territorial Policy (2022) *Cooperación Multilateral o Sectorial* [online], Available from: https://www.mptfp.gob.es/portal/politica-territorial/autonomica/coop_autonomica/Conf_Sectoriales.html

Moreno Fuentes, F. J. (2015) Retos y reformas de las políticas de cuidado de larga duración en España, in F. J. Moreno Fuentes and E. del Pino Matute (eds) *Desafíos del Estado del Bienestar en Noruega y España, Nuevas Políticas para Atender a Nuevos Riesgos Sociales*, Madrid: Tecnos.

Muñoz Díaz, C., Aceituno Nieto, P., and Ramiro Fariñas, D. (2021) ¿Cuán concertadas son las residencias de personas mayores concertadas en España?, *EnR? Envejecimiento en Red* [online], Available from: https://envejecimientoenred.es/cuan-concertadas-son-las-residencias-de-personas-mayores-concertadas-en-espana/

Navarro, C. and Velasco, F. (2022) From centralisation to new ways of multi-level coordination: Spain's intergovernmental response to the COVID-19 pandemic, *Local Government Studies*, 48(2): 191–210.

Novoa Jurado, A. J., Martínez Monreal, D., Pérez de los Cobos, E. M., Gutiérrez, J., López Román, F. J., Luzón Oliver, L., and Aguiran Romero, L. M. (2022) COVID-19: cómo debería cambiar la atención sanitaria en las residencias de mayores para evitar otra crisis, *The Conversation*, 13 March.

Organisation for Economic Co-operation and Development (OECD) (2020) *Who Cares? Attracting and Retaining Care Workers for the Elderly*, Paris: OECD.

Organisation for Economic Co-operation and Development (2021) *Health at a Glance 2021: OECD Indicators* [online], Available from: https://www.oecd.org/health/health-at-a-glance/

Parrilla, F. (2022) La gestión de la pandemia de COVID-19 en las residencias geriátricas de Cataluña, *Vacunas*, 1–12.

Pérez-Raya, F., Cobos-Serrano, J. L., Ayuso-Murillo, D., Fernández-Fernández, P., Rodríguez-Gómez, J. A., and Almeida Souza, A. (2021) COVID-19 impact on nurses in Spain: a considered opinion survey, *International Nursing Review*, 68: 248–55.

Riquelme, S. F. (2021) Historia interminable de la crisis del Coronavirus en España: entre olas y vacunas, *Revista Hispanoamericana de Historia de las Ideas*, 51: 1–15.

Sáez-López, P., and Arredondo-Provecho, A. B. (2021) Experiencia de colaboración entre hospital y centros sociosanitarios para la atención de pacientes con COVID-19, *Revista Española de Salud Pública*, *95*(1): e1–e15.

Sagan, A., Webb, E., Azzopardi-Muscat, N., de la Mata, I., McKee, M., and Figueras, J. (2021) Health systems resilience during COVID-19. Lessons for building back better, *Health Policy Series*, 56, UK: WHO [online], Available from: https://eurohealthobservatory.who.int/publications/i/health-systems-resilience-during-COVID-19-lessons-for-building-back-better

SATSE (2020) 5.500 enfermeras y enfermeros graves por la COVID 19, *SASTE*, 16 June [online] https://www.satse.es/comunicacion/sala-de-prensa/notas-de-prensa/5.500-enfermeras-y-enfermeros-graves-por-la-COVID-19

Sociedad Española de Geriatría y Gerontología (2020) *Resumen Normativa de Residencias* [last updated 17 June 2020], Madrid: SEGG [online], Available from: https://www.segg.es/media/descargas/Cuadro_resumen_SEGG_Normativa_Residencias_Rev.17junio2020.pdf

Spijker, J. and Zueras, P. (2020) Old-age care provision in Spain in the context of a new system of long-term care and a lingering economic crisis, *Journal of Population Ageing*, 13(1): 41–62.

Spijker, J., Devolder, D., and Zueras, P. (2022) The impact of demographic change in the balance between formal and informal old-age care in Spain. Results from a mixed microsimulation–agent-based model, *Ageing & Society*, 42(3): 588–613.

World Health Organisation (2020a) *Investing in and Building Longer-Term Health Emergency Preparedness During the COVID-19 Pandemic*, Geneva: World Health Organisation [online], Available from: https://pesquisa.bvsalud.org/global-literature-on-novel-coronavirus-2019-ncov/resource/pt/grc-741226

World Health Organisation (2020b) *Preventing and Managing COVID-19 Across Long Care Services*, Geneva: World Health Organisation [online], Available from: https://www.who.int/publications/i/item/WHO-2019-nCoV-Policy_Brief-Long-term_Care-2020.1

World Health Organisation (2021a) *Implementing Telemedicine Services during COVID-19: Guiding Principles and Considerations for a Stepwise Approach*, Geneva: World Health Organisation [online], Available from: https://apps.who.int/iris/handle/10665/336862

World Health Organisation (2021b) *COVID-19 Strategic Preparedness and Response Plan: Monitoring and Evaluation Framework*, Geneva: World Health Organisation [online], Available from: https://www.who.int/publications/i/item/WHO-WHE-2021.07-eng

15

Swedish long-term care for older people in the shadow of the COVID-19 pandemic

Lennarth Johansson and Pär Schön

Introduction

In the spring of 2020, the COVID-19 pandemic shocked Swedish society and put unprecedented pressure on the Swedish health and long-term care (LTC) system for older people. The pandemic functioned as a stress test of how prepared, robust, resilient, and well-organised the Swedish welfare system was to confront a crisis of this magnitude. The handling of the pandemic seriously challenged the Swedish self-image as an efficient and well-organised welfare state.

During the very first phase of the pandemic, Sweden had similar ambitions and strategy as most other countries: slowing down the spread of the virus (flattening the curve) and protecting older people. However, it soon became clear that the Swedish COVID-19 strategy stood out among European countries and most of the world. Unlike most EU countries, Sweden did not respond with a general lockdown or harsh restrictions. Instead, the Swedish strategy was based on voluntary measures, emphasising individual responsibility to follow government recommendations. As a result, Sweden was considered an international outlier at this time, where the efforts to stop or slow the spread of infection were few, weak, and late.

The first months of the pandemic were in fact chaotic. The healthcare system was ill-prepared and had not yet reorganised and adapted to the situation, or developed routines and effective treatments for COVID-19. There was a severe shortage of personal protective equipment (PPE), hospital beds, and care personnel. The situation in the LTC and care homes was even worse: lack of PPE and insufficient knowledge of basic hygiene routines among care personnel.

As in most EU countries, COVID-19 related mortality in Sweden primarily occurred among older people receiving LTC services, especially those living in care homes. In December 2020, more than 7,000 people died from the COVID-19 outbreak, of which almost 90 per cent were 70 years and older. Half of them were living in care homes, and around 30 per cent were receiving home help. Occasionally, during the first phase of the pandemic, Swedish death rates were among the highest in Europe. The infection spread to many care homes. Many sick older people had their care needs assessed by distance or not at all, and sometimes did not receive hospital treatment that could have helped them. Due to restrictions imposed, especially the visit ban at care homes, many older people died with no family member or any other person by their side (Swedish Government, 2020: 80).

How Sweden coped with COVID-19 has been continuously debated and has dominated the public debate. Consequently, in June 2020, the Swedish government appointed an independent inquiry committee – the Corona Commission – to review the Swedish COVID-19 strategy. The commission worked for over a year and a half, collected and analysed facts and assessed how Sweden handled the COVID-19 pandemic. As a result, the Commission has published several reports, which will be summarised and discussed in this chapter (Swedish Government, 2020, 2022a).

Swedish long-term care system at a glance

Sweden has a well-developed welfare system, providing health, social care services, and other social protection programmes to the citizens over the life course. The Swedish LTC policy aims to provide publicly subsidised, widely available services (in kind) based on the individual's needs, regardless of economic means and family resources (Sipilä,1997). Adult children have no legal obligations to provide care or economic security for their older parents. The underlying philosophy is to promote maximum independence from the family. However, given the public responsibility to cater to older people's service and care needs, it is still the family and next of kin who are the major providers of help to older people in Sweden (Ulmanen & Szebehely, 2015; Johansson et al, 2018). Following the universalist ambition of Swedish welfare provision, services should be affordable for the poor but attractive for the wealthier (Szebehely & Trydegård, 2012).

The governance structure of the Swedish (and the other Nordic countries) LTC system stands out in comparison with most other European countries at both policy and operational levels. The responsibility for health care and social services is highly decentralised and divided between three tiers of government: the national level, the regions, and the municipalities. Another aspect of the Swedish system, which differs from many other European countries, is that care homes do not constitute care facilities regulated within the Health and Medical Services Act; they are regulated within the Social Services Act. Consequently, the care homes are not equipped, staffed, or managed as healthcare facilities.

Ageing in place – from care homes to home care

Since the 1950s, ageing in place has been a key and guiding strategy, shifting direction in old age care from 'care homes to home care'. Publicly funded home-based care services were introduced and expanded rapidly through the 1960s and 1970s, peaking at the beginning of the 1980s.

In 1992, the Community Care Reform was implemented, consolidating the ageing-in-place policy and establishing the current structure of the Swedish LTC. The core of the reform was that the municipalities were given the statutory responsibility for all types of institutional care, including the responsibility to provide health care (up to the nurse level) in institutions. However, the responsibility to provide health care did not include medical care that still had to be provided by primary care doctors. Transferring some 31,000 nursing home beds from the regional *health and medical care* sector to the municipal *social services* sector implied a significant change in policy direction. The hospital-like nursing homes (*långvård*) were abolished, and the new ideal was home-like care homes inspired by a 'social care model' (Johansson, 1997).

The 1992 Community Care Reform triggered a dramatic reduction in the number of hospital beds, and in the ensuing 30 years, hospital bed numbers declined by more than half (NBHW, 2015). Sweden currently has the lowest per capita hospital bed rate in the European Union: 2.1 beds per 1,000 persons, compared to the EU average of 4.4 beds per 1,000 persons (OECD, 2021). The low number of hospital beds has led to shorter lengths of stay at hospitals.

From 2000 until 2021, one-third (33 per cent) of all municipal care home beds have been closed (NBHW, 2020a). Coverage ratios, 65 years and older, have correspondingly decreased by 53 per cent. In addition, the downsizing of care homes has increased the turnover rate among residents. National data show that 10 per cent of those admitted to care homes die within 2 months, 31 per cent within 12 months, and 50 per cent within 24 months. The mean length of stay in institutional care is 730 days (SALAR, 2020; NBHW, 2022).

The decreases in care home provision are not due to legislative changes or to the official policy of allocating care for older people according to need (Szebehely & Trydegård, 2012). Nor can the reduction be explained by health improvements among the oldest older people (Johansson et al, 2018). Instead, the cutbacks have been driven by financial restrictions, with tighter budgets, more restrictive local guidelines, and a subsequent raising of the 'eligibility threshold' for being admitted to a care home.

Going to the market

The 1990s brought forward a strong marketisation trend in Swedish LTC provision, including privatisation, competition, freedom of choice, and diversity. The increased reliance on the market was the result of an intense debate regarding the need for improved efficiency of public services. The marketisation was further reinforced by introducing a tax subsidy in 2007 for purchased help with household chores.

In 2009, the Act on System of Choice in the Public Sector (LOV) gave municipalities the option of contracting providers. This model was introduced in about half of Sweden's municipalities. After a needs assessment, the entitled person can choose between different (accredited) providers. In the contracting-out and customer-choice model, the municipality can set quality standards and prices, and inspect providers (Meagher & Szebehely, 2013).

Since 2010, LOV has been obligatory for primary health care in Sweden. LOV allows free establishment for accredited primary health care providers (Johanson et al, 2018. The regions cannot decide where the clinics should be located, for example, according to the needs of the area. Living alone at home, older people with complex health problems and severe needs often depend on service and care around the clock. The backbone of primary care consists of the country's more than 1,100 health centres. In 2020, more than 40 per cent of these were operated by private companies.

A consequence of the marketisation of LTC has been a rapid increase in the number of health and social care providers. Many private providers use (several) subcontractors to be able to provide the necessary services. When someone needs help around the clock, this will necessarily result in help by many care personnel, which in turn challenges continuity, security, and patient safety.

The Swedish LTC system is governed at three levels. Parliament and the government set out policy aims and directives at the national level using legislation and economic incentives. The 21 regions are responsible for the provision of health and medical care. The 290 municipalities are legally obliged to provide social services, home health care, and institutional care for older people at the local level. Regions and municipalities have a very high degree of autonomy vis-à-vis the central government.

The provision of LTC is based on a single-entry system; persons in need of help turn to the municipality where they live in order to claim help. Need is determined through a need assessment process by a municipal care manager. Eligibility to services, home-based and institutional care, is not means-tested, and there are no national regulations. The municipality decides the service level, eligibility criteria, and service range.

Taxes almost totally finance LTC services. The user only pays a fraction of the cost (≈4–6 per cent). Local taxes cover the most significant cost share (≈90 per cent). National taxes cover the remaining part of the cost (≈5 per cent).

The role of the care home sector

The outlook of most municipal care homes is quite like regular apartment houses, something that is also reflected in the housing standard. Typically, a care home apartment has one or 1½ rooms, with cooking facilities (kitchenette), a WC, and a shower (NBHW, 2020b). The residents furnish their apartments themselves to make them as home-like as possible. The resident pays rent for the apartment, and costs for food and care. Nevertheless, compared with the old nursing home wards, with multi beds rooms, bedside tables, and medical equipment for oxygen treatment, today's institutions have few similarities with senior care home facilities.

Nurses and assistant nurses provide health care. The caring personnel (mainly assistant nurses and care aids) cater to daily personal care, social activities, and companionship. The caring personnel tries to engage the residents in baking, cooking, setting the dinner, doing lighter gymnastics exercises and, if possible, taking a walk. The institutions generally have an operating manager, often with social worker training, that caters to the administrative tasks, economy, scheduling, and rostering of care personnel. Medical care is provided by doctors in the primary health care system. During non-office hours, there are nurses on call as well as doctors if needed.

The average age for moving to institutional care is 86 years. Two-thirds of the residents suffer from various degrees of cognitive impairment, which is the main reason for admittance to institutional care (Sköldunger et al, 2019). The remaining third of the residents are often suffering from severe medical conditions and functional decline, needing constant support and supervision.

The LTC system under attack

In Sweden, the so-called principle of responsibility is the basis for how the responsibility for health and social services is divided between different authorities, both in normal circumstances and in crises. It means that under normal circumstances, the authority or party responsible for a particular service is also responsible for those services in a crisis. It could be seen as a simple principle in theory, but the more institutions have to share the responsibility, the more difficult it becomes to make the system as a whole work well in practice. Sweden's decentralised LTC system divides responsibility, between 21 regions and 290 municipalities. Many regions and municipalities also have a large number of private providers. On top of this, central government agencies with a national responsibility are in LTC of older people.

Poor crisis preparedness

Sweden's crisis preparedness changed radically in the early 2000s. Previously, there were large emergency stocks of food, medical equipment, and supplies. However, since 2002, there are no national guidelines for healthcare equipment or medicines stocks. According to the responsibility principle, it is up to each region to be responsible for this.

In 2006, a new law on crisis preparedness was introduced, which prescribed municipalities and regions to take measures before and in the event of extraordinary events that may lead to severe disturbances in society. According to the law, risks, and vulnerabilities in one's operations, for example, hospital care, home care services, and care homes, must be analysed and prevented in contingency plans. Vulnerability analyses and contingency plans are a prerequisite for coordinating and collaborating between government agencies, regions, municipalities, organisations, and companies in crisis situations. However, the law does not provide precise instructions on what vulnerability analyses and contingency plans should look like.

The Agency for Civil Protection and Emergency Planning has the national responsibility, while the County Administrative Board has the coordinating responsibility for emergency preparedness for the regions and municipalities. A central part of the contingency plans is the extent to which they can be helpful when preparing society for a pandemic. For example, a municipality, region, and company must be able to show how much damage a pandemic risks causing to people, property, and businesses, how various effective countermeasures could be, and the necessary resources to be prepared for a pandemic.

As there is no national compilation or transparency in the municipal contingency plans, it is impossible to say whether the municipal contingency plans contain any analyses of the vulnerability of the municipal LTC. However, during the spring of 2020, it was evident that relevant vulnerability analyses were lacking, and contingency plans were often elementary and standardised. In a review carried out in February 2020 before the pandemic started, it was found that (only) 43 per cent of the municipalities had updated contingency plans (NBHW, 2020a).

Lack of personal protective equipment

There was no national coordination regarding purchasing PPE. It was up to each of the 21 regions to handle this. Given the poor preparedness for crises, the pandemic became an abrupt awakening for Swedish regions and municipalities during the spring of 2020. The PPE shortage became the very first stress test for health and social care when it was shown that the regions and municipalities lacked sufficient stocks of protective equipment such as face masks, visors, and protective coats for care. One explanation for the lack of access to PPE at the beginning of the pandemic was that many regions do not have large stocks at all, but usually acquire equipment 'just-in-time' in line with consumption in healthcare. When infected patients were hospitalised, the consumption of PPE increased more than a hundredfold in many hospitals. When the regions and municipalities tried to buy new PPE, they were forced to compete with national purchasing players from other countries, making it difficult to get opportunities to buy PPE.

In the regions, the shortage also applied to medical equipment such as respirators, and medicines, which was a significant shortcoming during the initial months of the epidemic. However, the major problem was the shortage of hospital bed capacity, especially intensive care beds. Two military hospitals were hastily built in Stockholm and Gothenburg but were never used when completed, as the first wave of the pandemic was over. The next problem was to staff the expansion of intensive care, which forced most hospitals to go up into staff mode. It enabled the hospital management to order the staff for more extended work shifts and to redeploy the staff from other parts of the hospital to the intensive care units. Then, the hospitals needed to recruit more staff who took over tasks in other hospital areas.

When the Swedish Public Health Agency recommended that the regions rapidly expand the test capacity for COVID-19, new problems arose. The regions required the central government to finance the increased testing activities before they started. That was also decided, but before the test activities expanded in the regions more than a month had passed.

The situation in the municipalities was even more difficult, especially concerning the care home sector. Again, the first major problem was the lack of protective equipment, clothing, face masks, and visors. There was also a lack of knowledge on how to act to meet this historically new situation. It emerged that the staff's knowledge of basic hygiene routines was in many cases insufficient, not least in care homes. Knowledge of organising the care of the infected in care homes was also low, as they had never confronted a similar situation before. It relates to the fact that in many municipalities, care personnel – especially hourly employees – worked both in-home care and in care homes, which meant an increased risk of bringing the infection into care homes and vice versa. Some municipalities hired additional staff to counteract this risk and started special corona teams in-home care, serving infected persons in their homes. Later in spring, they tried to organise the so-called cohort care in care homes to separate older people who were infected from those who were not. In response to problems with knowledge of and compliance with hygiene routines, a national e-training program developed by the National Board of Health and Welfare, was made available as a support to municipal care workers in home care and care homes.

Older people with multiple health problems and severe needs live and are cared for in care homes. To protect this vulnerable group from becoming infected and learn how to act if and when the residents became infected, the municipalities and care homes needed support from the regions and the doctors responsible for the resident's health status. During the spring of 2020, there were recurring problems and shortcomings in medical support in care homes. When the infection spread to care homes and the visit ban was introduced, and staff testing started, there were additional problems with staffing the care homes and replacing infected staff.

Fragmented governance structures

The regions and municipalities are dependent on the central government, and the municipalities, in turn, depend on the regions. For example, the municipalities depend on the regions for testing, although some municipalities, and private providers purchased their tests. The work of dealing with the pandemic was led at the national level by the Ministry of Social Affairs, under the strong influence of the Swedish Public Health Agency. A strong national player was SALAR (The Swedish Association of Local Authorities and Regions), an employers' organisation that advocates for local governments, representing the country's 21 regions and 290 municipalities. Other central actors were the National Board of Health and Welfare, the government's expert agency in health care and social services, and The Agency for Civil Protection and Emergency Planning, which is responsible for society's preparedness for major accidents, crises, and the consequences of war.

The operational government of healthcare in the regions consists of a multiple-layer structure. First, the management of each hospital, then the management of each clinic, and then the management of the primary health centre. The operations were governed separately in privately run hospitals and primary health care centres. Crisis groups were organised at the hospital level and primary health centres to lead, support, and coordinate the work during the pandemic.

In the municipalities and in the care homes, the work with the pandemic was led by the head of the care home, with the support of the medically responsible nurse (MRN), in charge of ensuring that the municipality health care is appropriate and safe, as well as with the doctor attached to the respective care home. In addition, many municipalities organised local crisis groups to support and coordinate the work during the pandemic. Also, in many municipalities, voluntary local production of protective coats, visors, and the manufacture of hand sanitiser, started to help to compensate for the most significant shortcomings.

Intersectoral collaboration

The effects of the pandemic on care homes must be seen because care homes in Sweden are not health care facilities but housing alternatives provided by municipalities to older people after a need assessment process. It means there are no nurses on duty around the clock, only during weekdays. Mobile care teams cater to interventions that require medical expertise at the nurse level or by doctors in the evenings, nights, and weekends. Care homes generally do not have medical equipment to respond to eventual medical interventions and/or to provide palliative care. A prerequisite is that there are nurses on duty, for example to give oxygen treatment, which is not the case in care homes around the clock.

The regions are responsible for medical care provided by doctors, and municipalities have no legal right to employ doctors. Consequently, this responsibility cannot be transferred to the municipalities. Moreover, it makes municipal eldercare dependent on the region's priorities for the medical assessments provided by doctors. It also means that doctors cannot be involved in the planning of healthcare in the municipality, not even in the crisis management that the municipality must perform during a pandemic.

The COVID-19 pandemic has shown that the coordination and cooperation between health care and social services in the care of older people have significant shortcomings. For the risk groups and those with LTC, there were general recommendations and instructions – care at home – avoid seeking hospital care. Doctors have a crucial role in assessing the patient and initiating the proper treatment, but the support from doctors in care homes varies. In the primary care sector, the regions recommended that doctor's visits to care homes be limited. It was especially problematic when it came to whether the sick person was to be sent to the hospital, cared for at home, or in their care home. Prescriptions and treatment instructions were given by telephone. If palliative care becomes relevant, this requires, according to the instructions from the National Board of Health and Welfare, an assessment by two doctors (who know the patient), in addition to the patient and his/her relatives, conditions that were often not met. This is the background behind the discussion about palliative care for COVID-19 patients being initiated too quickly on an uncertain basis. It has most likely resulted in some patients receiving incorrect care and, thus, inevitable death.

The Health and Social Care Inspectorate has shown marked reduction in the number of referrals to hospitals from care homes for older people during the spring of 2020. It is hard to establish whether the guidelines led to doctors failing to make individual assessments of care needs as dictated by guidelines issued by the National Board of Health and Welfare and, for example, the Stockholm Region. However, such guidelines – combined with the lack of equipment and partly staff needed for on-site medical treatment in residential care facilities – may have contributed to decisions to administer palliative care instead of hospital care or other active disease-related treatment.

Reviews of how the pandemic was handled

In the report from the first wave of the pandemic, the Corona Commission, focusing on and evaluating the Swedish strategy to protect 'the old and frail', stated:

> The Commission's overarching assessment can be simply summed up as follows: apart from the general spread of the virus in society,

> the factor that has had the greatest impact on the number of cases of illness and deaths from COVID-19 in Swedish residential care is structural shortcomings that have been well-known for a long time. These shortcomings have made residential care unprepared and ill-equipped to handle a pandemic. Staff employed in the elderly care sector were largely left by themselves to tackle the crisis. (Swedish Government, 2020)

Further about responsibility for the shortcomings:

> We have found that elderly care was unprepared and ill-equipped when the pandemic struck and that this was founded in structural shortcomings that were known long before the virus outbreak. The ultimate responsibility for these shortcomings' rests with the Government on power and the previous governments that also possessed this information. The Government governs the Realm and should therefore have taken the necessary initiatives to ensure that elderly care was better equipped to deal with a crisis of this nature. (Swedish Government, 2020)

In short, the Corona Commission found that the measures were implemented too late, too little, and were poorly coordinated. Furthermore, 'although we were in some sense theoretically prepared for a crisis, we were not mentally, logistically, and practically prepared for the crisis'.

In a review study of how the frontline care staff were exposed during the Swedish Municipal Workers' Union pandemic, several shortcomings were reported regarding the staff's working environment and conditions in elderly care (Huupponen, 2021). The report stated that the Swedish LTC was in crisis before COVID-19. The sector is underfunded and understaffed, and the Swedish population is aging. There is a shortage of trained care staff. The pandemic planning was insufficient. Although some improvements have been introduced during the pandemic, municipalities and regions will need additional resources to finance growing care needs and improve the sector's working environment. Elderly care needs to be prioritised politically and allowed to raise the standard (Huupponen, 2021).

In a study of how Medical Responsible Nurses (MRN) (over 200) and nurses in municipal LTC experienced the pandemic in the spring of 2020, most MRNs stated that they had good opportunities to participate in the municipality's management. But it also emerged that there had been a lack of cooperation within the municipality and between the municipality and the region, for example, at the beginning of the pandemic in terms of access to and distribution of protective equipment. In addition, their answers highlight a lack of health and medical competence among managers at various levels in the municipalities, which had a negative effect during the pandemic.

The nurses (over 900) who answered the questionnaire were more critical and pointed out additional shortcomings in the care of older people. They stated that the quality of care, both nursing and medical, had been negatively affected during the pandemic. Many pointed out shortcomings in support from managers and MRNs, which affected their work to combat the spread of the infection. The nurses described problems with providing information to the care staff, which they related to a lack of competence and the fact that managers within the organisation essentially do not have the competence to lead health and medical care work.

There was a consensus on the need for better competence of care staff and increased staffing of care staff and nurses. Furthermore, there was a need for management with health and medical care competence to guarantee excellent and safe care following the Health and Medical Care Act. Furthermore, the support from the region's doctors needs to become more transparent and have an increased continuity. Finally, according to the nurse, geriatricians are needed in municipal LTC systems (Boström et al, 2020).

From 2019 to 2021, the Health and Social Care Inspectorate (IVO) conducted an in-depth national inspection of medical care and treatment in care homes. IVO reviewed nearly 54,000 municipal healthcare patient records from 1,985 care homes in 283 municipalities. In addition, patients and relatives, as well as health and care staff, were asked about their experiences. The inspection revealed severe deficiencies in several areas, such as end-of-life care, medication management, information transfer, and documentation in care homes. In summary, IVO's supervision shows that the care homes have serious shortcomings. Even though Swedish care stands relatively well in international comparisons, the inspection shows that the minimum level of care at care homes is unacceptably low. IVO also states that there is significant variation across the country, but none of the municipalities examined fully meet the requirements that apply (IVO, 2022).

The care home sector before, during, and after the pandemic – lessons learned?

As highlighted by the Corona Commission, the structure of the LTC has direct consequences for collaboration between different authorities, principals, and services.

There is a recurring political discussion about the need for changed responsibilities between the central government and the regions' health care responsibilities. Repeated opinion polls show support for a central government takeover of health care. Some political parties also push for this issue in their critique of how the pandemic was handled. It is a consequence of the decentralised structure with a solid regional and municipal self-government, which significantly limits the central government 's opportunities to control the LTC system. However, to materialise such a takeover, extensive changes in responsibilities and forms of financing would be required, something that is not likely to happen shortly.

The Corona Commission criticised the central government, the regions, and municipalities for their lack of preparedness, late reaction and how they failed to protect older people. However, unclear responsibilities in the Swedish LTC system also make it challenging to identify which party in the system is to blame for the shortcomings in pandemic management.

Since 2020 and 2021, the government raised funds, partly to cover the direct COVID-19 costs, partly earmarked state subsidies for training during working hours and related full-time employment in eldercare. In addition, in April 2021, the Parliament decided to supplement SEK 4.3 billion to the municipalities in the 2021 budget.

In June 2022, a government inquiry presented a white paper proposing new legislation to counteract structural shortcomings, clarify tasks, responsibilities, and content, and create conditions for equal-quality eldercare. The proposals for the Elderly Care Act will supplement the Social Services Act and state what applies particularly to the care of older people. The law also contains new goals, for example, a preventive and health-promoting perspective and support for older people's functional ability.

Further, it is proposed that there must be health and medical competence at the municipal management level to ensure the municipality's responsibility for excellent and safe care. In the regions, there shall be, in a corresponding manner, management responsible for the planning and coordinating of health care interventions at the municipality level. The region is responsible for securing the availability of a doctor's assessment all around the clock and, correspondingly, the municipality for an assessment by a nurse on 24/7. The law also introduces requirements for two new functions; a quality manager for nursing and a quality manager for rehabilitation. The proposal has now been sent out for comments (Swedish Government, 2022a).

Since 2021, work has been underway to jointly purchase medicines, medical, and protective equipment and build warehouses to supply regions and municipalities in future crises. However, there is no overall picture of what is happening in the 21 regions and 290 municipalities regarding learning from the pandemic and implementing improvements in healthcare and elderly care. Contingency plans are being updated, and the municipalities are also trying to improve preparedness for protective equipment. The regions and municipalities are also reviewing existing agreements regarding support by doctors and medical care in care homes.

The future of the care home sector

At the beginning of 2022, the public debate was about managing the consequences of a more than 2-year-pandemic. Work had begun on the queues for postponed operations – the care debt – as well as on how to take care of the estimated 30,000 people affected by the post-COVID-19 syndrome. However, since the end of February 2022, all previous priorities have been overshadowed by the situation in Ukraine.

To a great extent, future prospects in municipal LTC are decided by demographic developments. In the coming 10 years, almost 50 per cent of the large post-war generation will reach the age of 80, with a corresponding increase in the need for health and social care. During the same period, the number of people of working age is expected to increase by only 4 per cent. In almost six out of ten municipalities, the working-age fraction of the population is declining. This development highlights that the labour shortage is one of the biggest challenges for municipalities and regions (SALAR, 2022).

The development of the care home sector in the years before the pandemic was characterised by specific trends. As mentioned earlier, the most significant was that the number of places in the care home sector for the elderly had fallen sharply. From 2000 to 2021, there were almost 40,000 fewer people aged 65 and older living in care homes, a decrease of about 33 per cent. In addition, service coverage, for example the proportion of people aged 80 years and older in care homes, almost halved (49 per cent) during that period (NBHW, 2001, 2022).

Previously, the municipalities owned the majority (79 per cent) of all care homes (Erlandsson et al, 2013). In recent decades, private companies have increasingly owned and operated care homes. It is often arranged through a sale-leaseback solution: municipalities sell their care homes to private companies and then rent care home beds from the company that bought the care home. As a result, the number of privately owned facilities (primarily for-profit institutions) has increased. According to a recent report, 55 per cent of the care homes started between 2018 and 2020 were owned by private companies (Ershammar, 2022).

A new concept is that private companies build average apartment houses, senior housing, and care homes for older people close to each other. The concept is a kind of hybrid housing alternative for older people consisting of condominiums, tenancies, and care homes.

In some cases, private companies can also offer places in care homes for those who can pay the entire cost out of their pocket. As access to publicly funded care home accommodation is becoming increasingly scarce, some older people will likely be interested in moving to a private care home and be able to bear the total costs on their own.

Lowering the costs and increasing the effectiveness of digital technology for care is now seen as necessary in-home care and care homes. As a result, welfare technology is now available in various forms in most care homes in the country (NBHW, 2021). The technology is used in residents' daily care and as an aid for the staff in the care work. These include passive alarms, webcams, and sensor surveillance.

The main problems the regions and the municipalities struggled with before the pandemic have been recruiting and retaining care personnel. Hospitals and primary care have significant recruitment needs of nurses, doctors, and other medical staff – especially specialist nurses in hospitals. These problems mean that hospitals cannot keep beds open, must postpone operations, and the queues for doctor visits in primary care are extended.

In the municipalities, the recruitment needs are enormous, both from a short and a long-time perspective. As a result, the prospects of increasing staff density and training levels and improving working conditions for staff in old age care are limited, which negatively affects the quality of care for the care recipients.

To conclude, it can be stated that there are currently no indications of a change in the structure, responsibilities, or financing of the LTC system and the care homes for older people. Likewise, it is unlikely that there will be any general expansion of the municipally funded care home sector in terms of the number of places. On the other hand, the supply of private senior housing and care homes is likely to increase. Therefore, the overall guiding principle for the care home sector will rather be consolidation: to maintain its role, function, and service levels in the best possible way.

References

Boström, A.-M., Marmstål Hammar, L., and Swall, A. (2020) *Vårdkvaliteten Inom den Kommunala Hälso- och Sjukvården under Pandemin: Medicinskt Ansvariga Sjuksköterskors och Sjuksköterskors Perspektiv [Quality of Care in the Municipal Health Care During the Pandemic: The Perspectives of Medical Responsible Nurses and Nurses]*. Karolinska institutet, Svensk sjuksköterskeförening, Mälardalens Högskola & Örebro Universitet.

Erlandsson, S., Storm, P., Stranz, A., Szebehely, M. and Trydegård, G-B. (2013) Marketising trends in Swedish eldercare: competition, choice and calls for stricter regulation, in G. Meagher and M. Szebehely (eds) *Marketisation in Nordic Eldercare: A Research Report on Legislation, Oversight, Extent and Consequences*, Stockholm: Department of Social Work, Stockholm University, pp 23–83.

Ershammar, M. (2022) *Det Tysta Övertagandet. En Kartläggning av Ägandet av Särskilda Boenden för Äldre [The Silent Takeover. Mapping Ownwership of Care Homes for Older People]*, Kommunal, Available from: https://www.kommunal.se/nyhet/det-tysta-overtagandet-en-kartlaggning-av-agandet-av-sarskilda-boenden-aldre#

Huupponen, M. (2021) *On the Corona Frontline. The Experiences of Care Workers in Sweden. Kommunal & Arena Idé*. Friedrich Ebert Stiftung, Available from: https://library.fes.de/pdf-files/bueros/stockholm/17690.pdf

Johansson, L. (1997) Decentralisation from acute to home care settings in Sweden, *Health Policy*, 41(Suppl.): 131–43.

Johansson, L., Malmberg, B., and Sundström, G. (2018) Ett halvt århundrade svensk äldreomsorg [Half a century of Swedish old-age care], *Tidskrift for Omsorgsforskning*, 4(1): 62–68 [in Swedish].

IVO, Health and Social Care Inspectorate (2022) *Tillsyn av Medicinsk Vård och Behandling vid Särskilda Boenden för Äldre. Delredovisning av Resultat på Nationell Nivå Avseende Kommunernas Hälso-och Sjukvård. [Inspection of Medical Care and Treatment in Municipal Care Homes. Interim National Results Report Regarding Municipal Health Care*, Available from: https://www.ivo.se/globalassets/dokument/publikationer/rapporter/rapporter-2022/sabo/ivo-tillsyn-av-medicinsk-vard-och-behandling-vid-sarskilda-boenden-for-aldre.pdf

NBHW, National Board of Health and Welfare (2001) *Statistik - Socialtjänst. Äldre - Vård och Omsorg År 2000 [Statistics – Social services. Elderly service and care 2000]*. Socialstyrelsen (in Swedish).

NBHW, National Board of Health and Welfare (2020a) *Vård och Omsorg om Äldre. Lägesrapport 2020 [Services and Care for Older People. Report of the Situation 2020]*. Socialstyrelsen (in Swedish).

NBHW, National Board of Health and Welfare (2020b) *Statistik om Äldre och Personer med Funktionsnedsättning Efter Regiform 2019 [Statistics on Older People and People with Disabilities According to Management form 2019*], Socialstyrelsen (in Swedish).

NBHW, National Board of Health and Welfare (2021) *E-Hälsa och Välfärdsteknik i Kommunerna 2021: Uppföljning av Utvecklingen Inom e-Hälsa och Välfärdsteknik i Kommunerna [E-health and Welfare Technology in the Municipalities: Review of the Development of E-health and Welfare Technology in the Municipalities]*. Socialstyrelsen (in Swedish).

NBWH, National Board of Health and Welfare (2022) *Vård och Omsorg om Äldre. Lägesrapport 2022 [Services and Care for Older People. Report of the Situation 2022]*. Socialstyrelsen (in Swedish).

OECD (2021) *Health at a Glance 2021: OECD Indicators*, Paris: OECD Publishing.

SALAR, The Swedish Association of Local Authorities and Regions (2020) *Vård och Omsorg i Hemmet 2019 – Svårigheter och Framgångsfaktorer [Homebased Care and Services 2019 - Difficulties and Success Factors]*. SKR, Stockholm (in Swedish).

SALAR, The Swedish Association of Local Authorities and Regions (2022) *Ekonomirapporten Maj 2022 [The Economy Report May 2022]*. SKR, Stockholm (in Swedish).

Sipilä, J. (1997) *Social Care Services: The Key to the Scandinavian Welfare Model*, London: Routledge.

Sköldunger, A., Wimo, A., Sjögren, K., Björk, S., Backman, A., Sandman, P-O., and Edvardsson, D. (2019) Resource use and its association to cognitive impairment, ADL functions, and behavior in residents of Swedish nursing homes: results from the U-Age program (SWENIS study), *International Journal of Geriatric Psychiatry*, 34(1): 130–6.

Swedish Goverment (2020) *Äldreomsorgen Under Pandemin. Delbetänkande från Coronakommissionen SOU 2020:80 [Elderly Care During the Pandemic. Interim Report from the Corona Commission SOU 2020:80]*, Available from: https://www.regeringen.se/rattsliga-dokument/statens-offentliga-utredningar/2020/12/sou-202080/

Swedish Goverment (2022a) *Sverige under Pandemin Volym 1 & 2. Slutbetänkande av Coronakommissionen SOU 2022:10 [Sweden During the Pandemic Volumes 1 & 2*. Final report from the Corona Commission, SOU 2022:10], Available from: https://www.regeringen.se/rattsliga-dokument/statens-offentliga-utredningar/2022/02/sou-202210/

Swedish Goverment (2022b) *Nästa Steg. Ökad Kvalitet och Jämlikhet i Vård och Omsorg för Äldre Personer. Betänkande av Utredningen om en Äldreomsorgslag och Stärkt Medicinsk Kompetens i Kommuner SOU 2022:41 [Next Step. Increased Quality and Equality in Care of Older People SOU 2022:41]*. White paper from the Inquiry on a new eldercare act and strengthened medical competence in the municipalities, Available from: https://www.regeringen.se/contentassets/bf57c17d12804992acf4b31349f0df75/sou-2022_41.pdf

Szebehely, M. and Trydegård, G. B. (2012) Home care for older people in Sweden: a universal model in transition, *Health & Social Care in the Community*, 20(3): 300–9.

Ulmanen, P. and Szebehely, M. (2015) From the state to the family or to the market? Consequences of reduced residential care in Sweden, *International Journal of Social Welfare*, 24(1): 81–92.

16

Cross-case analysis and conclusion

Eloísa del Pino and Francisco Javier Moreno-Fuentes

Introduction

This chapter provides a discussion on how European governments responded to the challenges posed by the Coronavirus (COVID-19) crisis in nursing homes. Particularly, it focuses on the integration of health and social service sectors and the coordination of different intergovernmental levels in the system for the care of institutionalised elderly individuals.

From the beginning of 2020, the coronavirus pandemic represented a highly intricate policy issue for European nursing homes, due not only to the characteristics of the affected population, but to the preexisting circumstances of these homes, and the nature of this multifaceted crisis. Additionally, governments had to take into account the intrinsic complexity of the relationship between the diverse actors involved in the long-term care (LTC) of the elderly, further exacerbated by the stressful context of the initial phase of the pandemic. Governments were faced with what we have called an 'intersectoral intergovernmental complex problem' (CIIP) (Paquet & Schertzer, 2020).

It is a reasonable assumption that governments which are required to address the management of a CIIP that cuts across two or more policy areas and two or more territorial jurisdictions will adopt an integrated policy approach, that is to say, a 'set of formal and informal rules, norms, procedures, as well as values, beliefs, knowledge and skills, enabling the reconciliation of composite policy goals, harmonisation of multiple policy instruments and coordination of relevant policy actors' (Domorenok et al, 2021a). However, our analysis of the initial responses to the challenges posed by the COVID-19 pandemic in nursing homes in 15 European governments during the first months of the crisis indicates that this assumption may have been overoptimistic.

This chapter analyses the extent to which European governments had or have developed initiatives and mechanisms for the integration of policy responses to the public health emergency associated with this pandemic in Europe. As previously discussed in the introductory chapter, the implementation of integrated policies that effectively address cross-sectoral and intergovernmental management issues necessitates the development of institutional capacities at three distinct levels: systemic, organisational, and individual (Wu et al, 2015; Domorenok et al, 2021a, 2021b).

As we will see, the challenges of policy integration that arose during this period of crisis were only (and only partially) addressed after a considerable time had elapsed. Analysing what happened during this period is key to better defining European governments' preparedness and response plans before such a circumstance occurs again, as experts warn will undoubtedly happen (Lenharo, 2023). This chapter therefore provides valuable insights into the initiatives and mechanisms developed, and the difficulties encountered by different levels of government and policy sectors to integrate policy responses during the pandemic in different European countries. It also explores the institutional capacities needed to support this integration in public health emergencies.

The initial section of this chapter serves to reacquaint readers with the initial period of uncertainty surrounding the impact of the pandemic on nursing homes. The next section then goes on to analyse the governmental response to the pandemic in the context of the adoption of integrated policy measures, in view of the complex nature of crisis management. In particular, at the systemic level, it analyses the existence of mechanisms for preparedness and response to a possible pandemic and security forecasts in the health and social care field; and the policy integration at the organisational level, including coordination at the political-administrative level and at the operational level, and policy integration at the individual level. Finally, we conclude with some remarks on the overall findings.

Understanding the impact of the pandemic on nursing homes and the type of government response that was necessary

By the end of 2019 or the beginning of 2020, some nursing home managers in Western Europe started to notice the growing incidence of a flu-like virus before it was officially identified as COVID-19. Some of them notified the regional social services managers that some type of virus was affecting their residents. Many started to adopt more or less drastic measures to counteract this illness (from the purchase of material to deal with an epidemic that was then associated with influenza, to the restriction of visits to their centres) long before they received any instruction from health or social services authorities about how to proceed to confront this disease.

On 30 January, the World Health Organisation (WHO) declared the outbreak of the new coronavirus a Public Health Emergency of International Importance (PHEIC), the highest level of alert under the International Health Regulations. Numerous articles appeared in the press speculating on the seriousness of a virus emerging in China and its possible spread to Europe. On 28 February, WHO recommended drastic containment measures. But residence managers really began to realise the dramatic consequences of COVID-19 for their centres as it became clear that, 40 days after the virus jumped from China to Italy, this European country, with a strong healthcare system (ninth in The Lancet 2016 global Healthcare Access and Quality Index), and reasonably well placed in the Global Health Security Index measuring the capacities of 195 countries to prepare for epidemics and pandemics (31st in the 2019 Index), was unable to control the effects of this coronavirus. The first case of COVID-19 in Europe appeared in Italy on 30 January 2020, when a Chinese tourist couple from Wuhan was admitted to the Spallanzani Hospital in Rome. Soon, the death toll in Italy was above 12,000 cases and more than 800 deaths, particularly among the elderly. Italy adopted the first national lockdown measures on 11 March, the most radical lockdown restrictions outside China. On the same day, the WHO declared the existence of a pandemic.

When nursing home managers became aware of the devastating effects that COVID-19 could have on their institutions, they became increasingly aware of two additional problems. On the one hand, nursing homes were incapable of dealing with this problem on their own (they were not prepared, and did not have the resources to deal with such a catastrophe). On the other hand, it was not going to be easy to make the authorities aware of the fact that nursing homes needed all kinds of measures to deal with a problem of this magnitude. Virtually in all countries, care homes 'were left on their own', as reflected in a quotation from the Austrian chapter, a statement that could be reproduced in most other European countries, maybe with only the exception of Finland.

Throughout the first wave of the pandemic (January to April 2020) European countries adopted a large number of public policy measures, from revising existing laws, to launching hundreds of public programmes in all sectors. The first of these measures were health related. Policymakers implemented an extensive range of measures to alleviate immediate pressures on healthcare systems, to gain control of the epidemic, and to try to ensure adequate treatment for the disease. But the scope of many of these measures, and the gravity of the situation, in turn generated the need for new decisions on areas as varied as transportation, employment, production, bureaucratic constraints on businesses, fundamental human rights and freedoms, and many others.

Some of these new regulations were specifically intended to facilitate the management of nursing homes. In most countries, existing general epidemic or pandemic regulations did not include specifications for care homes, and had to be modified to do so. Specific measures also had to be adopted, for example, to allow more workers to be employed on a less demanding basis, or to reduce the rights of workers and residents to handle the difficulties associated with the lockdowns.

These complex decisions forced governments to form new cross-sectoral and intergovernmental committees, and the relations within these newly created commissions were not always straightforward. The tension was partly due to the difficult context experienced by nursing homes, affected by a lack of resources, the extremely severe consequences of the disease among its residents, the particularly complex situation experienced by residents with dementia and other mental conditions, and the inexperience and uncertainty generated by such major challenges. But those strained relations had also to do with the fact that, although governments enjoyed an initial atmosphere of 'closing ranks' for a certain period in which societies uncritically supported them, soon they became subject to criticism, particularly as the situation of nursing homes turned more complex. During the first few weeks, the pandemic placed LTC into the forefront of public opinion awareness as the crisis in nursing homes unfolded. This led to discussions, for example, on the extent to which confinement measures taken in the residences should, or should not be, extended throughout the country, or to what extent the civil rights of residents and workers could be limited.

In general terms, the intervention of European governments in the first stages of the pandemic was largely reactive. Existing mechanisms (regulations, policy tools, arrangements, and institutional structures) in all countries were clearly insufficient to face the dramatic consequences of the pandemic. Policymakers had to look for innovative and creative solutions to problems that had not been confronted before. If this is a statement that can be made about crisis management in general, it is even stronger and truer in the case of the effects of the pandemic on nursing homes.

The response to the impact of the pandemic on European nursing homes as an example of complexity in crisis management

Policy integration at the systemic level: preparedness and response for a possible pandemic and with forecasts on safety in the socio-sanitary field

This section analyses the extent to which countries had a comprehensive long-term policy framework in place prior to the outbreak of COVID-19, establishing coherent policy goals and consistent policy instruments for dealing with a pandemic situation (Table 16.1). From a systemic point of view, the existence of global and specific regulations, previous interoperable information systems to monitor health in nursing homes, or plans on how to act during a pandemic, or socio-sanitary coordination mechanisms prior to the coronavirus pandemic could have served as a reference and may have been used during the management of the COVID-19 pandemic.

Existing general epidemic or pandemic regulations in European countries were weak to non-existent before the advent of COVID-19, and when the pandemic hit they required all sorts of adaptations. In a small number of countries epidemic laws existed (Luxembourg, Austria) but they needed an important update. In other countries the regulation was not able to adapt to the needs of the pandemic in certain territories. On the other end of the spectrum, countries like Finland were better equipped to deal with the contingencies of the pandemic thanks to the existence of the Emergency Powers Act, which proved critical to the government's ability to carry out rapid measures to respond to the pandemic. Pre-planning provided some help to professionals, although none of them foresaw a situation like COVID-19. As no one was prepared to protect the elderly in a pandemic situation, decisions had to be made on the go at all levels. This resulted in contradictory guidance, leading to inadequate and reactive leadership.

In the vast majority of countries, thanks to the WHO recommendations, and to the need to respond to health concerns in previous years, plans were in place to combat certain epidemics such as SARS, influenza virus, MERS-CoV coronavirus, Ebola virus disease, Dengue, or Zika, but in all cases, forecasts were insufficient to anticipate the characteristics and effects of this new coronavirus.

In a number of countries, the general or sectoral Emergency Preparedness Strategies and Plans in place before the pandemic included provisions regarding how to intervene in residential institutions, including notably care homes for the elderly (Germany, France, Italy, UK, or The Netherlands). However, in these cases too, forecasts proved insufficient or ineffective for a virus of such magnitude, and some of them even had negative consequences when responding to the pandemic in the care homes environment.

In the German case, the National Pandemic Plan had to be revised. The plan contained explicit planning aids for inpatient LTC, although there were also problems of articulation between the health and social services sectors in the case of residential care homes. In France, recent general health plans, reflecting previous learning from other types of health contingencies not just those related to viruses, were in turn deployed in white and blue plans (since 2005). These blue plans were instrumental in acting (in particular through individual and collective preventive measures, such as awareness raising on hand washing and social distancing, possible division of the residence premises, limitation/suspension of visits, interruption of collective activities, stock management, monitoring of the implementation of the planned measures, or increasing staff). In particular, the blue plan, which is revised annually to reflect experience and feedback from residential care homes, was activated soon in France, on 6 March 2020. In some other countries, these types of recommendations took several weeks to arrive to the managers of care homes.

In other countries (Finland), even though there were national, local, and even care unit-level contingency plans, part of this regulation was relatively new legislation and had not been sufficiently internalised by organisations. A study from 2014 found that the planning was carried out quite adequately by municipalities. However, it discovered statistically significant differences in the quality of the preparedness plans between small and large service areas, and how they took the elderly into consideration.

The case of England is worth a closer look. In October 2016, the UK government had conducted a simulation exercise, Operation Cygnus, on readiness for a pandemic. This exercise modelled the impacts of a seasonal influenza pandemic, from which COVID-19 differed in important respects, including its speed of transmission, the vulnerability of normally healthy people to severe illness, and the availability (at that time) of a vaccine. Operation Cygnus concluded that both preparedness and responses were inadequate. Significantly, residential care was considered only in respect to its role in relieving pressure on hospitals (in Italy a similar disposition existed). Little attention was paid to the potential pressures and challenges within the sector that could arise as a result of residents' infection, illness and/or mortality. Local authority Directors of Adult Social Care which responded with proposals to improve pandemic planning were not aware of whether government departments had adopted any of their recommendations.

In The Netherlands, the government had been previously advised on several occasions about the need to pool knowledge and expertise in relation to a possible pandemic, as well as to seek international cooperation, and to create buffers for ICU capacity, ventilators, and medicines. A crisis expert pointed out that disaster exercises, and the 2018 influenza epidemic, had shown that the available capacities would quickly fall short in the event of a pandemic. The main objection to the implementation of the improvements that had been pointed out would have been the costs.

The lack of foresight on nursing homes may have had to do with the fact that sometimes healthcare officials were involved in the elaboration of these plans, but not responsible officials from the social services. In the Spanish case, despite the fact that the Preparedness Plans provided for the express participation of both the regions and authorities related to social services in the committees that prepare these documents, the plans drafted at the initiative of the Ministry of Health before the pandemic did not specify how to act in care homes for the elderly in the event of a pandemic. However, they did contain specifications on how to act in companies' premises, for example.

Despite the shortcomings of preparedness and response plans, or the poor leadership, the pre-existence of clear plans for health and social services coordination in normal times could have been helpful in addressing the pandemic. However, in most countries it became clear that this is a challenge that remains to be addressed, probably due to the still central role of families in the domain of LTC, and to the fact that the healthcare sector is comparatively much more powerful than the social services one.

The pandemic also highlighted the serious problems of data management from a cross-sectoral and intergovernmental point of view. Some of the difficulties that decision-makers encountered were clearly related to problems prior to the arrival of the pandemic, such as, for example, the insufficient information that existed, not only at the national level, but also at the regional level, on the nursing home sector, including the number of existing nursing homes, their location and also their characteristics (for example, the number of beds occupied, the profile of the residents, or the staff of those centres). In all countries, social and health authorities made significant efforts to collect information on the impact of the pandemic on residents in care homes, or other useful data related to the effects of the disease, by putting information systems in place at an accelerated pace. However, in some countries, several months after the beginning of the pandemic, this data was still not made public, and until long after the beginning of the pandemic they did not begin to be published periodically, as it was the case in France for example.

Throughout the pandemic, there were discussions about the level of government or the ministries that should assume the sectoral and territorial leadership of the response to the emergency in many countries (Austria, Germany, and Spain). Most countries opted to entrust their health officials with the leadership of the response to the pandemic, which clearly biased the initiatives towards prioritising health measures, leaving other measures in the background, at least in the initial stages of the emergency crisis. This health sector bias, and the fact that in most countries this ministry was generally overburdened, may have affected the delay in taking decisions related to nursing homes and the high number of deaths that took place in those centres. For example, in some countries, the first protocols drawn up to intervene in nursing homes did not include experts from the LTC sector, and the same was true of the first committees that were set up during the crisis (Spain and the Netherlands).

Moreover, mainly for political reasons (it would have been difficult to explain that the government inhibited itself in these circumstances), in some countries central governments (Germany, Austria, Finland, or Spain) saw their role strengthened during the first wave even in social services competencies that were already in the hands of sub-national governments. There was a general debate across all of Europe about whether decisions to manage the pandemic should be homogeneous throughout the national territory (as the pandemic went beyond the borders of any specific territory), or if these decisions should be adapted to the peculiarities of each territory (for example, regions where the incidence of the virus was lower). In the case of France, the centralised administrative system seems to have had its advantages in terms of coordination. Numerous national recommendations were transmitted daily via each regional health agency, who also had the task of gathering information from care homes on a daily basis (through questionnaires to identify the number of people infected, the number of deaths, and any equipment and staff accommodation requirements) and accompanying directors in making choices to apply health protocols. In countries such as Austria or Spain, although some initiatives (such as bans or limitations) for visitors in care homes were introduced during the first months, a general code of action on how to deal with COVID-19 infections among residents in care homes was not introduced until May 2021.

In some countries with particularly privatised and fragmented systems, there were problems in imposing and controlling regulations (The Netherlands in the healthcare system, or Italy in the social services system). Moreover, in some countries, such as Sweden and Spain, the pandemic revealed that the compulsory and poorly controlled contingency plans in the case of the nursing homes themselves had resulted in these plans being elementary, standardized, and unanalysed. However, in the French case federations of residential care homes were mobilised from the very beginning of the health crisis in close association with the Ministry for Health, and contributed to the decisions taken by the government and transmitted the information to residential care homes. In countries such as Germany, the importance of regulation and control of residential homes, both public and private, also seems to have grown as the pandemic evolved. Particular attention should be paid to understand the circumstances experienced by residents with dementia and other mental conditions, since the situation of these groups was particularly challenging during the periods of confinement.

An overview on the functioning of the systemic level of policy integration to respond to the COVID-19 pandemic suggests a series of relevant conclusions:

- The need to improve preparedness and response mechanisms, specifically in collective accommodations (such as residences for the elderly, for people with disabilities, minors, or penitentiary infrastructures), as already suggested by preparedness exercises previously implemented in some countries.
- Before and during a pandemic, this would have been facilitated by involving, alongside public health specialists, experts from the social services sector and from sub-national governments with growing competencies in the management of care homes for the elderly.
- With regard to leadership in the health crisis, shared leadership between those responsible for the sector, and other affected sectors, is key to avoid saturation of the leader, and to achieve decisions where all needs have to be taken into consideration.
- When a crisis hits, no foresight is enough, but foresight is essential to guide the first steps of the response to a pandemic. In countries where the system of governance is highly fragmented, divided between different levels of governments, ministries and between private care providers and

regulators, these plans seem all the more necessary. Also, regulations need to allow for flexibility to adapt to the peculiarities of each crisis.

- More generally, there is still a challenge to be met in terms of socio-health coordination, which, in the absence of, or in the case of deficiencies in, preparedness plans, could have been very useful. In order to increase collaboration between sectors, intersectoral coordination plans have been proposed in some countries and in specific regions. These cross-sectoral coordination plans included: better data sharing, pooling of resources, contingency plans and protocols establishing the onus of different tasks, control mechanisms of implementation.
- With respect to the perception of a need to increase regulation of the residential care sector, in particular towards the private sector, governments now face the challenge of oversight and control of a very fragmented system.

Policy integration at the organisation level: coordination in the political-administrative sphere and at the operational level

A lack of general coordination among different levels of government and, especially, between healthcare and social services in relation to the care of older people, even within the same level of government as just mentioned, was apparent at the organisational level across Europe in the early stages of the pandemic. The passage of time, however, led to some mutual adaptation between the different policy sectors and levels of government.

In many countries, the lack of coordination between organisations linked to different public policy sectors was apparent on at least two spheres. Firstly, in the politico-administrative sphere (Ministries and Regional Ministries), in some countries there were 'tensions that lasted for weeks' or at least a 'lack of dialogue' between the Health and the Social Services Departments due to disagreements related to priority setting, or the extent to which each should be involved in the management of the pandemic.

The incorporation of care experts into the committees created ad hoc to address the crisis occurred late, while the predominant group of experts belonged to the healthcare sector, or even to other sectors (employment, economy, foreign affairs), as in the case of Spain or Sweden. In some countries, such as Germany, there existed a lesser capacity of influence of the professional nursing associations that were not represented in crisis committees, in contrast to doctors and representatives of residential home operators.

On a more operational level, although formal relationships between health care organisations (hospitals or primary care centres) and nursing homes existed in many countries before, the lack of coordination between them was also evident in the day-to-day operations during the first months of the pandemic. This lack of coordination covers a wide range of situations.

Table 16.1: Limited policy integration in the management of nursing homes in the context of the COVID-19 pandemic

Levels	Definitions	Indicators in the pandemic	Main findings
Systems and instruments	Comprehensive long-term policy framework, establishing coherent policy goals and consistent policy instrument	Laws, strategies and plans for preparedness and response to epidemics that would allow coordinated interventions between the health system and the social services system and among levels of government Socio-health coordination plans and exercises prior to the pandemic and during the pandemic, which consider all levels of government Clear rules on an integrated sectoral and territorial leadership in the pandemic crisis. Rules about how to manage territorial or sectoral differences Interoperable information systems to monitor health in nursing homes	Several countries had rules for emergencies and some specifically for epidemics, but no detailed measures for nursing homes There were some specific health plans to deal with epidemics but few of them had explicit provisions for care homes. Only in some countries were simulation exercises about the resilience to a pandemic There were discussions about sectoral and territorial leadership and management during all different stages of the crisis. Difficulties in coordinating public and private actors; plans were elementary, standardised and unanalysed Insufficient basic information about the number and features of nursing homes and very poor coordination among jurisdictions, public and private sector and social/health sectors
Organisation structures	Vertical and horizontal coordination mechanisms to ensure synergies and complementarity within and between the administrations involved	At the political-administrative level of the organisation, sectoral or territorial coordination structures ensuring information exchange and support for action Ad hoc expert committees At an operational level, administrative procedures and tools introduce and systematise to manage the pandemic	In general, lack of stable inter-sectoral structures at the organisational decision-making level Tensions at the organisational level between the political-administrative decision-makers in health and social policies about who should be responsible for managing the pandemic in nursing-homes In some countries and regions, expert committees did not include care systems experts until well into the pandemic There were shortcomings in the established coordination tools and mechanism between healthcare and nursing homes, evident in hospitals but also in the daily healthcare of elderly people living in residential homes, with some instances of neglect
Individual	Qualified staff capable of designing and managing cross-sectoral and intergovernmental integrated strategies	Empathy and perception of shared objectives between policy sectors and policy levels Professional background, specific training, on cross-sectoral skills Collaborative initiatives encouraging change in mind-sets and administrative practices	Significant contrasts between the organisational cultures of the health and social sectors, with a lack of awareness of the distinctive features of each other's work. Different levels of social recognition for their work during the pandemic Remarkable disparity in personal and professional status between managers of care homes and nursing homes. Different levels of social recognition for their work during the pandemic Throughout the pandemic, intersectoral spaces were established at both political and technical levels through formal and informal channels

Source: Own elaboration based on Wu et al (2015); El-Taliawi & Van Der Wal (2019); Domorenok et al (2021a, 2021b); Tosun & Lang (2017).

Regarding contingency plans and protocols at the organisational level:

- In some countries, protocols drawn up at the beginning of the pandemic by other authorities took a few months to reach nursing homes (England, Spain, Italy), sometimes several months (Austria, Greece, Ireland). In some countries, nursing homes received protocols from different authorities (central, regional, local, as well as from their companies in the case of privately-run care homes), in addition to drawing up their own specific contingency plans for each centre. Some of these plans were contradictory on many occasions. In most countries, the protocols changed over the months. Sometimes this was due to new information about the virus behaviour, but other times the changes were due to deficiencies in the functioning of nursing homes.
- The lack of intersectoral dialogue was also clear in the implementation of protocols that had not been properly coordinated between healthcare and social services, so that they did not show sufficient understanding of the functioning of the nursing homes, or of their characteristics, and consequently it was not always possible to apply them. They were, for instance, unaware of issues such as the architectural limits of the centres, or the criteria for arranging residents with mental problems (that could not be isolated, as the protocols sometimes required), or of residents with different degrees of dependency and the tasks that had to be developed by the staff of the care homes.
- Nursing home managers often complained about the large amounts of time spent each day reporting data to a large number of public actors and different public administrations (healthcare system, justice administration, municipalities and other administrations, safety officials, its own company, among others) who requested very similar information in different formats.
- In all countries, even in those where the protection of nursing homes was a priority from the beginning (Finland), most facilities had very low initial stocks of PPE at the start of the coronavirus crisis. In the vast majority of countries, healthcare facilities were prioritised for the allocation of these scarce and vital resources during the first weeks, and even months, of the pandemic.

With respect to the working conditions of the staff employed in the care homes sector:

- In most countries, there was a significant delay in protecting nursing home workers from contagion with respect to healthcare workers, due to very limited resources available and the prioritisation of needs in other sectors perceived to be more urgent. This led to infections among staff, an increase in sickness-related absences from work, and to abandonment of work due to fear of infection, family pressures, difficulties to balance work and family (many workers are immigrant women, sometimes without much family support), or trauma.

- In all countries chronic shortages of well-trained staff in LTC systems were compounded by casualties during the pandemic. These scarce staff had to cope with an enormous increase in resident needs, from communication with relatives, to palliative care, and a wide range of administrative tasks (Austria, France, Finland, Germany, Spain, England).
- The training of nursing home staff was inadequate for some of the healthcare tasks specified in the new protocols. In some countries, however, they were specifically trained to deal with these tasks and even to interact cross-sectorially, with other professionals such as healthcare professionals.
- In most countries extraordinary recruitment plans for the healthcare sector had to be implemented. Sometimes, these plans had a negative 'draining effect' on the nursing home care sector. Doctors and nurses opted to leave their jobs in nursing homes to be employed by hospitals, where contractual conditions and salary levels are more generous (Italy, England, Germany, Ireland). As a consequence, in some countries (Finland, Spain, Germany) staff were sought, sometimes using workers from other public facilities that were shut (such as nurseries, early child education, libraries), but also army personnel, retired care staff not belonging to the risk groups, medical students and foreign professionals were also recruited where necessary. In almost all countries, care home workers were asked to work significantly longer hours.

As regards care and assistance to residents:

- In some countries there was a perceived growing disinterest in caring for residents on the part of regular primary care physicians, who prioritised care for the general population, or substituted physical care by telephone calls (Spain, Austria, and the UK). In other places, such as in Ireland, private nursing homes do not have a formalised clinical governance relationship with the health system.
- Hospitals and primary care also had significant recruitment needs for nurses, doctors, and other medical staff – especially specialist nurses in hospitals. These problems mean that hospitals cannot keep beds open, must postpone operations, and the queues for doctor visits in primary care significantly grow.
- The lack of testing material for nursing homes was experienced in most countries in the early stages of the emergency, and in all of them there were changes in the criteria as to when residents and workers should

be tested: until around April, it was only for those with symptoms. In some countries, testing for residents and care home workers came even later. Sometimes, intergovernmental disagreement about which level of government should buy or pay for the tests was the cause of this delay (Sweden). Moreover, in some countries, there were different criteria for testing in hospitals and nursing homes, showing a lack of knowledge about how their centres worked and, according to some, a clear disregard for the older-age adults, treating them indiscriminately. Now we know that 'greater surveillance testing of staff members at skilled nursing facilities was associated with clinically meaningful reductions in COVID-19 cases and deaths among residents, particularly before vaccine availability' (McGarry et al, 2023).

- In the vast majority of countries, hospitals played a leading role in the handling of the consequences of the pandemic. They were the first to be protected, saw an increase in financial, personnel, and material resources, both ICUs and PPE, and in some cases played an important role in decision-making. In part, this was determined by the hospital-centric nature of the system in some countries (such as France), but it was also due to the fact that in most countries the pandemic was tackled with an approach that tried to alleviate the symptoms, rather than an approach that sought to prevent or eliminate contagion, that would have given much more joint leadership to both the primary healthcare centres and public health structures. Perhaps a telling anecdote that sums up the situation is the case where nursing homes were even asked to hand over some of their protection material to hospitals (UK, Italy). In some countries this hospital-centric approach is attributed to lobbying behind private hospitals (as in The Netherlands), however, this was also the case in countries with national healthcare systems where public primary care (and not so much hospitals) constitute the backbone of the healthcare system. It is quite possible that this was due to the practical difficulties of using a surveillance approach once the number of cases got out of control, and to the fact that it was very difficult to follow up each case. In any instance, this prevailing approach greatly affected the relationship between the healthcare system and nursing homes.
- The hospital-centric approach was also behind the insufficient reinforcement of healthcare centres. Sometimes, nursing homes had problems for the ordinary care of their residents by their assigned primary healthcare centres (Spain). This situation was particularly acute in those cases where nursing homes had no doctors, or where doctors decided to leave their jobs for different reasons (mainly belonging to a risk group, contagion, or fear). Only in a minority of countries, care homes seem to have had sufficient resources to take care of their residents' health (The Netherlands).

- The capacity to ensure care services in nursing homes was severely affected by the COVID-19 crisis. The priority was to protect residents from contagion. But this disrupted the organisation and functioning of the nursing homes, severely altering routines and activities that are fundamental to the health, quality of life and to the guaranteeing of the residents' rights. Alterations in the daily functioning of nursing homes occurred in many different ways, related to the conversion of common spaces into COVID-19 patient care areas or the application of hospital management criteria to residents, the isolation of residents in their rooms, the lockdown of residential centres, the radical reduction of social life inside and outside the rooms, the cancellation of visits from relatives, or the ceasing to treat non-COVID-19 illnesses. In general, residents' opinions and preferences were no longer sufficiently considered. One of the most dramatic circumstances of the pandemic, which was widely reported in most countries, affected residents' rights, in particular the limitation of movement and family visits for months.
- In some countries, such as Ireland or England, there was no state regulatory oversight of most private/voluntary sector LTC providers, and no routine inspections of care homes. In some other countries, the pandemic exposed the existence of unlicensed care homes, which often were among the most severely affected by the disease (Portugal, Spain).
- During the pandemic, some nursing homes showed problems of financial sustainability, as some residents preferred to move in with their families, others simply died, and the care homes were forced to accept fewer residents. This caused many care homes to raise their fees in a context in which the quality of the care they were providing had significantly deteriorated due to the adjustment of their protocols to the pandemic context, and their public image had experienced a serious hit due to the high mortality rates among their residents.

In several countries there was a suspicion that in the early stages of the pandemic hospital admission decisions were not based on an individualised assessment of each patient's state of health (trying to discern from among all applicants for a hospital bed who would benefit most in terms of health status from receiving such treatment), but on a generic categorisation whereby all residents in geriatric facilities were considered irrecoverable. This was considered morally unacceptable and provoked outrage in broad sectors of European societies and public opinion (Anand et al, 2022). Moreover, the criteria of hospital administration varied throughout the pandemic. In some countries, such as Spain, restrictions on hospitalisation in some regions caused great social alarm. In many countries, hospitalisation in nursing homes themselves was adopted. In other countries, the criteria remained the same as before the pandemic. In Italy, in this attempt to locate beds outside hospitals, the possibility of discharging hospitalised patients to nursing homes (including those affected by COVID-19 but in a less critical condition) was explicitly introduced.

As weeks went by, the authorities tried to find solutions to these organisational coordination problems, involving a substantial modification of the situation of relative disconnection between the healthcare and social services policy areas. Some of these solutions could be regarded as innovative, and would certainly have taken years to be pursued under normal circumstances. Some governments established or reinforced monitoring and support units for nursing homes. In some countries, mobile geriatric teams were established from hospitals to nursing homes, a 'coordinating doctor' (France) or a community nurse was appointed as responsible for nursing homes (Austria, Spain), or specific care 'lines' were designed for nursing homes (Luxembourg). Sometimes the nurse acted as a case manager in the nursing home itself, or simply provided a direct channel of communication between the nursing homes and the healthcare centres. This helped to reduce the sense of abandonment felt by nursing home managers at the beginning of the pandemic. The nurses were advised on how best to deal with the consequences of the pandemic, developing contingency plans, coordinating action for infected or symptomatic patients, and facilitating access to tests or medical supplies. The most intensive interventions involved the 'medicalisation' of the nursing homes, and thus the secondment of new staff to replace or supplement the nursing home personnel.

Most countries made progress in the application of healthcare technologies (remote consultations, prescriptions, and communication systems based on ICTs), and de-bureaucratisation that, where it not for the pandemic, would have taken years to implement (Austria, Germany). Epidemiological surveillance systems were put in place, or intensified, for care homes. Working groups with members from different territories on the specific field of care were promoted, sometimes to share best practices about contingency plans, or about obtaining evidence. Some of these groups have evolved towards spaces for institutional cooperation and dialogue on how to improve the residential model and the quality of care.

Policy integration at the individual level

In many countries, it has been clear for a long time that issues of 'mutual understanding' between people in the healthcare and the social sectors long predate the pandemic. There exist clear and deep differences between the organisational cultures of the healthcare and social sectors, as well as differences in professional status between care home and healthcare managers. In comparative terms, it is a highly feminised sector, with a strong presence of immigrants, a low socio-economic level of origin and low wages (in some countries, such as the UK, zero hours contracts are mentioned), and therefore poor resources of influence and family support during the period of the pandemic, much poorer training, and low social status make the care profession unattractive to potential workers, especially when compared to the healthcare sector, which is often an alternative. In several countries, both political and media attention was directed, at least in the first few months, at health care workers rather than caregivers in nursing homes. This situation has even been acknowledged in some official reports (Sweden). Finally, even in countries, such as France and Germany, which before the pandemic had strengthened their elderly care systems, all analyses in this book suggest the lack of personnel qualified to care for increasingly elderly and vulnerable residents.

These differences were exacerbated during the pandemic, and became evident both at the political-administrative level, and at the more operational one. On the one hand, political-administrative decision-makers in the care sector were slow to be listened to by their counterparts in the healthcare sector. On the other hand, professionals in the residential sector claimed to suffer from the consequences of a lack of knowledge of the peculiarities of the nursing home sector and its peculiarities on the part of the health authorities. In many instances, this may have had a negative impact on the living conditions of the elderly residing in care homes when healthcare professionals were assigned to take decisions on the structuring of these nursing homes to respond to the pandemic. This often implied a radical reduction of the social interactions of the residents, both inside and outside the facility, which resulted in a significant reduction in the physical, emotional, and cognitive abilities of the elderly residing in care homes. As an example of this type of situation, in one nursing home, following the intervention of the facility by the health authorities, healthcare staff who took over the nursing home and tried to re-organise it to function as a hospital, left many residents in bed all day, or sitting in an armchair, and in their pyjamas. From the point of view of the LTC professionals, and with a consideration of the nursing home as a place to live, the home of the residents, this was interpreted as neglect. In other cases, the healthcare authorities called for the confinement to their rooms of people with mental disorders, without considering the specificities of these residents (they may self-harm or even attempt suicide). At the same time, the care workers admitted that they did not have the necessary knowledge to care for sick residents. Finally, staff employed in the elderly care sector largely felt abandoned to their fate during those early stages of the pandemic. In the aftermath of the coronavirus crises, they felt little recognition from society for their efforts and sacrifices, in any case much less than the one shown to healthcare workers.

Throughout the pandemic, a process of mutual adaptation occurred, forced by the need to address the serious problems that affected nursing homes. It also became evident that a process of integrating healthcare and social policies cannot happen in a casual manner, since it requires a significant and deliberate effort of empathy and training from all parties involved. The establishment of intersectoral coordination spaces, both at political and technical level, through formal and informal channels (chats, email or instant messaging groups such as Whatsapp), was very useful for sharing the knowledge needed to deal with the pandemic and its consequences.

Concluding remarks

The challenge of the impact of COVID-19 on care homes during the first wave of the pandemic was colossal, and in many countries, it risked collapsing the critical capacities of the healthcare and social care systems. The generally weak, and in some cases direct absence, of coordination mechanisms between the healthcare and the social sectors aggravated the lack of strategies and plans to address an epidemic emergency, thus making it extremely difficult to implement an efficient response to the crisis in the first weeks of pandemic. The large number of deaths in European countries in general, and in care homes in particular, during those first months of the pandemic, have been considered by scholars as a focusing event (Beland & Marier, 2020). The dramatic and striking death toll and infection rates in nursing homes drew the general population's attention to the LTC sector, and very much in particular to the structural situation of the care homes, their infrastructures, their staff, and obviously their residents.

In this book we have emphasised the importance of the concept of policy integration to account for the complex intersectoral and intergovernmental articulations that would have been necessary to provide a more efficient response by care homes to the challenges posed by the pandemic. The problems derived from the low levels of policy integration occur in the day-to-day management of public administrations, but are more pronounced and visible during periods of crisis or polycrisis (Dinan et al, 2024). Adapting an existing multilevel conceptual framework (systemic, organisational, and personal) through which to achieve the integration of public policies in different sectors, we have analysed the management of nursing homes during COVID-19 in a series of European countries, showing the seriousness of the challenges posed by the pandemic to our societies in general, and to our social protection systems in particular, as well as the complexity of the institutional responses articulated to address such challenges.

Governments' actions faced with the crisis produced in the care homes sector by the pandemic were largely reactive. In all countries it is described that although the authorities saw how the pandemic affected their neighbouring countries at the initial stages of the pandemic, they trusted that they would know how to solve the problem better if they came to be affected. Despite varying degrees of development of LTC systems, even in countries where there were forecasts and emergency plans, governments ended up lagging well behind the consequences of the pandemic. Existing mechanisms (regulations, policy tools, arrangements and institutional structures) were insufficient in all countries, and policymakers had to look for innovative and creative solutions to problems they had not confronted before. If this is a statement that can be made about crisis management in general, it is even stronger and truer in the case of care homes and the COVID-19 pandemic.

LTC systems in Europe comprise a significant number of stakeholders. In all countries, regulatory, financing, monitoring, and service delivery competencies are distributed across the two or three levels of government. Furthermore, in all countries, public, private, and third sector actors are involved in the management of care homes. Finally, both the social services and the health sector are involved in these services. This multiplicity of actors contributes to the complexity of coordinating the needs that arise in the event of a crisis. Consequently, it is imperative that the protection of citizens who reside in these facilities on a permanent basis be a priority in national security regulations.

The deficiencies in information systems and the intricate flow of data between the numerous actors involved in LTC policy constituted significant impediments to the effective management of the pandemic. The aforementioned difficulties about the relationship among different actors are also evident in the multitude of activities that were undertaken in response to the pandemic, ranging from the procurement of equipment to the formulation and implementation of plans and protocols.

From a territorial perspective, some studies have indicated that countries with a centralised territorial model of power demonstrated a more expedient response to the pandemic, whereas countries with a more decentralised model exhibited greater flexibility in adapting to the distinctive characteristics of the COVID-19 pandemic across different territories (Carroll et al, 2023). With the available data, it is difficult to corroborate these findings for nursing homes across all the countries examined in this study. However, there are indications that this may have been the case. In any case, even in the decentralised countries, the basic coordination mechanisms between the different levels of government in each of the sectors functioned reasonably smoothly, but these mechanisms were activated more efficiently in the healthcare sector than in the social sector during the first months of the pandemic. It is also worth noting that from May 2020 onwards, criticism of the management of the pandemic from other levels of government of a different political colour began to become more obvious.

Decision-makers, and sometimes citizens themselves, are accustomed to hearing about conflicts, duplication, coordination problems, or lack of coherence between measures adopted by different levels of government. However, all these phenomena are less visible, although just as present and relevant in the relations between different public policy sectors within the same level of government (or between several levels of government). The COVID-19 crisis revealed numerous management problems related, in particular, to intersectoral management. As months passed, some of these difficulties were gradually overcome. Progress was clearly made in the design of intersectoral and interterritorial plans and measures and social-health information systems. Future analyses will have to assess whether that progress was significant and altered the patterns of fragmentation and lack of data intelligence, procedures and other shared policy tools. It remains to be seen to what extent some of these challenges will be efficiently and structurally addressed in order to make progress in the necessary social and health coordination, which continues to be one of the great unresolved issues for our social protection systems, even in times of normality.

This book also presents some evidence of the importance of the role played by individuals in the functioning of services involving different policy sectors. Different professional backgrounds, training and experience, professional recognition, organisational cultures and patterns of professional socialisation can represent a difficult hurdle to overcome when people are put to work together. These difficulties are more important in high-pressure contexts and, in particular, when there are no spaces and institutional mechanisms and procedures that have made this possible before by establishing rules and patterns of interaction that help to build interpersonal and inter-institutional trust. An additional factor in this dimension is the widespread perception among LTC professionals that their activity is poorly recognised, notably in comparison with that of the healthcare sector professionals in particular.

The great media attention received by this health crisis, and the importance attributed by citizens to the impact of the pandemic on care homes, created a 'policy window' to reform the LTC sector, to improve care workers' labor conditions, and to re-think the LTC system's governance to address the increasing risks derived from an older-age population. Given the current growing demand for care, which will only increase in the future, it is necessary to open a debate on the financing of the LTC system and infrastructures, its scope and coverage (Leichsenring & Sidorenko, 2024; Simmons et al, 2024). The increasing ageing of the population, combined with the growing demand for care services, calls attention to stop the underfunding of the LTC sector, and to correct the precarious labour market conditions of caregivers (promoting full-time, permanent employment with an adequate salary, grant proper occupational leave, minimum criteria for care workers' education and continuous training, enhance the training of care homes staff, and so on).

It is also a priority to ensure effective cross-sectoral coordination between care homes (social services system), and the healthcare system. As we have seen, there are institutional, organisational, and even psycho-sociological obstacles for such a reform. The analysis presented in this book illustrates that an integrated policy approach to pandemic management (encompassing the systemic, organizational, and individual actors levels), would have resulted in reduced response times and a more effective provision of care to citizens. This book demonstrates that crises facilitate integrated decision-making in order to resolve complex public policy issues. It is yet to be determined whether the conscious effort to improve the integration of the health and social sectors, which was evident during the pandemic, has been consolidated in its aftermath and has served to enhance the resilience and robustness of the system.

The question now is to what extent will the lessons learned during the pandemic be integrated in the reform of the LTC system. This reform should build on the trends established in recent years aimed at keeping the elderly population at home for as long as they wish and it is feasible while responding to the coverage of their daily needs. Beyond vague notions of 'care in the community' that may reflect a scaling down of public intervention in the LTC and a devolution of responsibility for care to the family (which in most cases is not able to face the implications derived from that trend), public administrations shall explore more individualised and autonomous formats of institutionalisation (serviced apartments with social and/or medical support, individual rooms in care homes, decrease in rules and restrictions for residents in nursing homes, and so on).

There are, of course, financial aspects to consider as well, when imagining a reform of the LTC sector in general, and of the nursing homes in particular. Most of the changes considered to be necessary and previously mentioned would imply increasing the resources (human, but notably financial) allocated to this policy domain. Again, the sustainability of the increase in spending associated with the response to the pandemic in the care home sector will question the functioning of the model as it operated before the coronavirus outbreak (Caracciolo di Torella, 2023).

The European Pillar of Social Rights (principles 9 and 18), as well as the EU Care Strategy (EC, 2022), propose to fully extend the social investment approach to the domain LTC. According to the EU Care Strategy, the development of high-quality care services should benefit the wellbeing, health and social inclusion of people in need of care and (in)formal caregivers, while providing good employment opportunities and making the care system more efficient and sustainable through increased fiscal revenues and social contributions. Based on the assumption that better job quality is a precursor to good care, this Strategy stresses that good quality of work is essential for the resilience and attractiveness of the sector as well as for gender equality and fair treatment of migrant workers. Although great expectations are placed on both 'social innovation' and 'care technologies' to simultaneously reach the four key objectives of LTC reforms (care affordability and accessibility, quality of care, quality of care work, and financial sustainability), while insuring the provision of 'integrated care' that adequately balances the social and healthcare components of an adequate LTC attention, it remains to be seen to what extent those developments manage to materialise balance progress in all those dimensions.

References

Anand, J., Donnelly, S., Milne, A., Nelson-Becker, H., Vingare, E., Deusdad, B., Cellini, G., Kinni, R.-L., and Pregno, C. (2022) The COVID-19 pandemic & care homes for older people in Europe – Deaths, damage & violations of human rights, *European Journal of Social Work*, 25(5): 804–15.

Béland D, and Marier P. (2020) COVID-19 and Long-Term Care Policy for Older People in Canada, *Journal of Aging and Social Policy*, 32(4–5): 358–64.

Caracciolo di Torella, E. (2023) Re-thinking care after the pandemic: a European care strategy for caregivers and care receivers, *ERA Forum*, 24: 55–67.

Carroll, B. J., Brummel, L., Toshkov, D., and Yesilkagit, K. (2023) Multilevel governance and responses to the COVID-19 pandemic: a systematic literature review, *Regional & Federal Studies*, DOI: 10.1080/13597566.2023.2292997

Dinan, S., Béland, D., and Howlett, M. (2024) How useful is the concept of polycrisis? Lessons from the development of the Canada Emergency Response benefit during the COVID-19 pandemic, *Policy Design and Practice*, 7(4): 430–41.

Domorenok, E., Graziano, P., and Polverari, L. (2021a) Introduction: policy integration and institutional capacity: theoretical, conceptual and empirical challenges, *Policy and Society*, DOI: 10.1080/14494035.2021.1902058

Domorenok, E., Graziano, P. and Polverari, L. (2021b) Policy integration, policy design and administrative capacities: evidence from EU cohesion policy, *Policy and Society*, 40(1): 58–78.

El-Taliawi. O- G. and Van Der Wal, Z. (2019) Developing administrative capacity: an agenda for research and practice, *Policy Design and Practice*, 2(3): 243–57.

European Commission (2022) European Care Strategy, Brussels, Available from: https://ec.europa.eu/commission/presscorner/api/files/document/print/en/ip_22_5169/IP_22_5169_EN.pdf

Leichsenring, K. and Sidorenko, A. (eds) (2024) *A Research Agenda for Ageing and Social Policy*, Cheltenham, UK: Edward Elgar Publishing.

Lenharo, M. (2023) Global plan for dealing with next pandemic just got weaker, critics say, *Nature*, 1 June [online], Available from: https://www.nature.com/articles/d41586-023-01805-4

McGarry, B. E., Gandhi, A. D. and Barnett, M. L. (2023) COVID-19 surveillance testing and resident outcomes in nursing homes, *New England Journal of Medicine*, 388: 1101–10.

Paquet, M. and Schertzer, R. (2020) COVID-19 as a complex intergovernmental problem, *Canadian Journal of Political Science/Revue Canadienne de Science Politique*, 53(2): 343–7.

Simmons, C., Ilinca, S., Comas-Herrera, A., Champeix, C., Southard, L., and Zonnenveld, N. (2024) Strengthening social infrastructure in long-term care for older people: coordinated action and local empowerment in Europe, in A-T. Renner, L. Plank, and M. Getzner (eds) *Handbook of Social Infrastructure*, Cheltenham: Edward Elgar Publishing, pp 39–56.

Tosun, J. and Lang, A. (2017) Policy integration: mapping the different concepts, *Policy Studies*, 38(6): 553–70.

Wu, X., Ramesh, M., and Howlett, M. (2015) Policy capacity: a conceptual framework for understanding policy competences and capabilities, *Policy and Society*, 34(3–4): 165–71.

Index

References to figures appear in *italic* type; those in **bold** type refer to tables.

D

E

F

G

L

M

N

T

U

V

W

Z